Fundamentals of Clinical Ophthalmology:

Cataract Surgery

Fundamentals of Clinical Ophthalmology series

Cornea
Edited by Douglas Coster

Glaucoma
Edited by Roger Hitchins

Neuro-ophthalmology
Edited by James Acheson and Paul Riordan-Eva

Paediatric Ophthalmology
Edited by Anthony Moore

Plastic and Orbital Surgery
Edited by Richard Collin and Geoffrey Rose

Scleritis
Edited by Paul McCluskey

Strabismus
Edited by Frank Billson

Uveitis
Edited by Susan Lightman and Hamish Towler

Fundamentals of Clinical Ophthalmology:

Cataract Surgery

Edited by
ANDREW COOMBES
St Bartholomew's Hospital and The Royal London Hospital, London, UK

DAVID GARTRY
Moorfields Eye Hospital, London, UK

Series editor
SUSAN LIGHTMAN
*Department of Clinical Ophthalmology,
Institute of Ophthalmology/Moorfields Eye Hospital,
London, UK*

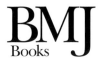

BMJ Books

First published in 2003
by BMJ Books, BMA House, Tavistock Square,
London WC1H 9JR

www.bmjbooks.com

British Library Cataloguing in Publication Data

A catalogue record for this book is available from the British Library

ISBN 0 7279 1201 1

Typeset by SIVA Math Setters, Chennai, India
Printed and bound in Malaysia by Times Offset

Contents

Contributors

Charles Claoe
Consultant Ophthalmologist
Harold Wood Hospital
Essex, UK

Andrew Coombes
Consultant Ophthalmologist
St Bartholomew's Hospital and The Royal London Hospital
London, UK

Jack Dodick
Chairman of the Department of Ophthalmology
Manhattan Eye, Ear and Throat Hospital
New York, USA

Jonathan Dowler
Consultant Ophthalmologist
Moorfields Eye Hospital
London, UK

David Gartry
Consultant Ophthalmologist
Moorfields Eye Hospital
London, UK

Peter Hamilton
Consultant Ophthalmologist
Moorfields Eye Hospital
London, UK

Colm Lanigan
Consultant Anaesthetist
Lewisham Hospital
London, UK

Thomas Neuhann
Consultant Ophthalmologist
Munich, Germany

CONTRIBUTORS

Marie Restori
Consultant Medical Physicist
Moorfields Eye Hospital
London, UK

Paul Rosen
Consultant Ophthalmologist
The Radcliffe Infirmary
Oxford, UK

Helen Seward
Consultant Ophthalmologist
Croydon Eye Unit
Surrey, UK

Hamish Towler
Consultant Ophthalmologist
Whipps Cross Hospital
London, UK

Sarah-Lucie Watson
Specialist Registrar
Moorfields Eye Hospital
London, UK

David Yorston
Specialist Registrar
Moorfields Eye Hospital
London, UK

Preface to the
Fundamentals of Clinical Ophthalmology series

This book is part of a series of ophthalmic monographs, written for ophthalmologists in training and general ophthalmologists wishing to update their knowledge in specialised areas. The emphasis of each is to combine clinical experience with the current knowledge of the underlying disease processes.

Each monograph provides an up to date, very clinical and practical approach to the subject so that the reader can readily use the information in everyday clinical practice. There are excellent illustrations throughout each text in order to make it easier to relate the subject matter to the patient.

The inspiration for the series came from the growth in communication and training opportunities for ophthalmologists all over the world and a desire to provide clinical books that we can all use. This aim is well reflected in the international panels of contributors who have so generously contributed their time and expertise.

Susan Lightman

Preface

Cataract surgery is a dynamic and complex field and is, without doubt, a fundamental part of ophthalmology. This book aims to cover the subject comprehensively, particularly the technical aspects of learning, performing, and teaching phacoemulsification. The inclusion of chapters on the Third World and the future of cataract surgery provide the reader with a broader perspective.

The structure of the text, cross-referencing between chapters, and a detailed index minimise repetition. For example, intraoperative complications are discussed within the relevant individual chapters on technique (although vitreous loss and the dropped nucleus have a chapter devoted to them), whereas postoperative complications are grouped together. For those who would like more detail, the text has been thoroughly referenced.

Inevitably, some knowledge has been assumed and some detail omitted, but we hope that this book will be useful to both trainees and established cataract surgeons.

Andrew Coombes and David Gartry

Acknowledgements

We must first acknowledge the contributing authors, without whom this book would not exist. Professor Susan Lightman and all at BMJ Books, particularly Mary Banks, must also be thanked for their part (and patience).

Many individuals have contributed photographs and their help has been very much appreciated. These include David Anderson (Figures 2.14, 3.3, 3.5, 5.3, 5.6, 5.14, and 7.20), Bill Aylward (Figure 10.21), Caroline Carr (Figure 9.2a–f), Emma Hollick (Figures 7.4, and 12.21), Alex Ionides (Figure 10.29), James Kirwan (Figure 8.13b, 10.23, 10.24, 10.26, 12.13, and 12.22b), Frank Larkin (Figure 12.14), Graham Lee (Figure 7.3a,b), Ordan Lehmann (Figures 8.14, 12.12, 12.15, 12.18, 12.22a, 12.24, and 12.26), Martin Leyland (Figure 10.16), and Chris Liu and Babis Eleftheriadis (Figure 7.13). The staff in the day surgery unit at Chelsea and Westminster Hospital should also be thanked for their help with many of the photographs.

A large number of companies have allowed their equipment, instruments, and lenses to be photographed, and we are grateful for their involvement. This book was originally developed from the Moorfields Eye Hospital phacoemulsification courses, and Alcon (and their wet laboratory facilities) deserve particular mention for their support of these courses over many years.

We should like to take this opportunity to thank those cataract surgeons who have taught us in the past and those who continue to inspire us. Finally, we thank our families (especially Sarah) for the support and tolerance that has been essential in completing this book.

1 Teaching and learning phacoemulsification

The change in cataract surgery to phacoemulsification over the past 10 years has been well documented by Learning,[1] who has conducted an annual survey of the practice styles and preferences of US cataract surgeons. In the UK a similar shift toward phacoemulsification has occurred[2] and is likely to continue. For the surgeon in training, phacoemulsification is no longer an option but an essential surgical skill to acquire. For the trained surgeon the ability to teach phacoemulsification in a structured manner has also become necessary.

Structured training and phacoemulsification courses

Phacoemulsification acquired an undeservedly poor reputation in the past. Surgeons did not spend sufficient time on structured training programmes and there was a lack of suitably qualified surgeons to supervise. Complications during the learning curve have been reported,[3] but with better training and a wider availability of simulated surgery these can be reduced. Structured training for phacoemulsification requires time that may not be readily available in a busy eye department, but provision must be made for both trainer and trainee if safe surgery is to be provided for our patients. Teaching and learning phacoemulsification should be an enjoyable, if challenging, experience and should not increase morbidity.

The success of the structured training plan described below depends on the trainee having already mastered microscope skills, including the ability to use the microscope foot control with the non-dominant foot. It also assumes knowledge of instrument handling and the ability to carry out delicate procedures using a microscope. For the teacher it is easy to forget what learning phacoemulsification was like. Teaching is a skill like any other; it requires patience and insight into the learning process. Courses designed to teach the trainer to teach are becoming more widespread, and these can help to improve the effectiveness of teaching and minimise the stress it can involve.

Teaching and learning phacoemulsification can be divided into three sections:

- Phacoemulsification theory (see Chapter 4)
- Simulated surgery practice (wet lab)
- Surgical learning programme (in vivo).

Where possible the trainer should be involved at each stage. For the trainee, each section should be mastered before progressing to the next. A well organised course that combines theory with an introduction to phacoemulsification surgery using a wet lab is an interesting and effective entry point. An introductory course should consist of several key lectures, including the following:

- The physics of phacoemulsification
- Phacoemulsification incisions (corneal and scleral)
- Capsulorhexis

- Principles of nuclear sculpting
- Nuclear management
- Aspiration of soft lens matter following phacoemulsification
- Rigid, folding, and injectable lens insertion
- Management of complications.

All trainees should leave a phacoemulsification course with a training plan based on their existing surgical skills.

Simulated surgery practice

Equipment

A well equipped surgical wet laboratory (wet lab) (Figure 1.1) is an ideal environment in which to practice phacoemulsification, and this should be supervised by an experienced surgeon. A wet lab station should consist of the follwing items:

- Microscope
- Phacoemulsification machine with phaco, and irrigation and aspiration hand pieces
- A mannequin's head, for example the Maloney head or a polystyrene head
- Plastic eyes with disposable cataracts and corneas (Figure 1.2), or fresh animal eyes
- Irrigating solutions
- Disposable knives
- Cystotome and forceps for capsulorhexis
- Spatula to use in the non-dominant hand
- Rigid, folding, or injectable intraocular lenses and instruments.

Neither postmortem animal eyes nor plastic model eyes are able to simulate all the attributes of the human cataractous eye. Each represents a compromise, and their advantages and disadvantages are summarised in Table 1.1. Although postmortem human eyes can be used, ethical and legal restrictions exist.

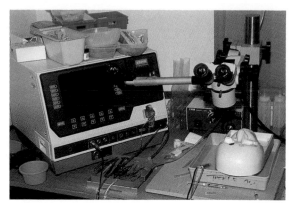

Figure 1.1 A typical wet lab. Note the use of the Maloney head (Iatrotech) to hold the artificial eyes.

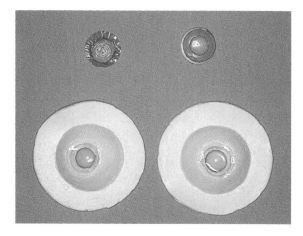

Figure 1.2 Artificial eyes (bottom) with disposable cataract (top left) and cornea (top right; Karlheinz Hannig Microsurgical Training Systems Company).

Animal eyes (most commonly from the pig) are ideal for practicing incisions and suturing, but because the anterior capsule is thick and elastic they do not always simulate capsulorhexis well. Also, the lens is soft and not ideal for practicing nuclear fracture techniques. Attempts have been made to harden the pig lens by injecting the eye with a mixture of formalin and alcohol,[4] using a microwave oven,[5] or replacing the lens with vegetable matter.[6] Animal eyes have the disadvantage that they are not always available and need to be refrigerated for storage. They are

Table 1.1 Comparison of plastic model and animal eyes

Eye type	Advantages	Disadvantages
Plastic model eyes	Relative sterility (can be used in the operating theatre) Consistent nucleus density (stimulates sculpting well) Capsular bag for practising capsulorhexis/intraocular lens implantation Readily available	Plastic cornea poorly simulates incision Air bubbles are trapped within the anterior chamber during phacoemulsification Lens cannot easily be rotated Nucleus difficult to crack
Animal eyes	Excellent for incision and suturing practice "Normal" lens capsule for capsulorhexis, hydrodissection and nucleus rotation	Non-sterile (cannot be used in operating theatre) Soft nucleus, which is mainly aspirated Variable availabilty and require refrigerated storage

non-sterile and may potentially be infected with, for example, prions. In the absence of a dedicated wet lab, the operating theatre, with its microscope and phaco machine, is often used to provide a wet lab facility out of hours. Unlike plastic model eyes, animal tissue should not be used in this environment. Plastic model eyes consistently simulate the human cataract during sculpting,[7] and some systems have the facility to vary the density of the "nucleus". In contrast, rotating and cracking the lens are less like they are in surgery in vivo. The artificial cataract is contained within a capsule (that may be supplied as coloured) that allows capsulorhexis and intraocular lens implantation to be practised. Unfortunately, the thin plastic cornea of the model eye does not behave like the human eye when attempting incisions and is prone to trapping air bubbles.

Wet lab training

The set up sequence for the machine and equipment should be understood before commencing simulated surgery practice in the wet lab. The following is a suggested programme for wet lab learning and teaching.

Foot pedal control

Trainees should spend time familiarising themselves with foot pedal function and control (also see Chapter 4).

- Foot position 1 engages irrigation only.
- Foot position 2 engages irrigation together with aspiration (the sound of aspiration can be heard from the machine).
- Foot position 3 engages phacoemulsification as well as irrigation and aspiration (the hand piece emits a high pitched sound).

Additional audible cues may be generated by some machines, which act as a guide to the surgeon's foot position. The trainee should be able to move comfortably from one foot position to the next without watching the screen and should know which foot pedal position has been engaged. It is important to explain and understand the need to remain consistently in foot position 1 while the phaco tip is in the eye. This maintains the anterior chamber depth throughout the procedure. When the three foot positions have been mastered, the use of reflux should be taught (usually a kick to the left once the foot is taken off the pedal). The use of the vitrectomy foot position should also be explained, as should the use of the bipolar pedal. Before moving to the next step, it is essential that the trainer observe the trainee using the foot pedal. The trainee needs to be able to simulate sculpting by engaging foot position 3 for a few seconds and then move comfortably back to foot position 1 or 2. The use of complex pedal

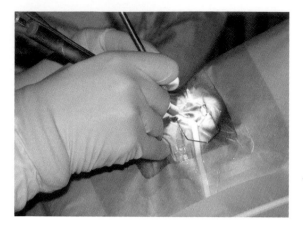

Figure 1.3 Holding the phacoemulsification hand piece.

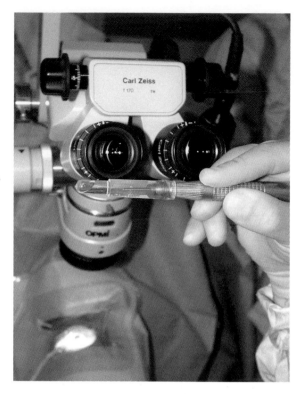

Figure 1.4 Balancing irrigation and aspiration before inserting the phacoemulsification tip into the eye (the plastic test chamber should collapse at approximately the level of the microscope eyepieces).

movements, such as those required for dual linear control, is best reserved for the more accomplished surgeon.

Holding the phacoemulsification hand piece

The hand piece should be held like a pencil, and it is important to bring the index finger quite close to the tip (Figure 1.3). This gives good control of the phacoemulsification hand piece in the eye (in the USA many surgeons hold a phaco hand piece like a screwdriver). It is important that the tubing and lead rest over the arm to prevent kinking of the irrigation and aspiration lines. The trainer should emphasise the importance of relaxing the hand and maintaining the horizontal position of the wrist at this stage.

Balancing infusion and aspiration

Before inserting the phacoemulsification tip into the eye, the trainee should check that the hand piece is working and that the level of the infusion is matched to the rate of aspiration. This is achieved by putting the plastic test chamber (the "condom") over the phacoemulsification needle and filling it with irrigation fluid using foot position 1. The hand piece is then held

horizontally and foot position 2 is engaged while the hand piece is raised. The chamber should collapse at approximately the level of the microscope eyepiece (Figure 1.4). If it collapses at the level of the patient's eye, then the aspiration rate is too high for that level of infusion or the infusion bottle is too low. Conversely, if the chamber does not collapse until well above the level of the microscope eyepiece, then either the infusion bottle is too high or the aspiration level is too low and this should be rectified. The sound of the phacoemulsification hand piece should be heard and should be vigorous when the foot pedal is fully depressed. If, for example, the needle is loose, then the sound will not be normal. This process is a quality control procedure that ensures that the phaco hand piece is in working order before the tip is inserted into the eye.

Inserting the phaco tip into the eye

Before inserting the phaco tip into the eye the correct position of the plastic sleeve should be checked. This may vary depending on the nuclear disassembly technique employed, but usually approximately 1 mm of the phacoemulsification needle will be exposed beyond the irrigation sleeve. The infusion apertures in the sleeve should be directed laterally to ensure that fluid is not directed against the endothelium or the capsule. Foot pedal position 1 is engaged as the phacoemulsification tip is inserted into the eye, with the bevel down to prevent the sharp edge of the needle catching the iris. Once the tip is in the eye, the non-dominant hand turns the hand piece through 90° while the dominant hand supports the hand piece.

Simple "Divide and conquer" (Figure 1.5)

Sculpting the nucleus   The plastic cataract is ideally suited for learning sculpting. The phaco tip is used to sculpt or "shave" the surface of the nucleus. Sculpting commences within the capsulorhexis, starting close to the incision. As the phaco tip touches the lens surface the foot pedal is depressed to position 3, and at the end of the stroke the foot pedal is moved back to position 1. The sequence is then repeated. The tip of the phaco needle should never be completely occluded, although the amount of the lens engaged by the phaco needle depends on the density of the nucleus. In a soft nucleus up to half of the needle can be engaged and the phaco tip can be moved reasonably quickly. Conversely, in a hard nucleus only about one fifth of the needle should be engaged and it must be moved slowly. This avoids pushing the nucleus, which may apply stress to the zonules. If the needle moves the nucleus, then increasing the phaco power should prevent this. For the learning surgeon using a relatively soft plastic nucleus, the phaco power should be set to

20–30%. Hence, when foot position 3 is engaged 20–30% phaco power will result. With more experience, linear power should be used so that the surgeon may vary the power between 1 and 100%, depending on the density of the nucleus.

A groove, approximately one and a half phaco tips in width, should be sculpted from the nucleus. The surgeon should be encouraged to groove the nucleus to at least 75–80% of its depth. A clue to groove depth is the red reflex appearing in the groove base (even in a plastic eye). Also the depth can be gauged by comparison with the phaco tip diameter. When the surgeon feels a depth of at least 75% has been reached, the cataract should then be removed from the eye for inspection. If the surgeon successfully grooves two or three cataracts to 75% depth, then it is no longer necessary to remove the cataract from the eye while learning.

Rotating and cracking the nucleus   A second instrument should be inserted through a side port incision and time should be spent working with two instruments within the eye Although the plastic cataract may not rotate within the bag, the second instrument should be inserted and an attempt should be made to rotate it in order to familiarise oneself with this movement. Usually the cornea has to be removed to rotate the nucleus. Also, if air bubbles become a problem during the sculpting, then the remainder of the procedure can be performed without the cornea in place. A further groove should be made 90° from the original groove and sculpting should be continued until a cross has been made in the cataract. This usually requires the nucleus to be rotated several times through 90°. The trainee should ensure that the phaco tip is never buried within the nucleus and that it is always visible while using only short bursts of phacoemulsification. Once the two grooves have been made (at right angles to each other) an attempt is made to crack the

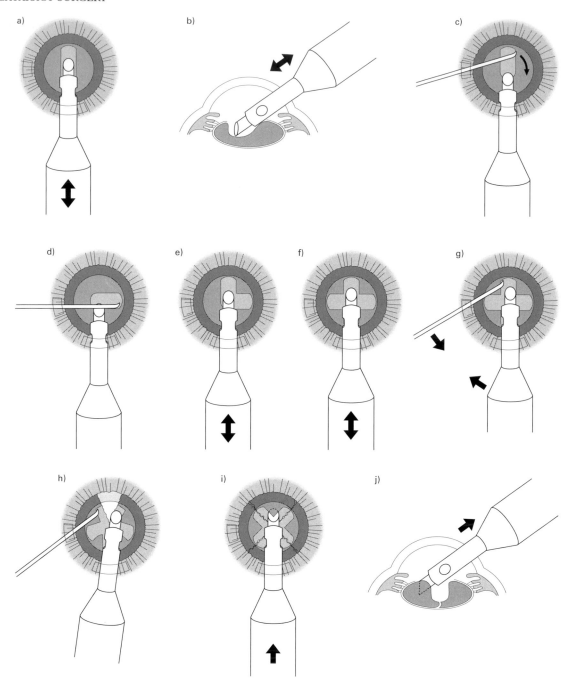

Figure 1.5   Basic elements of "divide and conquer" phacoemulsification. (a) Basic sculpting: microscope view. (b) Basic sculpting: cross-section of anterior segment. (c) Positioning the second instrument prior to nuclear rotation. (d) Rotating the nucleus through 90°. (e) Creating the second groove. (f) Further rotation and sculpting to create a cross. (g) Positioning the second instrument and phaco probe prior to cracking. (h) Bimanual cracking, generating two halves (repeated after 90° rotation to create four quadrants). (i) The phaco probe is driven into a quadrant of the nucleus. (j) Once the phaco tip is buried, suction is maintained to grip and extract the quadrant, allowing removal with phacoemulsification in the "central safe zone".

nucleus, ensuring that both instruments are deep within the groove. Even if the procedure is difficult to perform, this is an excellent learning experience in the simultaneous use of two instruments within the eye. Cracking is much more difficult in the plastic cataract and will take time. The plastic cataract will tend to break into smaller pieces rather than into four complete quadrants.

Nucleus quadrant removal To remove the quadrants higher aspiration rate and vacuum level are used. The consistency of the plastic cataract is often chalky, and this may cause the hand piece and the aspiration tubing to block. Despite the higher vacuum level, the hand piece may require regular washing through with water. To remove a quadrant it is first engaged with a short burst of phaco using foot position 3. Foot position 2 is then used to maintain aspiration, gripping the quadrant, to allow it to be drawn into the mid-pupil or safe area where it can be emulsified. During removal of the quadrants the trainee should be taught the use of pulsed phaco and the use of a higher vacuum level.

Irrigation and aspiration, and lens insertion

If the cornea has been removed it should then be replaced, and time should be spent becoming familiar with the various irrigation and aspiration hand pieces. Plastic cataracts do not usually leave any soft lens matter behind but it is still worthwhile inserting these hand pieces, in particular the angled hand piece that provides easier access to the subincisional cortex.

A complete capsular bag should remain and lens insertion can then be attempted. For the trainee surgeon, a variety of rigid, folding, and injectable lenses should be kept in the wet lab so that experience may be gained in their insertion techniques. The intricacies of the different folding instruments and systems can then be mastered in the wet lab before their use in vivo.

Surgical learning programme

The structure of a surgical learning programme will depend on whether the surgeon is a trainee or an experienced extracapsular cataract surgeon making the transition to phacoemulsification. Whatever the level of previous experience, an individually structured training plan should be drawn up, with specific goals for the training period agreed by trainer and trainee. This plan may need to be flexible and regular appraisal should take place, allowing problem areas to be identified and remedied.

During the transition from wet lab to operating theatre, it is important to involve all members of the theatre team, particularly because time will be required for training and the organisation of the operating list will have to reflect this. The choice of patients for the trainee to operate on must also be addressed. This all requires advance planning if it is to be successful.

For all levels of experience, video recording is an extremely effective and useful tool for learning and improving phacoemulsification surgery. Trainees can benefit from watching their own technique, and the trainer has the opportunity to emphasise good technique and discuss errors (constructive criticism). Recording every procedure should become a routine event.

Ever-increasing numbers of methods and surgical instruments are used for phacoemulsification. It is important that a trainee become competent and comfortable with one surgical technique using familiar instruments before moving on to trying different incisions, nucleus fragmentation techniques, and varying methods of intraocular lens insertion. Returning to the wet lab to practice specific surgical techniques in conjunction with time spent in theatre should be encouraged.

Surgeons in training

For the surgeon in training who has mastered a step in the wet lab, that step can then be put into action in the operating theatre under the supervision of an experienced surgeon. A period of 40–45 minutes dedicated to training, at the start of each operating list, enables the trainee to have regular teaching time. This also ensures that a patient is not subjected to a particularly long operation, both in terms of the need for them to lie still and of macular light exposure (turning the operating light off or only using axial illumination when it is required also minimises this). Trainees often find operating stressful, and the knowledge that the training will take a finite time can help to allay their fears. An alternative allocation of time is for the trainee to repeat the same step of an operation in a series of cases. For example, a trainee can perform the incision for each case on the list, with the trainer completing the remainder of the operation. This can be applied to the initial stages of a "reverse" training pattern (Table 1.2), in which the trainee performs the latter stages of the operation, the earlier stages having been performed by the trainer. Thus, the trainee first starts by aspirating the viscoelastic after lens insertion and then progresses to soft lens matter aspiration, perhaps combining this with lens insertion and removal of the viscoelastic. Phacoemulsification can then be practiced by performing hydrodissection, sculpting and, if appropriate, nucleus rotation. Capsulorhexis is left until later when the trainee has become competent with the other steps (see Chapter 3).

Experienced microsurgeons

For the extracapsular surgeon making a transition to phacoemulsification, a different training plan is suggested (Table 1.3). Capsulorhexis and hydrodissection are essential aspects of phacoemulsification techniques, and for the experienced surgeon they should become

Table 1.2 Reverse chain: sequence of steps for trainees

Step	Details
1	Viscoelastic irrigation and aspiration
2	Soft lens matter irrigation and aspiration
3	Intraocular lens insertion
4	Hydrodissection and nucleus sculpting
5	Nucleus rotation and cracking, and quadrant removal
6	Continuous curvilinear capsulorhexis
7	Incision
8	Complete case

Note that steps can be combined within a single case. For example, once step 1 has been learnt steps 2, 3, and 1 may be combined. Similarly once steps 4 and 5 are learnt, they can be combined with steps 1, 2, and 3 to build up to a complete case.

Table 1.3 Sequence of steps for experienced cataract surgeons

Step	Details
1	Continuous curvilinear capsulorhexis through extracapsular incision or paracentesis
2	Automated irrigation and aspiration for soft lens matter
3	Phaco incision (modified extracapsular cataract extraction) and nucleus sculpting
4	Nucleus rotation and cracking, and quadrant removal
5	Complete case

Note that steps can be combined within a single case. For example, step 1 combined with step 2, followed by steps 1, 2, and 3 together.

part of their extracapsular surgery. Following capsulorhexis, relieving incisions in the capsule opening allow expression of the crystalline lens, or it may be possible to simply viscoexpress or hydroexpress the nucleus.

Using automated irrigation and aspiration to remove soft lens matter familiarises the surgeon with the phaco machine and helps with developing foot pedal control. It also enables the nursing staff to practice machine set up. When capsulorhexis and automated irrigation and aspiration have been mastered, phaco incision and basic nucleus sculpting can be practised.

The surgeon can make a partial thickness incision, as for extracapsular surgery, and then use this as the first step in the construction of either a tri- or biplanar incision for the phaco hand piece. The nucleus is sculpted so that the surgeon can appreciate the difference between the plastic cataract and the human lens. Following initial grooving, if the surgeon still feels confident that the cataract is within his or her ability, then the nucleus can be rotated and further grooving performed. If difficulties are encountered then the phaco tip should be removed from the eye, the incision opened, and an extracapsular cataract extraction performed. Having sculpted three or four nuclei most surgeons will feel confident to continue with phacoemulsification and proceed to nuclear cracking with quadrant removal. The incision should always be constructed to enable the surgeon to perform an extracapsular extraction at any stage should this become necessary.

Case selection

Virtually all cataracts can be removed from the eye using phacoemulsification. The limiting factor is not the machinery but the surgeon's skill. It is important that the trainer and trainee select appropriate cases together at the preoperative assessment stage and arrange the theatre list accordingly.

There are a number of points to consider when selecting cases (Box 1.1). The eye should have a clear healthy cornea, a pupil that dilates well, and a reasonable red reflex. A deep-set eye or prominent brow/nose can make access difficult while learning. Axial length should be considered when selecting patients. Hypermetropic short eyes present problems with a shallow anterior chamber, whereas myopic eyes have a deep anterior chamber. Patients with potential zonular fragility such as those with pseudoexfoliation or a history of previous ocular trauma should be avoided, as should patients who will find it difficult to lie still for an appropriate length of

---

Box 1.1   Case selection: The ideal training case

- Healthy cornea
- Full pupil dilatation
- Good red reflex
- Moderate cataract density
- Easy surgical access
  (for example, no prominent brow)
- Average axial length
  (for example, 22–25 mm)
- Lack of ocular comorbidity
  (for example, pseudoexfoliation)
- Able to lie still and flat under local anaesthesia

---

time or who require awkward positioning on the operating table.

The team approach

Adequate training must be provided for all members of the team in the operating theatre. A surgeon learning phacoemulsification is highly dependent on the nurse who is setting up and controlling the machine. For example, when the nurse fully understands how the phaco machine works, the surgeon need only concentrate on the operation. However, trainees will find it less stressful if they are familiar with how to set up the tubing and hand pieces, and with selecting programmes for the phaco machine. This should be encouraged by the trainer at an early stage on the learning curve and may be achieved by the trainee acting as the scrub nurse, supervised by a member of the nursing staff. This is also an effective method of team building.

The team needs to have a full understanding of how training is to proceed and the time implications for surgery. This includes the nurses, the anaesthetist, and anaesthetic technicians. Each team member plays a role in the training process, and when the final piece of nucleus disappears into the phaco tip at the end of the surgeon's first "complete phaco" the team should feel that they have all shared in that success.

Trainer and trainee communication

Most cataract surgery takes place under local anaesthetic and beginners need to be taught that the patient beneath the drape is awake. Appropriate communication should be used between the trainer and trainee. It is particularly important to repress the desire for expressions of surprise or frustration.

It may be appropriate to inform the patient that a team of doctors is present at the operation and that discussion or description of various stages of the procedure may take place. This will help to prevent the natural anxiety that is experienced by patients who feel that a "junior doctor" is "learning" on their eye. A useful teaching technique is to use the first person, for example "I rotate the nucleus now", as an actual instruction and to use a pre-agreed word to indicate that instrument removal from the eye is desired.

References

1 Leaming D. Practice styles and preferences of ASCRS members: 1998 survey. *J Cataract Refract Surg* 1999; **25**:851–9.
2 Desai P, Minassian DC, Reidy A. National cataract surgery survey 1997–8: a report of the results of the clinical outcomes. *Br J Ophthalmol* 1999;**83**:1336–40.
3 Seward HC, Davies A, Dalton R. Phacoemulsification: risk/benefit analysis during the learning curve. *Eye* 1993;7:164–8.
4 Sugiura T, Kurosaka D, Uezuki Y, Eguchi S, Obata H, Takahashi T. Creating a cataract in a pig eye. *J Cataract Refract Surg* 1999;**25**:615–21.
5 van Vreeswijk H, Pameyer JH. Inducing cataract in post-mortem pig eyes for cataract training purposes. *J Cataract Refract Surg* 1998;**24**:17–18.
6 Mekada A, Nakajima J, Nakamura J, Hirata H, Kishi T, Kani K. Cataract surgery training using pig eyes filled with chestnuts of various hardness. *J Cataract Refract Surg* 1999;**25**:622–5.
7 Maloney WF, Hall D, Parkinson DB. Synthetic cataract teaching system for phacoemulsification. *J Cataract Refract Surg* 1988;**14**:218–21.

2 Incision planning and construction for phacoemulsification

Phacoemulsification is a significant advance in cataract surgery that reduces postoperative inflammation, with early wound stability, resulting in minimal postoperative astigmatism and rapid visual rehabilitation. Most of these advantages are directly attributable to the sutureless small incision. Accordingly, incision construction is a key component of modern cataract surgery. In each of the steps of phacoemulsification, the success of a subsequent step is dependent on that preceding it. The incision may be viewed as the first step in this process and hence is central to the overall success of the procedure.

In 1967 Kelman[1] demonstrated that phacoemulsification might allow surgical incisions to be as small as 2–3 mm in width. However, the subsequent widespread introduction and acceptance of intraocular lenses (IOLs) constructed of rigid polymethylmethacrylate necessitated an incision width of approximately 7 mm. The advantage of a small phacoemulsification incision, with low levels of induced astigmatism, was therefore substantially reduced. It has been recognised that if an incision is placed further from the optical axis, then it may be increased in width while remaining astigmatically neutral (Figure 2.1).[2] The need for a larger incision was therefore partly overcome by the development of posteriorly placed scleral tunnel incisions[3] and innovative astigmatic suture

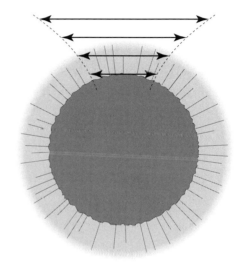

Figure 2.1 The "astigmatic funnel": a series of incisions have to shorten in width as they are placed closer to the optic axis in order to induce the same astigmatism.

techniques.[4] The advent of lens implants with an optic diameter of around 5 mm allowed these scleral tunnels to be left unsutured, and such incisions have been shown to be extremely strong.[5] The development of foldable lens materials has enabled the initial small phacoemulsification incision to be retained.[6] This has made it possible for a self-sealing incision to be placed more anteriorly, in the clear cornea, without increasing astigmatism or loss of wound stability. Further development in hand piece technology has seen a reduction in phaco tip diameter and hence incision width. Some lenses can be inserted through these incisions that measure less than 3 mm; however, it remains to be seen whether this further reduction in wound size confers a significant refractive advantage.

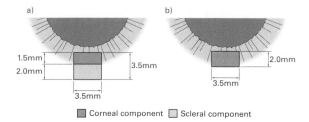

Figure 2.2 Incision shapes. (a) A "square" scleral tunnel incision. (b) A "rectangular" clear corneal incision.

Incision choice

The principal decision facing a surgeon is whether to perform a scleral tunnel incision (STI) or clear corneal incision (CCI). The refractive implications of these incisions are dealt with separately below, but there are several other factors that may influence the choice of incision.

The more anterior position and overall shorter tunnel length of a CCI increases hand piece manoeuvrability and allows the phaco probe more direct access to the anterior chamber and the cataract. Furthermore, a CCI may be less likely to compress the irrigation sleeve of the phaco probe and hence reduces the risk of heating the incision, or "phaco burn". However, the tunnel of a CCI extends further anteriorly than does that of a STI, and this may lead to corneal distortion or striae from the phaco hand piece. It has been demonstrated that incisions in which the tunnel width and length are approximately the same (square or near square; Figure 2.2a) are more resistant to leakage than are those in which the width is greater than the tunnel length (rectangular; Figure 2.2b).[5] Hence, when a polymethylmethacrylate or folding IOL that requires a larger incision is used, the comparatively longer tunnel of a STI may be more likely to provide a wound that can remain unsutured.

A STI requires a conjunctival peritomy and cautery to the episclera. This is time consuming and in patients with impaired clotting, for example those taking asprin or warfarin, it is best avoided. Disturbance of the conjunctiva may also compromise the success of subsequent glaucoma drainage surgery.[7] In addition, if a patient has a functioning trabeculectomy, then a CCI avoids an incision of the conjunctiva and

the risk of damaging the drainage bleb. Of course, a scleral tunnel is a prerequisite when performing a phacotrabeculectomy.

There is some evidence to suggest that endothelial cell loss may be lower when phacoemulsification is performed through a STI[8] and it may therefore be a preferable technique in patients with poor endothelial reserve, for example those with Fuchs' endothelial dystrophy or following a penetrating corneal graft. The possible need, identified before surgery, for conversion to an expression extracapsular technique may also influence the choice of incision. In favour of an enlarged STI is that it may be easier to express the nucleus and less detrimental to the endothelium. However, a CCI may be quicker and easier to enlarge, at the possible risk of greater, induced astigmatism.

Factors such as previous vitreous surgery, in which the sclera may be scarred, and disorders that predispose to scleral thinning and conjuctival diseases, for example ocular cicatrical phemphigoid, all favour a CCI. Histological analysis has demonstrated that phacoemulsification incisions placed in vascular tissue initiate an early fibroblastic response and rapid healing as compared with those in avascular corneal tissue.[9] This may be relevant to patients for whom rapid healing is advantageous (for example children and those with mental handicap) and to patients with reduced healing (for example diabetic persons and those taking corticosteroids).

Table 2.1   Comparative advantages of scleral and corneal incisions

Incision type	Advantages
Scleral tunnel incision	Minimal induced astigmatism
	Large sutureless incisions possible
	May be combined with trabeculectomy at single site
	Less endothelial cell loss
	Rapid wound healing
	Safe if converted to large-incision extracapsular technique
	Phaco hand piece less likely to cause corneal striae and distort view
Clear corneal incision	Induced astigmatism may be used to modify pre-existing astigmatism
	Reduced surgical time
	Less likely to compromise existing or future glaucoma filtration surgery
	No risk of haemorrhage; cautery not required
	Reduced risk of phaco burn (shorter tunnel)
	Increased ease of hand piece manipulation
	Avoids conjunctiva in diseases such as ocular cicatricial pemphigoid
	Avoids sclera when scarred and/or thinned
	Easy to convert to large-incision extracapsular technique

Table 2.1 summarises the comparative advantages of STIs and CCIs. It has been suggested that these advantages may be combined by placing the incision over the limbus.[10] However, the disadvantage is that bleeding still occurs and cautery may be required.

Incision placement

A STI is usually placed at the superior or oblique (superolateral) position, which ensures that the conjunctival wound is under the patient's upper lid. Surgeon comfort and ease of surgery are also factors in this decision, and these same factors influence the choice of position for a CCI. Aside from the refractive issues dealt with below, there may be a number of other considerations when selecting the placement of an incision.

Access via a temporal approach is often easier in patients with deep-set eyes or with a prominent brow. In these circumstances the use of a lid speculum with a nasal rather than temporal hinge may be helpful (Figure 2.3). Pre-existing ocular pathology, such as peripheral anterior synechiae, corneal scarring and pannus, or the position of a trabeculectomy filtering bleb may alter the selection of an incision site.

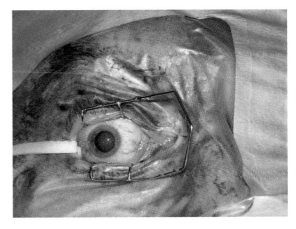

Figure 2.3 Lid speculum with nasal hinge (BD Ophthalmic Systems).

Surgically induced astigmatism

Scleral and corneal incisions both cause some degree of corneal flattening in the meridian (or axis) on which they are performed, with corresponding steepening in the perpendicular meridian, termed "surgically induced astigmatism". As previously stated, this effect is dependent on the size of the incision and its proximity to the centre of the cornea (Figure 2.1). Because a STI is performed further from the optic axis it induces less astigmatism than does a CCI of equivalent width. Various STI pregroove shapes

13

Table 2.2   Reported surgically induced astigmatism (SIA) in unsutured triplanar incisions at three months

Incision type	Incision site	Incision length (mm)	SIA (dioptres)	Reference
STI	Superior	3·2	0·63 ± 0·43	Oshika et al.[14]
		5·5	1·00 ± 0·59	
	Oblique	3·2	0·37 ± 0·28	Hayashi et al.[15]
		5·0	0·64 ± 0·39	
CCI	Superior	3·0–3·5	0·88 ± 0·66	Long and Monica[12]
	Temporal	3·0–3·5	0·67 ± 0·49	
		3·0	0·20 ± 0·32	Rainer et al.[18]
	Oblique	3·0	0·39 ± 0·73	

SIA vector analysis was conducted using the Jaffe method, except for Rainer et al.,[18] who used the Cravy method.

have been described that, by altering wound construction, attempt to minimise surgically induced astigmatism. These include straight, curved (limbus parallel), reverse curved (frown), and V-shaped (chevron) incisions. However, none of these has been clearly identified as inducing less astigmatism.[11]

The degree of induced astigmatic change and its stability over time varies with the meridonal axis on which the incision is placed. Both STIs and CCIs produce the least astigmatism when they are placed on the temporal meridian and most astigmatism when they are placed superiorly.[12–14] An oblique position has an intermediate effect.[15,16] These findings reflect the elliptical shape of the cornea and the greater proximity of the superior limbus to its centre. The surgically induced astigmatism reported by several authors using different unsutured triplanar incisions at three months is summarised in Table 2.2. Superiorly placed incisions are also associated with an increase in astigmatism over time and a change toward "against the rule" (ATR) astigmatism, with a steeper cornea in the 180° axis.[17,18] This effect, which is dependent on incision size, has been attributed to the effect of gravity and pressure from the lids.

The meridian on which an incision is placed is therefore an important factor in surgical planning, particularly with reference to a patient's pre-existing keratometric or corneal astigmatism. It should be noted that the spectacle refraction may be misleading because lenticular astigmatism is negated by cataract surgery. With increased age the majority of the population develop ATR astigmatism. Hence, a temporally placed incision may reduce or neutralise this astigmatism. In a few circumstances the incision may induce a small degree of "with the rule" (WTR) astigmatism, with corneal steepening in the 90° meridian. Although it is generally preferable to undercorrect pre-existing astigmatism and avoid large swings of axis,[19] WTR astigmatism is considered normal in younger individuals and may confer some optical advantage.

Reducing coexisting astigmatism during phacoemulsification

Naturally occurring astigmatism may be present in 14–50% of the normal population[20,21] and cataract surgery provides the opportunity to correct this astigmatism. This improves patients' unaided vision after surgery, reducing their dependence on spectacles and increasing their satisfaction. In patients with moderate levels of pre-existing astigmatism, a reduction in astigmatism without altering the axis may be achieved, by placing the incision on the steep or "plus" meridian. This is of particular importance when using multifocal lens implants, where astigmatism may substantially reduce the multifocal effect.[22] In these circumstances, modifying incision architecture may increase the astigmatic effect of a CCI. Langerman[23] described a triplanar CCI with a deep (750 μm) pregroove that was intended to create a limbal "hinge" and ensure a non-leaking incision even if pressure was applied to its posterior lip (Figure 2.4). The deep pregroove has been noted to have a keratotomy or limbal relaxing effect that induces more astigmatic change, which is more pronounced as the incision length increases.[24]

When attempting to reduce astigmatism by incision positioning, it is important to ensure

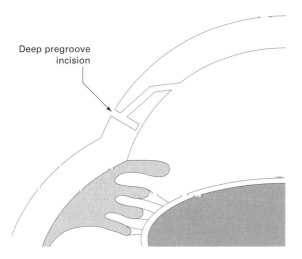

Figure 2.4 Wound profile of Langermann's hinge incision.

that it is accurately placed on the steep meridian. A 30° error will simply alter the axis of astigmatism without changing its power (if attempting a full correction). Smaller errors decrease the effect of the incision and change the axis of astigmatism, albeit less dramatically. Because torsional eye movement may occur despite local anaesthesia, the steep axis, or a reference point on the globe from which this axis can be derived, should be identified or marked before anaesthesia. The axis can also be confirmed with intraoperative keratometry at the start of surgery. When placing an incision on the steep meridian of astigmatism, there are some meridia that may necessitate the surgeon adopting an unusual operating position or operating with their non-dominant hand (Figure 2.5). In such cases it may be preferable to use a standard phacoemulsification incision in conjunction with an incisional refractive technique or a toric lens implant. It is relevant to note that, when correcting astigmatism with an incisional technique, coupling changes the overall corneal power and larger corrections may therefore alter the IOL biometry calculation (see

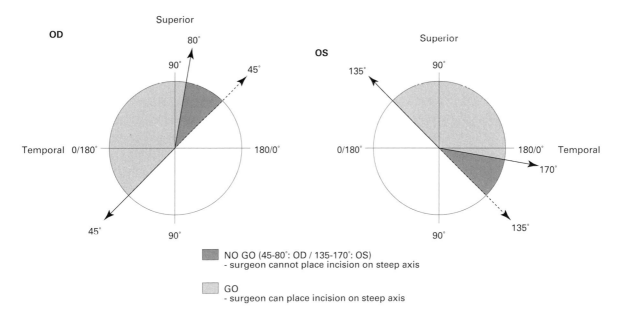

Figure 2.5 The "no go" meridia for a right handed surgeon.

Table 2.3   Unsutured small incision planning in relation to pre-existing astigmatism

Pre-exisiting keratometric astigmatism	Incision type and position
+ 0·75 D ATR + 1·00 D WTR or oblique	Temporal CCI (or STI)
>+ 0·75 D ATR >+1·00 D WTR or oblique	Langermann hinge CCI on axis

Note: if > +1·75 D (ATR, WTR, or oblique) then consider an incisional refractive technique or toric intraocular lens. ATR, against the rule; CCI, clear corneal incision; D, dioptres; STI, Scleral tunnel incision; WTR, with the rule.

Chapter 6). Table 2.3 suggests an approach to modifying incision type and placement in order to avoid increasing, and possibly reduce, pre-existing keratometric astigmatism. However, surgically induced astigmatism varies with the size of incision and from surgeon to surgeon, and it may be necessary to adapt this guide on the basis of an individual's experience with their preferred incision techniques.

Several techniques exist for modulating high astigmatism intraoperatively. These include astigmatic keratotomy, limbal relaxing incisions, opposite CCIs, and toric IOL implantation. Irrespective of the technique used, the astigmatic effect of the phacoemulsification incision also needs to be taken into account (unless it is astigmatically neutral). Corneal video topography should be performed before any refractive surgery is performed to exclude the presence of irregular astigmatism from, for example, a corneal ectatic disease. This reaffirms the axis of astigmatism, which should be identified or marked on the eye, as discussed above. The surgeon's principle aim should be to preserve corneal asphericity and reduce high preoperative astigmatism while maintaining its principal meridian.

Limbal relaxing incisions are partial thickness incisions at the limbus (the corneoscleral junction) and have been advocated as an effective and safe method of reducing astigmatism during cataract surgery.[25] Compared with astigmatic keratotomy they have the advantage of better preserving corneal structure with more rapid visual recovery and less risk of postoperative glare or discomfort. They are also easier to perform and do not require preoperative pachymetry. The

Table 2.4   Limbal keratotomy nomogram

Astigmatism (dioptres)	Incision type	Length (mm)	Optical zone
2–3	Two LRIs	6·0	At limbus
>3	Two LRIs	8·0	At limbus

Modified Gills nomogram for limbal relaxing incisions (LRIs) to correct astigmatism with cataract surgery. Modified from Budak et al.[25]

incisions can be performed at the start of phacoemulsification or after lens implantation (before removal of viscoelastic). With reference to a suitable nomogram (Table 2.4) or software program, single or paired, 6- to 8-mm long incisions are made at the limbus centred on the axis of corneal astigmatism. They are typically 550–600 μm deep, and preset guarded disposable blades are available that avoid the need for an adjustable guarded diamond blade. Astigmatic keratotomy nomograms usually use degrees of arc to define the incision length and require special instrumentation. With an optic zone of 12 mm (the corneal diameter), degrees of arc approximate to millimeters (for example, ~60° = ~6 mm), and this conveniently allows the length of a limbal relaxing incision to be marked along the limbus with a standard calliper. Opposite CCIs also do not require new instrumentation or new surgical skills.[26] The use of paired incisions (both on the steep meridian) increases the expected flattening effect of a single CCI, and a mean correction of 2·25 D has been reported (using 2·8 to 3·5-mm wide phaco incisions). Although simple to perform, opposite CCIs necessitate an additional penetrating incision that may have greater potential for complications when compared with an alternative non-penetrating incisional technique.[27]

Implantation of a toric IOL avoids the potential complications of additional corneal incisions and has no effect on corneal coupling. An example is the Staar foldable toric lens implant, which is identical to current silicone plate haptic lenses except on its anterior surface there is a spherocylindrical or toric refracting element.[28] Like all toric lenses, this requires accurate intraoperative alignment in order to correct astigmatism and relies on the IOL remaining centred. Although plate haptic lenses may rotate within the capsular bag immediately after implantation, they show long-term rotational stability as compared with loop haptic lenses.[29] Early postoperative reintervention may therefore be required with plate haptic toric lenses and the ideal toric lens design remains to be identified. A toric IOL also has the disadvantage that the astigmatic correction is limited to a narrow range of powers.

Incision technique

Scleral tunnel incision technique

A conjunctival peritomy is first performed with spring scissors and forceps (Figure 2.6a). This is approximately the same length as the proposed final incision width, and should be measured and marked using a calliper beforehand. The conjunctiva is blunt dissected posteriorly to expose the sclera 2–3 mm behind the limbus. It is important that this is fully beneath Tenon's fascia. If necessary, one or two radial relieving incisions may be made at the ends of the conjunctival wound to improve exposure. The minimum cautery required to achieve haemostasis is applied to the exposed episcleral vessels over the proposed incision site.

The width of the incision should be marked 2 mm behind the limbus using a calliper. The first step of the incision is to create a straight pregroove incision of around one third scleral thickness in depth (Figure 2.6b). Care should be

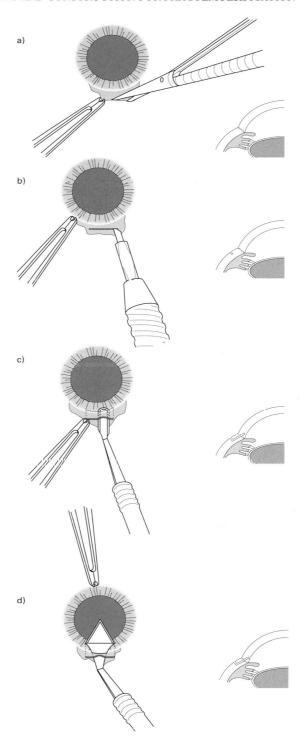

Figure 2.6 Microscope view and wound profile: steps in the construction of a scleral tunnel incision. (a) Conjunctival peritomy. (b) Pregroove incision. (c) Scleral and corneal tunnel. (d) Entry into the anterior chamber with a keratome.

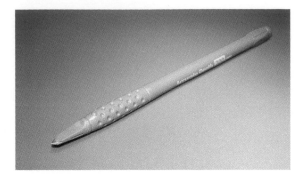

Figure 2.7 A disposable 300 μm guarded blade for pregroove incision (Beaver Accurate Depth Knife; BD Ophthalmic Systems).

taken not to cut too deeply and incise the ciliary body. This may be avoided by using a guarded blade with a preset cutting depth of approximately 300 μm (Figure 2.7). Disposable blades with a fixed cutting depth are widely marketed for this purpose. During this step, the globe can be stabilised, and counter traction applied, by forceps gripping the limbus near to the lateral edge of the peritomy.

In the second step a pocket or crescent blade is used to create the scleral tunnel. By pressing on the posterior edge of the pregroove with the flat base of the blade, its tip is placed into the anterior aspect of the groove. Initially this may require the blade to be directed relatively downward, but as soon as the tunnel is commenced the heel of the blade should be lowered to the conjunctival surface to ensure an even lamellar dissection through the sclera into the corneal plane. The lamellar cut should proceed smoothly and anteriorly, with a combination of partial rotatory and side to side motions. The lamellar dissection is continued until the tip of the pocket blade is just visible within clear cornea, beyond the limbus (Figure 2.6c). The tunnel can then be extended further laterally, to the full width of the pregroove and the desired incision width. During creation of the scleral pocket, counter traction can be improved by gripping the sclera adjacent to the lateral edge of the pregroove or its posterior lip. Neither the fragile anterior edge nor the roof of the tunnel

should be gripped. If an extremely sharp pocket or crescent knife is used, for example a diamond blade, then counter traction may not be required.

The final stage of the incision is then performed using a keratome blade, the width of which is matched to the diameter of the phaco tip. Counter traction is now best provided either by gripping the limbus directly opposite the incision with forceps or by using a limbal fixation ring. Limited side to side motions may facilitate full entry of the blade, without damage to the pocket. Once the blade tip is visible in clear cornea, at the end of the tunnel, it is angled posteriorly. The blade should enter the anterior chamber directly, avoiding contact between its tip and the lens or iris. The blade should be advanced so that the full width of the blade enters the anterior chamber (Figure 2.6d).

Clear corneal incision technique

Many techniques have been described that produce an effective self-sealing CCI. This may mimic a triplanar STI, with the creation of a pregroove, followed by a tunnel or pocket and then entry into the anterior chamber. In contrast, a uniplanar or "stab" incision may be performed with a keratome directly through the cornea. A biplanar incision is made by first creating a pregroove into which the keratome is placed. A bi- or triplanar incision is more likely to provide a reproducible self-sealing incision in terms of width, length, and overall configuration than is a uniplanar incision. Moreover, in the event of conversion to a non-phacoemulsification technique, enlargement of a uniplanar incision may cause difficulty in achieving an astigmatically neutral wound closure. For these reasons, a uniplanar incision is not recommended for surgeons with little experience in corneal tunnel construction. If the lens nucleus is hard and a higher level of ultrasound power or phacoemulsification time is anticipated, then the anterior wound edge may be prone to damage from either manipulation or

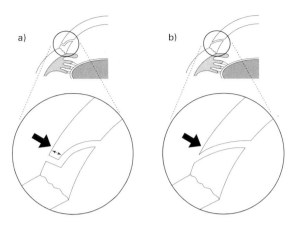

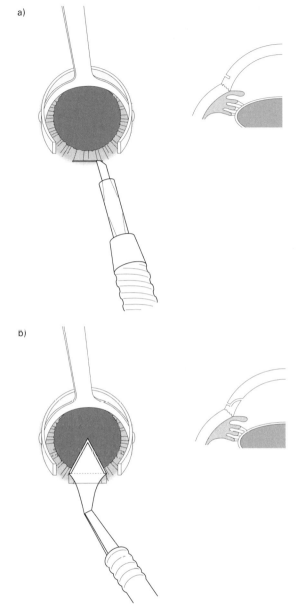

Figure 2.8 Clear corneal incision wound profiles compared. (a) Biplanar: detail of the anterior external wound edge highlights the pregroove. (b) Uniplanar: the anterior external wound edge is less robust.

phaco burn, and in these circumstances an incision with a pregroove may be favoured (Figure 2.8).

Before commencing the incision, the formation of a self-sealing paracentesis at the limbus in the plane of the iris will allow the anterior chamber to be filled with a viscoelastic. This provides a consistently firm eye on which the incision may be performed. If a pregroove is used, then its dimensions should first be marked with a calliper along the avascular limbus. The eye is stabilised using either a limbal fixation ring or toothed forceps at the limbus adjacent to the incision site. Some surgeons prefer to grip the paracentesis, which reduces the risk of a subconjunctival haemorrhage. The pregroove incision is then made perpendicular to the corneal surface, just inside the limbal vascular arcade, with a depth of around one third of corneal thickness (Figure 2.9a). The use of a guarded blade with a preset depth of approximately 300 µm ensures a consistent depth. The keratome is placed in the groove by depressing its posterior lip with the base of the blade flattened against the globe. Counter traction is now best provided by gripping or supporting the limbus, directly opposite the incision. The path of the keratome through the

Figure 2.9 Microscope view and wound profile: steps in the construction of a biplanar clear corneal incision. (a) Eye stabilised with a ring and pregroove performed with a diamond blade. (b) Corneal tunnel and entry into the anterior chamber with a keratome.

cornea is similar irrespective of whether a one or two step incision is used. The blade is first angled to create a lamellar dissection in the corneal plane. This is continued anteriorly

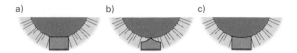

Figure 2.10 Internal incision shape depending on angle of anterior chamber entry with keratome. (a) Correct: corneal plane entry. (b) Incorrect: too steep. (c) Incorrect: too shallow.

within the cornea for approximately 2 mm. Some keratomes are marked in order to gauge this distance. If the anterior chamber is relatively shallow then a longer tunnel may be desirable. This ensures that the distance between the iris and the internal aspect of the incision is maintained, reducing the risk of intraoperative iris prolapse,[30] although possibly causing corneal distortion by the phaco hand piece.

Once the required incision length has been achieved the keratome is then directed posteriorly. This creates a dimple in the cornea overlying the blade, and it is then advanced so that the tip incises Descemet's membrane and enters the anterior chamber. The angle of the blade is subsequently returned to its original plane and the incision completed (Figure 2.9b). This creates a straight incision through Descemet's membrane (Figure 2.10a). If the blade remains steeply inclined, them the internal wound shape adopts a "V" pattern, the apex of which points toward the centre of the cornea (Figure 2.10b). In contrast, a shallow entry angle has the opposite effect (Figure 2.10c). The keratome should be fully advanced into the anterior chamber, so that the incision width is uniform along its length. This ensures that the manoeuvrability of the phaco tip and hand piece is not restricted by the internal aspect of the incision. It also reduces the risk of compression of the irrigation sleeve or iatrogenic detachment of Descemet's membrane when introducing the phaco tip into the anterior chamber.

The choice of keratome width is determined by that recommended by the manufacturer of the phaco tip and hand piece. There is evidence to suggest that a diamond keratome offers the advantage over a steel blade of a more regular and smoother incision.[31] However, a diamond keratome tends to be thicker than an equivalent metal blade and hence a slightly wider incision is created.

Incision complications: avoidance and management

Both STIs and CCIs have associated complications, which may appear during their construction or only become apparent during phacoemulsification. Table 2.5 identifies these complications and suggests both immediate and preventative actions. Complications that may occur during the postoperative period are discussed in Chapter 12.

Incision enlargement

It is frequently necessary to enlarge an incision surgically, either to facilitate IOL implantation or to convert to a non-phacoemulsification cataract extraction technique. To maintain, as far as possible, the advantageous features of the phaco incision, it is preferable that enlargement should preserve the three dimensional structure of the initial incision. When the desired incision width is anticipated to exceed that of the initial keratome, then the length of the pregroove and the width of the tunnel of a triplanar incision should be constructed to correspond with the expected final wound dimensions. This also applies to the length of the pregroove in a biplanar incision. If it is necessary to enlarge an incision later in the procedure, after marking with a calliper, then a pregroove should either be created or extended to the required width. The wound is usually, although not necessarily, enlarged equally on both sides of the pre-existing incision. To ensure that a single pregroove incision is made, the blade should be placed in the existing incision and cut outward from each side. When substantially enlarging a scleral tunnel, the peritomy should first be extended and cautery applied in order to achieve haemostasis.

Table 2.5 Incision complications

Incision	Problem	Immediate action	Prevention
Scleral	Incision of ciliary body during pregroove	Consider suturing incision and performing new incision at alternative or anterior site; if localised, a deep radial suture may allow incision to proceed	Care with pregroove depth; consider using a guarded blade with preset depth
	Anterior perforation through roof of scleral tunnel with pocket blade	New incision at alternative site or recommence with deeper lamellar dissection at same site	Maintain lamellar dissection with scleral pocket blade less "heel down"; confirm that the dissection is in sclera and not Tenon's fascia
	Anterior perforation at lateral edge of scleral tunnel with pocket blade	Proceed cautiously; if the wound leaks during phaco, consider new incision at alternative site	Remember that the dissection is part of a sphere not a flat plane; confirm that the dissection is in sclera not Tenon's fascia
	Premature AC entry with pocket blade	Proceed cautiously; wound may not self-seal and may require a suture; if the wound leaks during phaco or the iris prolapses, consider new incision at alternative site	Maintain "heel down" position with scleral pocket blade during lamellar pocket dissection
	Distortion of cornea with phacoprobe (excessively long tunnel)	Incise along the lateral aspect of the scleral tunnel	Place pregroove nearer to the limbus and/or extend tunnel less into clear cornea
	Haemorrhage within scleral tunnel ± hyphaema	Direct pressure over incision; cautery to posterior and internal aspect of wound	Adequate cautery (particularly posterior to the pregroove); ensure tunnel is not unnecessarily deep; consider CCI (patients with impaired clotting)
Corneal	Excessive leak of irrigation fluid during phaco (wound too wide)*	Temporary suture to partially close wound; increase irrigation bottle height; consider new incision at alternative site	Care to reduce any lateral movement of the keratome during incision; check size of keratome and phaco hand piece
	Tight fit around phaco probe (small internal incision)*	Repeat keratome incision ensuring full entry of blade shoulders into anterior chamber	Ensure full entry of keratome into anterior chamber; check size of keratome and phaco hand piece
	Corneal distortion and striae with phaco probe (anteriorly placed AC entry)	Consider new incision at alternative site	Shorten corneal tunnel length
	Iris prolapse during phaco (posteriorly placed AC entry)*	Check for alternative cause of iris prolapse; consider new incision at alternative site; consider peripheral iridectomy; the wound may not self-seal and may require a suture	Increase corneal tunnel length, particularly with a pre-existing shallow AC
	Conjunctiva "ballooning" with irrigation fluid (incision too posterior)	Grasp conjunctiva posterior to the incision with forceps and tear conjunctiva posteriorly away from wound	Place the external aspect of the incision further anteriorly into clear cornea

*Problem may affect both types of incision. AC, anterior chamber; CCI, clear corneal incision.

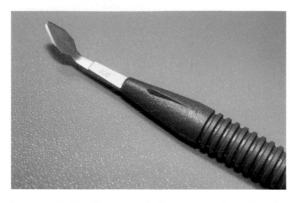

Figure 2.11 Truncated keratome for incision enlargement (Edge Ahead IOL knife; BD Ophthalmic Systems).

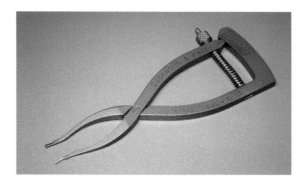

Figure 2.12 Pearce single diamond tipped calliper for wound enlargement (Duckworth and Kent).

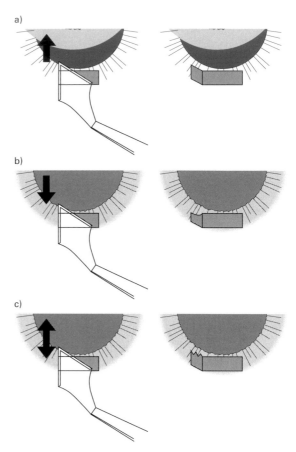

Figure 2.13 Wound profile following enlargement is dependant on direction of blade cut. (a) Correct: inward, resulting in a consistent tunnel length. (b) Incorrect: outward, resulting in a shortened tunnel length. (c) Incorrect: inward and outward, resulting in a varying tunnel length.

A specifically designed keratome with a truncated tip, of known width, can be used to complete the enlargement of an incision precisely and safely (Figure 2.11). Similarly, an adjustable diamond tipped cutting calliper can be used (Figure 2.12). However, a standard blade, pocket knife, or keratome may be employed. The anterior chamber should first be filled with a viscoelastic material in order to reduce the risk of inadvertent damage to the intraocular structures, in particular the anterior capsule. The blade is then introduced into the incision, ensuring that its edge is parallel to the lateral margins of the tunnel. Cutting on the inward stroke of the blade ensures that the sides of the tunnel remain a consistent length (Figure 2.13a). If the incision is cut on the outward stroke the tunnel length shortens (Figure 2.13b), and if a sawing action is used the wound adopts a zigzag pattern (Figure 2.13c). Placing the blade parallel to the internal lateral margin of the tunnel avoids creating a funnel shape and achieves a consistent width. When converting from phacoemulsification to an alternative extracapsular technique, an alternative is to close the initial temporal incision and revert to a different incision type at the superior meridian.

Several studies have demonstrated that the initial incision width enlarges during instrumentation.[32] Scanning electronmicroscopy has shown tearing of corneal structures following IOL implantation through small incisions.[33] It has been suggested that adequate surgical

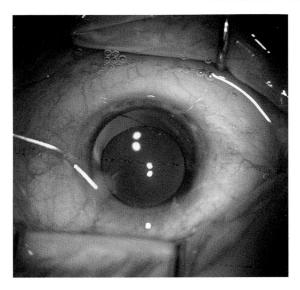

Figure 2.14   Corneal hydration to close a clear corneal incision.

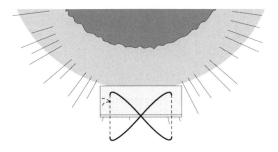

Figure 2.15   Detail of a cross ("X") suture.

enlargement of the primary incision, before IOL insertion, avoids deformation and lateral tearing of the wound, preserves incision structure, and reduces the risk of wound leakage. Enlargement or stretching of the wound during IOL implantation has been shown to vary with the type of lens implant used and, importantly, with its power.[34] High dioptre power lenses are usually thicker and therefore require more wound enlargement before implantation.

Incision closure

Following exchange of viscoelastic for balanced salt solution (BSS) at the end of surgery, the anterior chamber should be filled with BSS via the paracentesis. This allows the valve-like internal corneal lip of the incision to close. The security of the incision can then be examined by gentle pressure on the central cornea or the limbus. The incision and paracentesis (or paracenteses) can be dried with a surgical sponge, and if they are watertight then they will remain dry. It should be recognised that substantial pressure on the posterior aspect of the tunnel may cause leakage and does not necessarily imply a failure to self-seal.

Corneal hydration can be used to augment closure of a CCI. BSS in a syringe with a narrow-gauge blunt cannula is employed. The cannula tip is placed within the lateral aspect of the tunnel and directed laterally into the stroma. BSS is then gently injected to achieve localised oedema with loss of corneal clarity (Figure 2.14). A suture may be required to close a wound that has failed to self-seal or where a phaco burn has occurred. Both absorbable and non-absorbable sutures have been employed, although non-absorbable monofilament is more frequently used with corneal incisions. In cases where a large incision may induce astigmatism, a suture may also be desirable. However, this may delay stabilisation of postoperative astigmatism as compared with unsutured incisions.[35] A suture may be useful to reinforce the wound in patients who are likely to rub the eye, for example children or those with mental handicap.

In the past interrupted radial sutures have been widely employed to close large-incision cataract extraction wounds. Such sutures appose blocks of tissue and prevent aqueous leakage; however if tight they may induce corneal steepening and "plus" astigmatism. Conversely, loose sutures may result in corneal flattening and "minus" astigmatism. Suture techniques to close both scleral and corneal phacoemulsification incisions include the simple "X" suture (Figure 2.15), the Shepard horizontal suture,[4] and the Fine infinity suture.[36] They aim to oppose the floor and the roof of the incision and create anteroposterior wound compression, minimising radial forces on the cornea and hence reducing induced astigmatism.

References

1 Kelman CD. Phacoemulsification and aspiration: a new technique of cataract removal: a preliminary report. *Am J Ophthalmol* 1967;**64**:23–35.

2 Koch PS. Structural analysis of cataract incision construction. *J Cataract Refract Surg* 1991;**17**(suppl): 661–7.

3 Girard LJ, Rodriguez J, Mailman ML. Reducing surgically induced astigmatism by using a scleral tunnel. *Am J Ophthalmol* 1984;**97**:450–6.

4 Shepard JR. Induced astigmatism in small incision cataract surgery. *J Cataract Refract Surg* 1989;**15**:85–8.

5 Ernest PH, Lavery KT, Kiessling LA. Is there a difference in incision healing based on location? J *Cataract Refract Surg* 1998;**24**:482–6.

6 McFarland MS. The clinical history of sutureless surgery: the first modern sutureless cases. In: Gills JP, Martin RG, Sanders DR, eds. *Sutureless cataract surgery*. Thorofare, NJ: Slack Inc., 1992.

7 Broadway DC, Grierson I, Hitchings RA. Local effects of previous conjunctival incisional surgery and the subsequent outcome of filtration surgery. *Am J Ophthalmol* 1998;**125**:805–18.

8 Oshima Y, Tsujikawa K, Oh A, Harino S. Comparative study of intraocular lens implantation through 3·0 mm temporal clear corneal and superior scleral tunnel self-sealing incisions. *J Cataract Refract Surg* 1997;**23**: 347–53.

9 Ernest PH, Neuhann T. Posterior limbal incision. *J Cataract Refract Surg* 1996;**22**:78–84.

10 Ernest PH, Lavery KT, Kiessling LA. Relative strength of scleral corneal and clear corneal incisions constructed in cadaver eyes. *J Cataract Refract Surg* 1994;**20**:626–9.

11 Vass C, Menapace R, Rainer G. Corneal topographic changes after frown and straight sclerocorneal incisions. *J Cataract Refract Surg* 1997;**23**:913–22.

12 Long DA, Monica ML. A prospective evaluation of corneal curvature changes with 3·0–3·5mm corneal tunnel phacoemulsification. *Ophthalmology* 1996;**103**: 226–32.

13 Wirbelauer C, Anders N, Pham DT, Wollensak J. Effect of incision location on preoperative oblique astigmatism after scleral tunnel incision. *J Cataract Refract Surg* 1997;**23**:365–71.

14 Oshika T, Tsuboi S, Yaguchi S, *et al.* Comparative study of intraocular lens implantation through 3·2 and 5·5 mm incisions. *Ophthalmology* 1994;**101**:1183–90.

15 Hayashi K, Hayashi HHH, Nakao F, Hayashi F. The correlation between incision size and corneal shape changes in sutureless cataract surgery. *Ophthalmology* 1995;**102**:550–6.

16 Rainer G, Menapace R, Vass C, Annen D, Strenn K, Papapanos P. Surgically induced astigmatism following a 4·0 mm sclerocorneal valve incision. *J Cataract Refract Surg* 1997;**23**:358–64.

17 Roman S, Auclin F, Chong-Sit DA, Ullern MM. Surgically induced astigmatism with superior and temporal incisions in cases of with-the-rule preoperative astigmatism. *J Cataract Refract Surg* 1998;**24**:1636–41.

18 Rainer G, Menapace R, Vass C, Annen D, Findl O, Schmetter K. Corneal shape changes after temporal and superolateral 3·0 mm clear corneal incisions. *J Cataract Refract Surg* 1999;**25**:1121–6.

19 Guyton D. Prescribing cylinders: the problem of distortion. *Surv Ophthalmol* 1997;**22**:177–88.

20 Bear JC, Richler A. Cylindrical refractive error: a population study in Western Newfoundland. *Am J Optom Physiol Opt* 1983;**60**:39–45.

21 Hirsch MJ. Changes in astigmatism during the first eight years of school. *Am J Optom* 1963;**40**:127–32.

22 Ravalico G, Parentin F, Baccara F. Effect of astigmatism on multifocal intraocular lenses. *J Cataract Refract Surgery* 1999;**25**:804–7.

23 Langerman DW. Architectural design of a self-sealing corneal tunnel, single-hinge incision. *J Cataract Refract Surg* 1994;**20**:84–8.

24 Amigo A, Giebel AW, Muinos JA. Astigmatic keratotomy effect of single-hinge, clear corneal incisions using various preincision lengths. *J Cataract Refract Surg* 1998;**24**:765–71.

25 Budak K, Friedman NJ, Koch D. Limbal relaxing incisions with cataract surgery. *J Cataract Refract Surg* 1998;**24**:503–8.

26 Lever JL. Dahan E. Opposite clear corneal incisions. *J Cataract Refract Surg* 200;**26**:803–5

27 Nichamin LD. Opposite clear corneal incisions. *J Cataract Refract Surg* 2001;**27**:7–8.

28 Leyland M, Zinicola E, Bloom P, Lee N. Prospective evaluation of a plate haptic toric intraocular lens. *Eye* 2001;**15**:202–5.

29 Patel CK, Ormonde S, Rosen PH, Bron AJ. Postoperative intraocular lens rotation: a randomized comparison of plate and loop haptic implants. *Ophthalmology* 1999;**106**:2190–5.

30 Allan BD. Mechanism of iris prolapse: a qualitative analysis and implications for surgical technique. *J Cataract Refract Surg* 1995;**21**:182–6.

31 Radner W, Menapace R, Zehetmayer M, Mallinger R. Ultrastructure of clear corneal incisions. Part I: effect of keratomes and incision width on corneal trauma after lens implantation. *J Cataract Refract Surg* 1998;**24**: 487–92.

32 Steinert RF, Deacon J. Enlargement of incision width during phacoemulsification and folded intraocular lens implant surgery. *Ophthalmology* 1996;**103**:220–5.

33 Kohnen T, Koch DD. Experimental and clinical evaluation of incision size and shape following forceps and injector implantation of a three-piece high-refractive-index silicone intraocular lens. *Graefes Arch Clin Exp Ophthalmol* 1998;**236**:922–8.

34 Moreno-Montanes J, Maldonado MJ, Garcia-Layana A, Aliseda D, Munuera JM. Final clear corneal incision size for AcrySof intraocular lenses. *J Cataract Refract Surg* 1999;**25**:959–63.

35 Lyhne N, Corydon L. Two year follow-up of astigmatism after phacoemulsification with adjusted and unadjusted sutured versus sutureless 5·2mm superior scleral tunnels. *J Cataract Refract Surg* 1998;**24**: 1647–51.

36 Fine IH. Infinity suture: modified horizontal suture for 6·5mm incisions. In: Gills JP, Sanders DR, eds. *Small incision cataract surgery: foldable lenses, one-stitch surgery, sutureless surgery, astigmatic keratotomy*. Thorofare, NJ: Slack Inc., 1990.

3 Capsulorhexis

Capsulorhexis is not just a neat way to open the anterior capsule. It is fundamentally different from all previous techniques in that it maintains the mechanical and structural integrity of the capsular bag. It has therefore become the universally accepted standard method of opening the anterior capsule for the purpose of cataract extraction (Box 3.1). The continuous smooth edge to the capsulotomy provides a much greater degree of strength,[1] and as such it has contributed significantly to the development of today's safe and controllable phacoemulsification techniques. Moreover, it has made possible precise, reproducible, and permanent intracapsular fixation of the intraocular lens (IOL).[2]

In the past, the opening of the anterior lens capsule for the purpose of removing the cataract using an extracapsular technique was relatively uncontrolled. Toothed forceps were used to remove whatever could be grasped or a needle would be employed to create a slit opening in the anterior capsule. With the advent of modern extracapsular techniques better and more controlled anterior capsulotomy techniques were needed to aid manipulation of the nucleus and aspiration of cortex. The "can opener" and the "letter box" endocapsular techniques became the most widely used (see Chapter 8). The need for even better control arose with the realisation that the IOL should ideally remain in a physiological position within the capsular bag and that ragged peripheral radial tears in the capsulectomy margin can allow one or both

> **Box 3.1 Advantages of capsulorhexis**
>
> - No loose tags or jagged flaps of anterior capsule to interfere with surgery (especially during the aspiration of cortical remnants)
> - Forces exerted on the capsule and the zonules are minimal
> - The anterior capsule remains stretched horizontally, maintaining the intracapsular space for surgical manoeuvres
> - Radial tears cannot occur with an intact capsulorhexis
> - Secure, verifiable, reproducible, and permanent intracapsular implantation and fixation of lens implants
> - Secure intraocular lens implantation into the ciliary sulcus in the event of a posterior capsular rupture
> - It can be learned safely, without exposing the patient to any risk, during a standard extracapsular procedure

haptics to dislodge out of the bag. Capsulorhexis was developed to solve this problem. In 1984, simultaneously and independently, Howard Gimbel and Thomas Neuhann described the same technique, namely tearing a circular opening in the anterior capsule, instead of cutting or ripping the capsule, to obtain an aperture with a smooth continuous margin. The technique was demonstrated in 1985 in the form of video presentations, and the first formal publication was in 1987.[3] The new term "capsulorhexis" (capsule tearing) was proposed by Thomas Neuhann in order to emphasise the novel nature of the technique. Howard Gimbel originally termed his technique "continuous tear capsulotomy". By bringing together both terms, the abbreviation "CCC" for "continuous curvilinear capsulorhexis" evolved.

Surgical technique

The technique of capsulorhexis is based on the property of the anterior lens capsule to behave mechanically like cellophane. Whereas tearing from a smooth edge is very difficult, tearing occurs readily with a minimal amount of force when departing from a linear break. Following an incision in the capsule, tractional forces are applied using either a needle or forceps to propagate the rhexis tear. Stretching forces, applied perpendicular to the desired direction of the tear, will cause tearing but this may be sudden and uncontrolled (Figure 3.1a). Shear forces are applied in the direction of tear and are preferable because the tear direction and rate are more controllable (Figure 3.1b). In practice a combination of stretch and shear is used to steer the tear. An inward or centripetal vector is required to direct the tear centrally (Figure 3.2c), whereas an outward or radial vector is applied to tear in the opposite direction (Figure 3.2d). The more distant the point of engagement is from the leading edge of the tear, the more difficult it is to control the tear and the more centripetally it must be torn. In contrast, the closer the point of engagement is to the leading edge, the more directly the tear will follow the direction of traction (Figure 3.3). It is therefore advisable to regrasp the flap close to the leading edge of the tear frequently (a basic principle governing the entire technique and its variations). The intrinsic forces on the anterior capsule are largely determined by the tension of the zonules. Shallowing of the anterior chamber and forward movement of the lens–iris diaphragm causes a change in the normal vector forces, making it

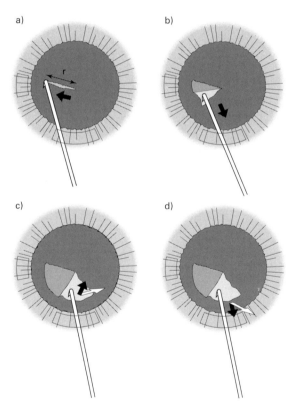

Figure 3.2 Capsulorhexis. (a) Initiating the capsulorhexis: central anterior capsule puncture is extended radially. Note: length r determines the radius (and hence diameter) of the rhexis. (b) Flapping over the tearing edge to facilitate shear tearing. (c) Steering the tear: centripetal vector (solid arrow) = tear directed inward (open arrow), decreasing rhexis diameter. (d) Steering the tear: radial vector (solid arrow) = tear directed outward (open arrow), increasing rhexis diameter.

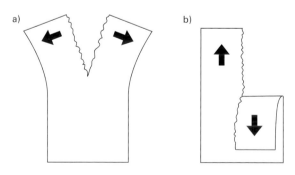

Figure 3.1 Comparison between tear propagation by shear and stretch forces illustrated using a sheet of A4 paper (try it for yourself). (a) Stretch: uncontrolled. (b) Shear: controlled.

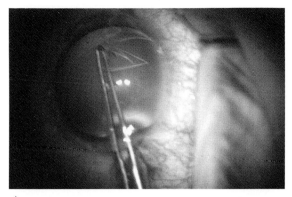

a)

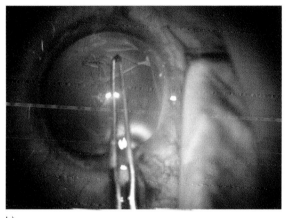

b)

Figure 3.3 Controlling the tear. (a) Grasping away from the tearing edge reduces control. (b) Grasping near the tearing edge maximises control.

more difficult to keep the tear from irretrievably running outward. Maintaining a deep anterior chamber during capsulorhexis is therefore essential, irrespective of the technique used.

There are three basic choices a surgeon has to make at the outset:

- The instrument used: a cystotome needle or capsulorhexis forceps
- The access: via the main incision or via a side port (paracentesis)
- The medium: irrigation with fluid, viscoelastic, or air.

These three options may be variously combined, for example using a cystotome through a side paracentesis under fluid irrigation, or forceps through the main incision using viscoelastic. Whichever technique (of the countless variations that have been described) the individual surgeon comes to prefer is not important. What is important is that the surgeon understands the basic underlying principle and adapts it to their individual surgical technique.[4] Capsulorhexis is not a technique in the sense of a cookbook recipe; it is really a principle that everybody can make work their own way. In that sense, the descriptions below are to be understood as "basic directions" rather than strict prescriptions.

Needle technique

Either a needle specifically designed for capsulorhexis is used or a 23-gauge needle may be bent to about 90° near the hub and its tip bent 45° away from the bevel (Figure 3.4). If viscoelastic is not used then the needle can be mounted on an infusion hand piece connected to a gravity-fed infusion at its maximum height. With the infusion continuously running, the anterior chamber is entered through the side port, the size of which should just permit passage of the needle. The chamber is therefore fully formed and maintained as deep as possible. When using viscoelastic it may be necessary to refill the anterior chamber during the rhexis, and by mounting the needle on the viscoelastic syringe this can be achieved without removing the needle from the eye (Figure 3.4).[5]

The anterior capsule is first perforated near its geometric centre with the needle tip, which is advanced to one side (right or left, depending on surgeon preference) to create a small curved incision in the capsule (Figure 3.2a). The desired radius of curvature (or diameter) of the rhexis is determined by the magnitude of this sideways movement. When this is reached, the capsule is lifted close to the leading edge of the

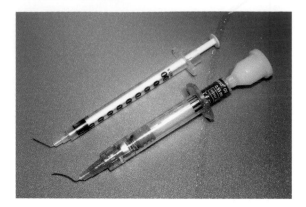

Figure 3.4 Capsulorhexis needles. Insulin syringe needle bent to act as a cystotome (top). Manufactured cystotome (BD Ophthalmic Systems) mounted on a viscoelastic syringe (bottom).

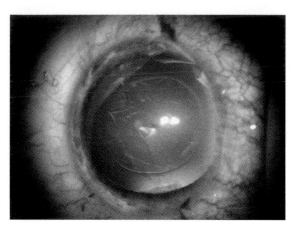

Figure 3.5 Completed capsulorhexis. Note that, by overlapping the start and finish points, it is completely circular and that the cortex is undisturbed.

incision and pushed (or pulled) upward in order to commence the tear. This lifting movement creates a small flap that is turned or flipped over on itself (Figure 3.2b). The rhexis tear is then propagated by engaging this capsule flap with the tip of the needle (i.e. engaging the side that had originally been in contact with the cortex but is now reflected back). Sufficient pressure is used to grip the flap without the needle tip perforating the capsule or disturbing the underlying cortex. (This is particularly important because disturbing the cortex can severely reduce visualisation of the flap and tear.) Having engaged the capsular flap, it is torn in a circular fashion using appropriately directed tear vectors. When brought around full circle, the tear is blended into itself from outside in to avoid a discontinuity. This inward spiralling manoeuvre, in which the final part of the rhexis is made to overlap the origin, to ensures that the rhexis forms a (near) perfect circle (Figure 3.5). If this is not carried out then a small triangular peak results that might interfere with subsequent elements of the phacoemulsification procedure.

When using viscoelastic to maintain the anterior chamber it is important to ensure that, as the capsular flap increases in size, the flap is kept reflected or spread out over its undersurface so that the torn edge is clearly identifiable. Disregarding this detail can lead to an irregular flap that is frozen in viscoelastic and possibly mixed with disrupted cortex, making identification of the tear edge difficult and leading to loss of control of the rhexis.

Forceps technique

When using a forceps technique for capsulorhexis a viscoelastic substance is typically used to maintain the anterior chamber, although an infusion with an anterior chamber maintainer may be used as an alternative. Forceps of the Utrata type (Figure 3.6a) require access through the main incision (approximately 3 mm in width) whereas vitrectomy-type forceps (Figure 3.6b), such as the Koch forceps, may be used through a paracentesis. To commence the forceps technique a small central puncture is first made in the anterior capsule, either with a needle or tip of the forceps. Some forceps are available with sharpened tips that are specifically designed for this purpose.[6]

Capsulorhexis using forceps allows the capsule to be grasped directly and has the advantage of making the technique more controllable for many surgeons. The forceps

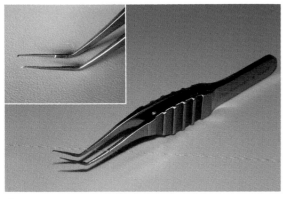

a)

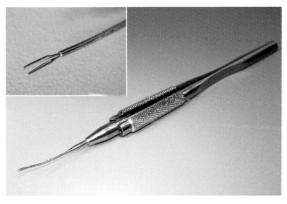

b)

Figure 3.6 Capsule forceps with close-ups of tips. (a) Utrata-type forceps for use through main incision (Duckworth and Kent). (b) Vitrectomy-type forceps for use through a paracentesis (Duckworth and Kent).

technique carries the disadvantage that as the rhexis proceeds, especially beneath the incision, deformation of the wound makes the loss of viscoelastic inevitable. As discussed previously, it is crucial to maintain a deep anterior chamber during capsulorhexis. Refilling the chamber with viscoelastic as loss occurs minimises the risk of loss of control over the capsule tear but is time consuming. Using instruments that open only at the tip (cross-action or vitrectomy-type capsulorhexis forceps) and that may be used through a paracentesis can help to tackle this problem.

Optimal diameter

The question of which diameter should ideally be attempted is best answered with respect to the size of the lens implant optic. Most surgeons prefer a diameter that will just cover the margin of the optical part of the IOL, completely sealing it into the capsular bag, which reduces posterior capsule opacification (see Chapter 12). There is no doubt that an asymmetrical opening, partly covering and partly not covering the optic margin, is to be avoided because for its potential of causing IOL decentration.

Learning capsulorhexis

A major advantage of capsulorhexis is that a surgeon familiar with extracapsular sugery can learn it without exposing the patient to additional risk. Whatever technique of anterior capsulotomy the surgeon normally uses, a capsulorhexis may first be attempted using the guidelines above. The key rule to follow is not to persist when control of the tear is lost. From this moment, the surgeon should continue by reverting to their standard capsulotomy technique. Therefore, during the learning period the patient, as well as the surgeon, will at least benefit from the surgeon's basic technique. For the new surgeon, artificial and animal eyes allow the capsulorhexis technique to be practised safely (see Chapter 1). Staining the capsule as discussed below can help the trainee during the early stages of learning to perform a rhexis.[7]

Complications: avoidance and management

There are three key intraoperative complications that can occur during capsulorhexis:

- A discontinuity of the capsule margin
- A tear into the zonules
- A diameter that is too small.

The causes, prevention, and management for each of these situations are discussed here. The two commonest postoperative complications following capsulorhexis are anterior capsule contraction and incarceration of viscoelastic, which are discussed in Chapter 7.

Discontinuity of the anterior capsule margin

The major causes of a discontinuity in the rhexis are finishing the capsulorhexis from inside outward or cutting an intact rhexis margin with the second instrument or the phaco tip during surgery. The most important rule when completing the capsulorhexis is always to close the circle from outside inward. If the flap breaks off during the course of the tear then the remaining flap created by the initial incision in the capsule can sometimes be used to complete the rhexis by going in the opposite direction (for example, clockwise instead of anticlockwise). If this is not possible then a deliberate incision at a separate site in the rhexis edge may be torn round to include the discontinuity (Figure 3.7). This can also be useful if the tear runs out during capsulorhexis. A break in the rhexis that is recognised during surgery should, if possible, be grasped with forceps and torn round to blend it into the main rhexis edge.

A break in an otherwise intact rhexis margin will in most cases cause a radial tear into the zonules. The risk of a radial tear extending around into the posterior capsule increases with friability of the zonules and manoeuvres that distend the anterior capsule opening. Nuclear fracturing techniques, which rely on pushing the nuclear parts widely apart, and IOL implantation must therefore proceed with caution. A radial tear in the rhexis margin is a contraindication to plate haptic lens implantation but it does not necessarily preclude the use of other folding IOL implants. The IOL should be carefully inserted and the haptics placed at 90° from the radial tear (a relaxing incision opposite the first tear may be considered).

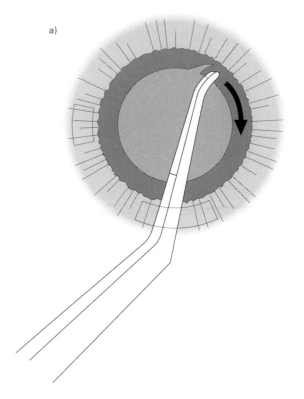

a)

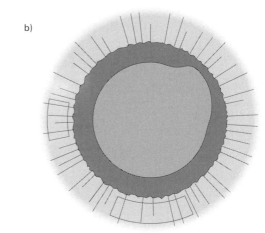

b)

Figure 3.7 Blending a break in the capsulorhexis margin into main rhexis. (a) Gripping the tear with capsule forceps. (b) Resulting complete but asymmetrical rhexis.

Tear into the zonules

If the tear involves zonular fibres, either because it is too peripheral or because the zonules insert abnormally centrally, then it cannot easily be continued. Persistent attempts to retrieve the rhexis may simply direct the tear along the zonule fibre into the periphery, like tearing paper alongside a ruler. With the help of high microscope magnification, careful focusing, and an optimised red or specular reflex, the relevant zonules may usually be identified and their insertions carefully removed from the capsule with a needle or forceps. The tear can then be directed centrally and continued. Sometimes this situation can also be managed by grasping the flap close to its tearing edge and briskly pulling it centrally. However, this manoeuvre carries a higher risk and is only advised when the more controlled approach does not seem possible.

Capsulorhexis with too small a diameter

If the surgeon realises that the diameter of the rhexis is getting smaller than desired, then the tear may be continued beyond 360° in an outward spiral until the desired diameter is reached. Alternatively, the diameter may be secondarily enlarged after phacoemulsification, as described below for the mini-capsulorhexis technique.

Difficult situations (troubleshooting)

Capsulorhexis is usually comparatively straightforward to perform under ideal conditions. When these conditions are not met capsulorhexis becomes more difficult but should not be unmanageable.

There are several difficult situations. Although these frequently occur in various combinations, they are discussed separately in order to make the basic principles of management clear. In all cases maintaining control of the capsule tear is essential. It is important that the anterior chamber be maintained as deep as possible, and the rhexis should progress slowly in small steps with frequent regrasping near the tearing edge.

No red reflex

When there is an inadequate reflex from the fundus to retroilluminate the surgical site, other clues and techniques can be used to visualise the capsule. First, slightly inclining the eye relative to the observation and illumination paths can sometimes produce enough of a red reflex to proceed safely. Increasing the microscope magnification is also often helpful. Oblique illumination, either in addition to or instead of coaxial illumination, can provide an "orange skin" like specular reflex on the capsule. Having switches on the microscope control pedal allows the two illumination types to be used to maximum effect. Alternatively, a vitrectomy endoilluminator, used through a paracentesis, can produce effective oblique illumination.[8] In the UK Mr Arthur Steele popularised capsulorhexis under air using a needle in a closed chamber when no red reflex is present. More recently capsule stains have been used to improve visualisation of the capsule (Figure 3.8). Fluorescein,[9] indocyanine green,[10] and trypan blue[11] have all been described, either injected directly intracamerally or under the capsule. Intracameral injection is usually preceded by injecting an air bubble into the anterior chamber, and the air and dye is then displaced by viscoelastic.[12] Capsule visualisation with fluorescein staining is improved by using a blue light source.

The small pupil

In addition to obscuring the anterior capsule, a small pupil may also reduce the red reflex. Therefore, the techniques described above may be needed. Measures to increase the pupil diameter are discussed in Chapter 10. Alternatively, the pupil can be retracted with a second instrument through a paracentesis, allowing the peripheral capsule to be viewed and the rhexis performed. As the tear progresses the second instrument is moved along the pupillary edge to maintain visualisation. Pulling the tear around behind the iris without seeing the tearing

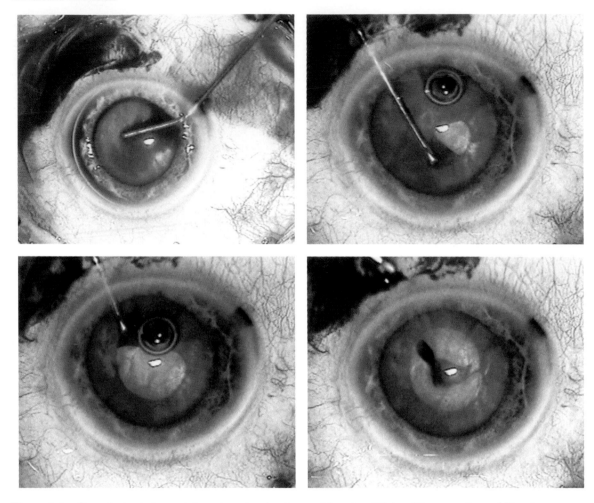

Figure 3.8   Capsulorhexis in a white cataract using trypan blue dye (Vision Blue; courtesy of Dorc)

edge is possible but requires considerable experience. It should be noted that the ideal capsulorhexis diameter should be larger than the "small" pupil in order to avoid synechiae between iris and rhexis margin.

Positive forward pressure

Positive forward pressure on the lens–iris diaphragm alters the forces on the anterior capsule and may cause loss of control of the rhexis with tearing out into the zonules. If possible the cause of the pressure should be identified. For example, is the speculum pressing on the eye, has a large volume of anaesthetic been used, or has a suprachoroidal haemorrhage occurred? If forward pressure cannot be relieved, then the capsulorhexis should commence with an intentionally small diameter using pronounced centripetally directed traction on the flap with frequent small steps, regrasping close to the tearing edge. Exerting counter pressure by pushing the lens back with a high viscosity viscoelastic is essential, and additional viscoelastic should be injected if loss of control of the tear occurs. If the forward pressure is relieved the rhexis can then be increased in width.

The intumescent white cataract

The intumescent lens combines the difficulties of forward pressure with those of a lack of red reflex. Logically, therefore, all of the above mentioned advice should be observed. A forceps technique is preferable because the cortex is often liquefied and presents no resistance to a needle tip. The lens can be decompressed using a small puncture in the anterior lens vertex and some of the liquid content aspirated,[13] but this carries a substantial risk of causing an uncontrolled capsule tear into the zonules. The fact that a wide variety of approaches are described to deal with the intumescent lens highlights the fact that there is no ideal method to tackle these technically difficult situations. Even the most experienced surgeon is aware that this remains a major challenge and from time to time will be confronted with an apparently unavoidable "explosion" of the capsule on perforation. Gimbel and Willerschcidt[14] suggested that a can opener capsulotomy may sometimes be successful, and its margin can then be secondarily torn out to form a rhexis (if it is still without radial tears). Rentsch and Greite described the use of a punch type vitrector to cut the capsule with communicating minipunches, which may occasionally be effective. A further option is diathermy capsulotomy, and if available this may be a wise choice in these cases.[15] However, the mechanical strength of a diathermy capsulotomy is significantly less that of a torn capsulorhexis.[16]

The infantile/juvenile capsule

Here the problem is due to the high elasticity of the lens capsule. Traction on the capsule flap stretches it before propagating the rhexis, and this creates a pronounced outward radial tear vector. To prevent the tear being lost into the zonules, the rhexis should be kept deliberately small using a pronounced inward centripetal vector (it will become wider by itself). Alternative techniques that have been suggested include radiofrequency diathermy capsulorhexis[17] and central anterior capsulotomy performed with a vitrector.[18] Although it is difficult to control the tear in a highly elastic capsule, it has the advantage that should a discontinuity in the rhexis margin occur it is less likely to extend peripherally.

Anterior capsule fibrosis

With experience, cases of minimal capsule fibrosis can still be torn in a comparatively controlled manner using pronounced centripetal tear vectors. In contrast, extensive dense anterior capsule fibrosis may make capsulorhexis practically impossible. Steering the rhexis around focal fibrosis may be a solution, but the tear can easily extend peripherally into the zonules. Instead, scissors can be used to cut the capsule, stopping at the margin of the fibrosis, from where the normal capsule opening is continued as a tear. Fortunately, rhexis discontinuities within areas of fibrosis caused by a scissor cut tend not to tear into the periphery during surgery.

Special surgical techniques

The basic principles of capsulorhexis have been applied to the development of techniques or "tricks" that may prove helpful in certain situations.

Posterior capsulorhexis

Leaving the posterior capsule intact is one of the aims and major advantages of extracapsular surgery. Nevertheless, this goal cannot always be attained. Intentional removal of the posterior capsule may be indicated in cases such as dense posterior capsular plaques or infantile cataract (in which postoperative opacification is inevitable).[19] Unintentional posterior capsule rupture, with or without vitreous loss, is a well recognised complication of surgery. Irrespective of the cause, the opening in the posterior capsule should ideally have the same quality as that in the anterior capsule, namely a continuous smooth margin. Although the posterior capsule is considerably thinner, this can be achieved by applying the same principles of anterior capsulorhexis. If the posterior capsule is intact, it is first incised with a needle tip and viscoelastic is then injected through the defect in order to separate and displace posteriorly the anterior vitreous face. The cut flap of the posterior capsule edge is next grasped with capsule forceps and torn circularly.

When an unintended capsular defect occurs, assuming it is relatively small and central, it can be prevented from extending using the same technique. This then preserves the capsular bag in the form of a "tyre", into which an IOL can securely be implanted, maintaining all of the advantages of intracapsular implantation.

"Rhexis fixation"

In the case of a posterior capsular rupture that cannot be converted to a posterior capsulorhexis, but the anterior capsulorhexis margin is intact, another "trick" may maintain most of the advantages of intracapsular implant fixation. The IOL haptics are implanted into the ciliary sulcus, but the optic is then passed backward through the capsulorhexis so that it is "buttoned in" or "captured" behind the anterior rhexis. This provides secure fixation and centration of the lens, and in terms of its refractive power the IOL optic is essentially positioned as if it were intracapsularly implanted.

"Mini-capsulorhexis" or "two or three-stage capsulorhexis" techniques

"In the bag" phacoemulsification can be performed through a small capsulorhexis that is

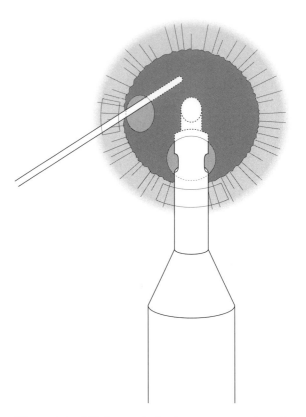

Figure 3.9   Mini-capsulorhexis to accommodate the phaco probe and second instrument.

just sufficient to accommodate the phaco probe.[20] Because the tip has its fulcrum in the incision, this mini-capsulorhexis should be ideally be oval to prevent distending the capsular opening. If a bimanual technique is used then a second mini-capsulorhexis may be produced for the introduction of the second instrument into the bag (Figure 3.9). After evacuation of the lens material, the capsular opening can either be enlarged to its full size or the capsule may be filled with a polymer (see Chapter 14). To enlarge the rhexis, the anterior chamber and the capsular bag are filled with viscoelastic, a cut is made in the margin of the mini-rhexis, and a "normal" (third) capsulorhexis may be formed with forceps, which is blended back into the mini-capsulorhexis.

References

1 Assia EI, Apple DJ, Tsai JC, Lim ES. The elastic properties of the lens capsule in capsulorhexis. *Am J Ophthalmol* 1991;**111**:628–32.

2 Colvard DM, Dunn SA. Intraocular lens centration with continuous tear capsulotomy. *J Cataract Refract Surg* 1990;**16**:312–4.

3 Neuhann T. Theory and surgical technique of capsulorhexis [in German]. *Klin Monatsbl Augenheilkol* 1987;**190**:542–5.

4 Gimbel HV, Neuhann T. Continuous curvilinear capsulorhexis. *J Cataract Refract Surg* 1991;**17**:110–1.

5 Teus MA, Fagundez-Vargas MA, Calvo MA, Marcos A. Viscoelastic-injecting cystotome. *J Cataract Refract Surg* 1998;**24**:1432–3.

6 Gimbel HV, Kaye GB. Forceps-puncture continuous curvilinear capsulorhexis. *J Cataract Refract Surg* 1997;**23**:473–5.

7 Pandey SK, Werner L, Escobar-Gomez M, Werner LP, Apple DJ. Dye-enhanced cataract surgery, part 3: posterior capsule staining to learn posterior continuous curvilinear capsulorhexis. *J Cataract Refract Surg* 2000;**26**:1066–71.

8 Mansour AM. Anterior capsulorhexis in hypermature cataracts. *J Cataract Refract Surg* 1993;**19**:116–7.

9 Hoffer KJ, McFarland JE. Intracameral subcapsular fluorescein staining for improved visualization during capsulorhexis in mature cataracts. *J Cataract Refract Surg* 1993;**19**:566.

10 Newsom TH, Oetting TN. Idocyanine green staining in traumatic cataract. *J Cataract Refract Surg* 2000;**26**:1691–3.

11 Melles GRJ, Waard PWT, Pamcyer JH, Houdijn Beekhuis W. Trypan blue capsule staining to visualize the capsulonhexis in cataract sugery. *J Cataract Refract Surg* 1999;**24**:7–9.

12 Pandey SK, Werner L, Escobar-Gomez M, Roig-Melo EA, Apple DJ. Dye-enhanced cataract surgery, part 1: anterior capsule staining for capsulorhexis in advance/white cataract. *J Cataract Refract Surg* 2000;**26**:1052–9.

13 Rao SK, Padmanabhan R. Capsulorhexis in eyes with phacomorphic glaucoma. *J Cataract Refract Surg* 1998;**882–4.

14 Gimbel HV, Willerscheidt AB. What to do with limited view: the intumescent cataract. *J Cataract Refract Surg* 1993;**19**:657–61.

15 Hausmann N, Richard G. Investigations on diathermy for anterior capsulotomy. Invest *Ophthalmol Vis Sci* 1991;**32**:2155–9.

16 Krag S, Thim K, Corydon L. Diathermic capsulotomy versus capsulorhexis: a biomechanical study. *J Cataract Refract Surg* 1997;**23**:86–90.

17 Comer RM, Abdulla N, O'Keefe M. Radiofrequency diathermy capsulorhexis of the anterior and posterior capsules in paediatric cataract surgery: preliminary results. *J Cataract Refract Surg* 1997;**23**:641–4.

18 Andreo LK, Wilson ME, Apple DJ. Elastic properties and scanning electron microscopic appearance of manual continuous curvilinear capsulorhexis and vitrectorhexis in an animal model of pediatric cataract. *J Cataract Refract Surg* 1999;**5**:534–9.

19 Gimbel HV. Posterior continuous curvilinear capsulorhexis and optic capture of the intraocular lens to prevent secondary opacification in paediatric cataract surgery. *J Cataract Refract Surg* 1997;**23**:652–6.

20 Tahi H, Fantes F, Hamaoui M, Parel J-M. Small peripheral anterior continuous curvilinear capsulorhexis. *J Cataract Refract Surg* 1999;**25**:744–7.

4 Phacoemulsification equipment and applied phacodynamics

Phacoemulsification cataract extraction was first introduced by Charles Kelman in New York in 1968.[1] In his original technique the nucleus was tyre-levered into the anterior chamber for subsequent removal with the phacoemulsification probe. His equipment was crude by modern day standards, not only being large in size but also requiring a technician to operate it. There were few advocates of phaco cataract surgery because of the limitations in technology and a lack of small-incision intraocular lenses.

With the development of posterior chamber phacoemulsification, capsulorhexis, and the introduction of foldable small-incision intraocular lenses, phacoemulsification cataract extraction became a real and potentially widespread method of cataract surgery. The combination of efficient ultrasound generation for phacoemulsification with sophisticated control of the vacuum pumps has taken phacoemulsification cataract surgery to a new era and, coupled with the latest in small-incision intraocular lenses and methodologies to control astigmatism, it has moved into the era of refractive cataract surgery, or refractive lensectomy.

Components of phacoemulsification equipment

The key components are of phacoemulsification equipment are as follows:

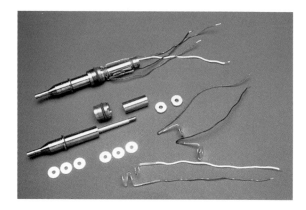

Figure 4.1   Exploded view of hand piece.

- A hand piece containing piezoelectric crystals, and irrigation and aspiration channels (Figure 4.1)
- Titanium tip attached to the hand piece (Figure 4.2)
- Pump system
- Control systems and associated software for the pump and ultrasound generator
- Foot pedal (Figure 4.3).

These principal components of the system allow for infusion of balanced salt solution into the eye, which has the triple purpose of cooling the titanium tip, maintaining the anterior chamber, and flushing out the emulsified lens nucleus. The irrigation system is complemented

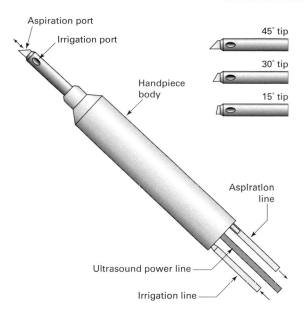

Figure 4.2 Hand piece with irrigation/aspiration channels and different tip angles.

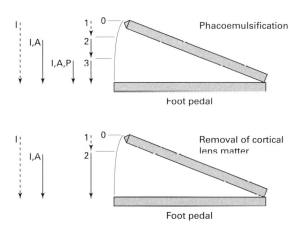

I = Irrigation; A = Aspiration; P = Phacoemulsification

Figure 4.3 Foot pedal positions.

by the aspiration channel, the control of which is discussed in greater detail below. The hollow titanium tip liquefies or emulsifies the lens nucleus, and these systems are all controlled by the foot pedal.

The foot pedal (Figure 4.3) in its simplest form has four positions. In position 0 all aspects of the phacoemulsification machine are inactive. On depressing the foot pedal to position 1 a pinch valve is opened that allows fluid to pass from the infusion bottle into the eye via the infusion sleeve surrounding the titanium tip. Further depression of the foot pedal to position 2 activates aspiration, and fluid flows up through the hollow central portion of the titanium tip. Depressing the foot pedal to position 3 activates the ultrasound component, causing the titanium tip to vibrate at 28–48 kHz and emulsify the lens nucleus. If the control unit has been programmed for "surgeon control", then the further the foot pedal is depressed the more phaco power is applied. If it is set on "panel control" then the maximum preset amount of phaco power is automatically applied when foot position 3 is reached. In some systems using this mode, further depression of the foot pedal increases the vacuum pressure.

"Dual linear" systems have a foot pedal that acts in three dimensions: vertically to control irrigation and aspiration, with yaw to the left or right to control ultrasound power. The actual position of the foot pedal and its associated action is usually programmable.

Mechanism of action of phacoemulsification

There are two principal mechanisms of action for phacoemulsification.[2] First, there is the cutting effect of the tip and, second, the production of cavitation just ahead of the tip.

Mechanical cutting

This occurs because of the jackhammer effect of the vibrating tip and relies upon direct contact between tip and nucleus. It is probably more important during sector removal of the nucleus. The force (F) with which the tip strikes the nucleus is given by F = mass of the needle (fixed) × acceleration (where acceleration = stroke length × frequency). Therefore, power is proportional to stroke length. Stroke length is the major determinant of cutting power, and increasing the programmed or preset power input increases the stroke length. The high acceleration of the tip (up to 50 000 m/s) causes disruption of frictional bonds within the lens material, but because of the direct action of the tip energy it may push the nuclear material away from the tip.

Cavitation

This occurs just ahead of the tip of the phaco probe and results in an area of high temperature and high pressure, causing liquefaction of the nucleus. The process of cavitation is illustrated in Figure 4.4. It occurs because of the development of compression waves caused by the ultrasound that produce microbubbles; these ultimately implode upon themselves, with subsequent release of energy. This energy is dispersed as a high pressure and high temperature wavefront (up to 75 000 psi and 13 000°C, respectively). During phacoemulsification a clear area can be seen between the tip and the nucleus that is being emulsified, and this probably relates to the area of cavitation.

Sound, including ultrasound, consists of wavefronts of expansion (low density) and compression (high density). With high intensity ultrasound, the microbubble increases in size from its dynamic equilibrium state until it reaches a critical size, when it can absorb no more energy; it then collapses or implodes, producing a very small area of very high temperature and pressure.

The determinants of the amount of cavitation are the tip shape, tip mass, and frequency of vibration (lower frequencies are best). Therefore, reducing the internal diameter will increase the mass of the tip for the same overall diameter and therefore increase cavitation for harder nuclei. A side effect of this component of phacoemulsification is the development of free radicals; these may cause endothelial damage

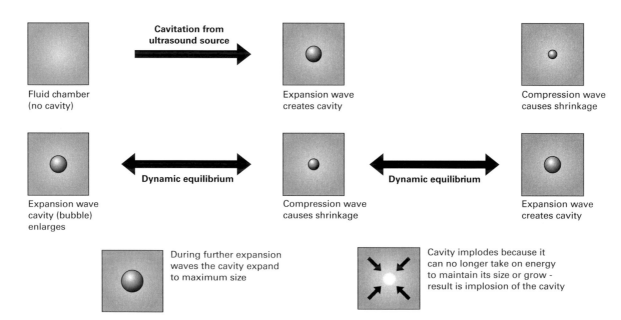

Figure 4.4   Cavitation.

but they may be also absorbed by irrigating solutions that contain free radical scavengers, for example glutathione.

Cavitation should not be confused with the formation of bubbles in the anterior chamber. These are from dissolved gases, usually air, coming out of solution in the anterior chamber in response to ultrasound energy or are sucked into the system (i.e. secondary to turbulent flow over the junction of the titanium tip and hand piece).

Tip technology and generation of power

Phacoemulsification tips are made of a titanium alloy and are hollow in the centre. There are a number of different designs with varying degrees of angle of the bevel, curvature of the tip, and internal dimensions.

The standard tip (Figure 4.5) is straight, with a 0, 15, 30, or 45° bevel at the end. At its point of attachment to the phaco hand piece there may either be a squared nut (Figure 4.5) or a tapered/smooth end that fits flush with the hand piece. The advantage of this latter design is that turbulent flow over the junction is avoided, and so air bubbles are less likely to come out of solution and enter the eye during surgery. Tips with 45° or 60° angulation are said to be useful

for sculpting harder nuclei, but with a large angle the aperture is greater and occlusion is harder to achieve. In contrast, 0° tips occlude very easily and may be useful in chopping techniques where sculpting is minimal. Most surgeons would use a 30–45° bevel.

Angled or Kelman tips (Figure 4.5) present a larger frontal area to the nucleus, and therefore there is greater cavitation. They have a curved tip that also allows internal cavitation in the bend to prevent internal occlusion with lens matter. Reducing the internal diameter but maintaining the external dimensions increases the mass of the tip and hence increases cavitation (Figure 4.6).

The "cobra" or flare tip is straight but there is an internal narrowing that causes greater internal cavitation and reduces the risk of blockage. These tips are useful in high vacuum systems in which comparatively large pieces of lens nucleus can become impacted into the tip. If internal occlusion occurs then there may be rapid variations in vacuum pressure, with "fluttering" of the anterior chamber.

Ultrasonic vibration is developed in the hand piece by two mechanisms: magnetostrictive or piezoelectric crystals. In the former an electric current is applied to a copper coil to produce the vibration in the crystal. There is a large amount

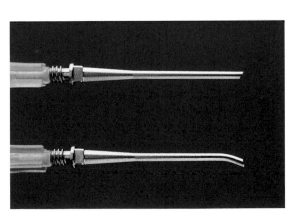

Figure 4.5 Kelman (top) and straight (bottom) phaco tips.

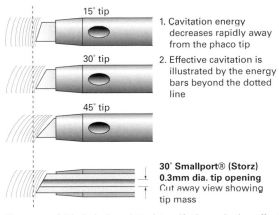

Figure 4.6 Effect of tip angle and mass on cavitation wave.

of heat produced and this system is inefficient. In the piezoelectric system power is applied to ceramic crystals to produce the mechanical output (Figure 4.1). The power is usually limited to 70% of maximum and, as previously mentioned, this is controlled by the foot pedal either in an all or none manner (panel control) or linearly up to the preset maximum (surgeon control).

It is usual to be able to record the amount of energy applied. This may simply be the time (t) for which ultrasound was activated, the average power during this period (a), or the full power equivalent time (t × a). It is then possible to calculate the total energy input to the eye (in Joules).

The application of phaco power to the tip can be continuous, burst, or pulsed. The latter is particularly useful toward the end of the procedure with small remaining fragments. In the pulsed modality, power (%) is delivered under linear (surgeon) control but there are a fixed series of ultrasound pulses with a predetermined interval and length. For example, a two pulse per second setting generates a 250 ms pulse of ultrasound followed by a 250 ms pause followed by a 250 ms pulse of ultrasound, and so on. This contrasts with burst mode, in which the power (%) is fixed (panel control) and the length of pulse is predetermined (typically 200 ms), but the interval between each pulse is under linear control and decreases as the foot pedal is depressed until continuous power is reached. Burst mode is ideally suited to embedding the tip into the lens during chopping techniques because there is reduced cavitation around the tip.[3] This ensures a tight fit around the phaco probe and firmly stabilises the lens.

Pump technology and fluidics

The pump system forms an essential and pivotal part of the phacoemulsification apparatus because it is this, more than any component, that controls the characteristics of particular machines.[4,5] The trend is toward phaco assisted

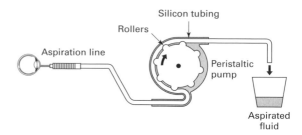

Figure 4.7   Peristaltic pump.

lens aspiration using minimal ultrasound power. This requires high vacuum levels that need careful control to prevent anterior chamber collapse. Four different pump systems are available: peristaltic, Venturi, Concentrix (or scroll) and diaphragm. The most popular type is the peristaltic pump followed by the Venturi system, although interest in the concentrix system is increasing. The diaphragm pump is now rarely used.

Peristaltic system (Figure 4.7)

In this system a roller pushes against silicone tubing squeezing fluid along the tube, similar to an arterial bypass pump for cardiac surgery. The speed of the rollers can be varied to alter the "rise time" of the vacuum. This parameter is known as the "flow rate" and is measured in millilitres per minute. The vacuum is preset to a maximum, with a venting system that comes into operation when this maximum has been achieved. Without this it would be possible to build up huge pressures depending on the ability of the motor to turn the roller, with the potential for damage during surgery. The maximum vacuum preset is usually between 50 and 350 mmHg, although it may be set as high as 400 mmHg when using a chopping technique. Once this level of vacuum is achieved and complete occlusion of the phaco tip has occurred, then a venting system prevents the vacuum from rising any further. This is a particularly useful parameter during phacoemulsification and is known as a "flow dependent" system.

An essential feature of the peristaltic system is that vacuum pressure only builds up when the tip is occluded. The aspiration flow rate, typically 15–40 ml/min, depends on the speed of the pump and, after occlusion occurs, this determines the vacuum "rise time". "Followability" refers to the ease with which lens material is brought, or drawn, to the phaco tip, and this is also dependent on the aspiration flow rate. Particularly when higher vacuum is used, it is possible for pieces of nucleus to block the tip and cause internal occlusion. When this is released there can be sudden collapse of the anterior chamber, known as postocclusion surge, caused by resistance or potential energy contained in the tubing. This has been reduced with narrow bore, low compliance tubing, and improved machine sensors/electronics.

Venturi system

This type of system differs considerably from the peristaltic pump, both in the method of vacuum generation and in terms of vacuum characteristics. Such systems are referred to as "vacuum based" systems. Air is passed through a constriction in a metal tube within the rigid cassette of the phacoemulsification apparatus, causing a vacuum to develop (Figure 4.8). This is similar to the Venturi effect used in the carburettor of a car. In this type of pump the maximum vacuum can be varied, unlike the aspiration flow rate, which is fixed. The advantage of the Venturi system is that there is always vacuum at the phaco tip, and so there is a very rapid rise time and followability is better than in peristaltic systems. The disadvantage is that there is less control over the vacuum because it is effectively an "all or none" process. These pump systems are declining in popularity because of this lack of control.

Diaphragm pump (Figure 4.9)

This system has significantly declined in popularity and has characteristics that are in between those of the Venturi and peristaltic systems. The principles of action are illustrated in Figure 4.9. On the "upstroke" fluid is sucked by the diaphragm through a one way valve into a chamber, and on the "downstroke" fluid is expelled from the chamber through another one way valve.

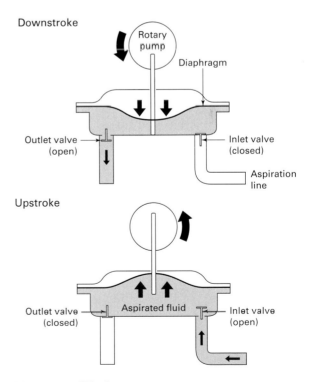

Figure 4.9   Diaphragm pump.

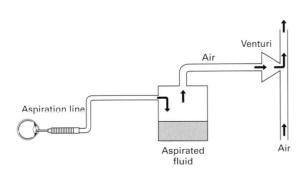

Figure 4.8   Venturi pump.

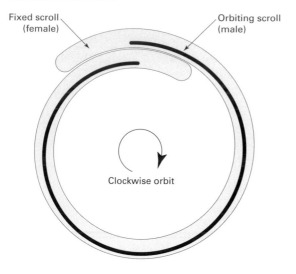

Figure 4.10   Cross-section through a scroll pump.

Scroll or Concentrix system

This pump system has more recently been introduced and consists of two scrolls (Figure 4.10), one fixed and the other rotating, producing a small channel through which fluid is forced. The scrolls are contained in a cartridge with a pressure sensor. To generate a flow based system, the scroll rotates at a constant speed and behaves like a peristaltic pump. If a vacuum based system is required then the pump rotates at a variable speed to achieve the required vacuum.

Phaco parameters

All phaco modules are controlled by complex, upgradable software that allows infinite control of parameters such as vacuum pressure, bottle height, aspiration rate, and power delivery. These can be varied to facilitate training and altered according to surgical technique (see Chapter 5), personal preference, and an individual surgeon's experience.

Aspiration flow rate

As previously mentioned, this parameter is related to the speed of the pump in peristaltic systems. The faster the pump speed, the greater the flow rate. As the flow rate increases the followability improves and the vacuum rise time decreases. A typical aspiration flow rate during lens sculpting is 18 ml/min. This may be increased to allow the lens quadrants to be engaged and then reduced during removal of epinuclear material to minimise the risk of accidental capsule aspiration. The minimum flow rate is usually 15 ml/min, with a maximum of approximately 45 ml/min.

Vacuum pressure

Vacuum pressure is preset between 0 mmHg and a maximum of 400 mmHg or more. This parameter is related to the holding ability of the phaco tip. With zero or low vacuum there is minimal force holding the nucleus to the tip, but this has the advantage of a reduced risk of capsule incarceration into the port. Low vacuum settings are usually used for the initial sculpting and nuclear fracture stages of phacoemulsification. Most current phacoemulsification techniques are biased toward phaco assisted lens aspiration, and therefore a high vacuum pressure is necessary to hold the lens during chopping and then aspirate pieces of nucleus from the eye.

Bottle height

This determines the rate of flow of fluid into the eye and is usually set between 65 cm and 105 cm above eye level. There must be a balance between input and output. If the infusion bottle is too high then the pressure head may cause abnormal fluid dynamics within the eye. After posterior capsule rupture and vitreous loss, the bottle must be lowered to prevent hydrostatic pressure forcing vitreous into the anterior chamber.

Memory

Most systems now have surgeon-determined memories for the vacuum and flow rate plus some other parameters, for example bottle height and foot pedal control. This enables the surgeon to switch easily from zero vacuum to high vacuum techniques during a procedure.

Postocclusion surge

This occurs in an unmodulated system after the occlusion breaks, particularly when using high vacuum or flow rates. During occlusion the vacuum generated causes the walls of the tubing to partially collapse. When occlusion breaks, the tubing re-expands and in peristaltic systems the pump restarts. This may result in fluctuations in the depth or collapse of the anterior chamber (Figure 4.11). Counteracting postocclusion surge has been addressed in several ways. First, narrow bore tubing that is less compliant and more rigid may be used. Second, a pressure sensor incorporated into the vacuum line detects rapid pressure variation and releases fluid into the line to neutralise the pressure differences. Third, sensors may detect when an occlusion break is about to occur and momentarily stop the pump. Finally, the phaco tip may be modified with a small hole in the side that allows a constant but very small flow of fluid through the tip even with occlusion (Aspiration Bypass, Alcon; Figure 4.12).[6] This also maintains flow around the phaco tip, which may reduce local tissue heating or phaco burn.

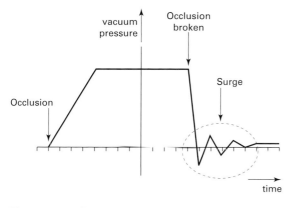

Figure 4.11   Graphical representation of postocclusion surge.

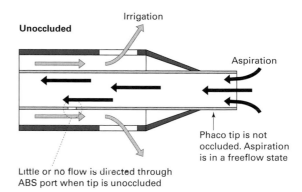

Little or no flow is directed through ABS port when tip is unoccluded

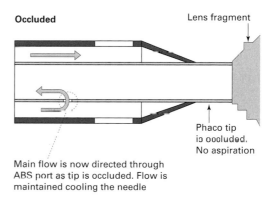

Main flow is now directed through ABS port as tip is occluded. Flow is maintained cooling the needle

Figure 4.12   Aspiration bypass tips.

New developments

The recent trend in phacoemulsification cataract surgery has been toward the use of "phacoemulsification assisted lens aspiration" to minimise the use of phaco power. The pump system then becomes the principal determinant of the phaco machine characteristics, controlling the parameters to allow initial central sculpting followed by aspiration with phaco of the segments of the lens nucleus. The latest phacoemulsification apparatus enables one to modulate the phaco power, to pulse it, and to control directly the relationship between the phaco power and the aspiration vacuum levels. Two recent developments are Neosonix (Alcon) and White Star (Allergan).

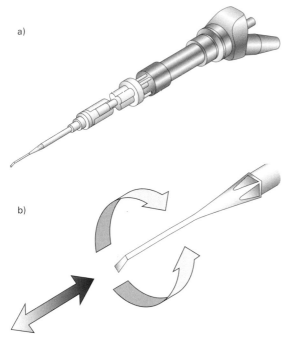

Figure 4.13 Neosonix (Alcon). (a) Hand piece: internal view. (b) Action: oscillatory motion in addition to conventional ultrasonic energy (± 2° at 100 Hz).

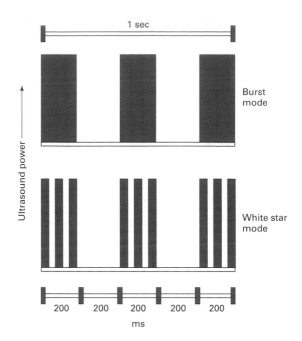

Figure 4.14 Burst mode versus Whitestar (Allergan; 600 ms duty cycle/400 ms rest).

Neosonix

The standard phaco tip oscillates essentially in a longitudinal direction (two dimensions). Neosonix adds a third dimension with a side to side movement of 2° from the central axis at 100 Hz. This is achieved using an electric motor within the hand piece (Figure 4.13), and its principal advantage is greater utilisation of phaco power for harder cataracts. The efficacy of this system is greatest with curved Kelman tips.

White star

Mechanical motion of the phaco tip is required to generate cavitation. This has the unwanted effect of developing heat and pushing nuclear fragments away from the tip. An irrigation sleeve around the phaco tip is required to provide cooling, and rest time is needed to allow dissipation of heat and regain contact with the lens fragment. The White Star system allows more rapid pulsing of phaco energy and significantly reduces energy requirements. This reduces heat generation and allows separate irrigation and phaco instruments to be used through 1 mm incisions.

This system is a refinement of burst mode, allowing pulsing of the phaco energy within a burst. A high "duty cycle" (for example, 600 ms burst/200 ms rest) is used for sculpting. Conversely, a low duty cycle with short bursts of energy and longer rest periods is useful for quadrant removal with good followability. It is this combination of pulse and burst modes that makes the use of ultrasound energy more efficient (Figure 4.14).

References

1 Kelman C. Phacoemulsification and aspiration. A new technique of cataract removal. A preliminary report. *Am J Ophthalmol* 1967;**64**:23–35.
2 Pacifico R. Ultrasonic energy in phacoemulsification: mechanical cutting and cavitation. *J Cataract Refract Surg* 1994;**20**:338–41.

3 Fine IH, Packer M, Hoffman RS. Use of power modulations in phacoemulsification. *J Cataract Refract Surg* 2001;**27**:188–97.

4 Masket S, Crandall AS. *An atlas of cataract surgery.* London: Martin Dunitz Publishers, 1999.

5 Seibel BS. Phacodynamics: Mastering the tools and techniques of phacoemulsification, 3rd ed. ThoroFare, NJ: Slack Inc., 1999.

6 Davison J. Performance comparison of the Alcon Legacy 20000 1·1 mm TurboSonics and 0·9 mm Aspiration Bypass System tips. *J Cataract Refract Surg* 1999;**25**:1386–91.

5 Phacoemulsification technique

Hydrodissection and hydrodelamination

Following capsulorhexis it is essential to mobilise the lens within the capsular bag. The ability to rotate the nucleus–lens complex is central to all phacoemulsification nuclear disassembly techniques. Cortical cleaving hydrodissection separates the lens from the capsule by injecting fluid between them.[1] This also has the effect of reducing the amount of residual cortical material at the end of phacoemulsification, the need for cortex aspiration, and the incidence of posterior capsular opacification.[2]

Hydrodelamination is achieved by injecting fluid between the epinucleus and the nucleus.[3] It is most useful when employing chopping techniques because it isolates and outlines the nucleus, it reduces the size of chopped lens fragments, and the epinucleus acts as a layer protecting the capsule.

Technique

The basic technique of hydrodissection and hydrodelamination employs a small syringe (typically 2·5 ml) filled with balanced salt solution attached to a narrow gauge cannula (approximately 26 G; Figure 5.1). Some cannulas have a flattened shape in cross-section that is designed to improve contact with the anterior capsule and distribute fluid in a fan-like manner. The substantial pressure generated

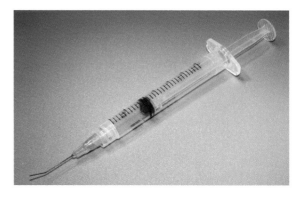

Figure 5.1 Cannula (BD Ophthalmic Systems) and 3 ml syringe with Luer-Lok (Becton Dickenson) for hydrodissection and hydrodelamination.

during injection may fire the cannula from the syringe, risking ocular injury. Syringes with Luer-Lok connections (Becton Dickenson) prevent this complication.

Hydrodissection is most easily commenced at a site opposite the main incision. The cannula is advanced through the main incision, across the anterior chamber, and under the capsulorhexis edge. To ensure that the injected fluid passes between the lens and capsule, the cannula tip should be advanced toward the lens periphery and at the same elevated so that the capsule is tented anteriorly. With steady injection, fluid is directed toward the equator of the capsule (Figure 5.2a). The fluid then passes posteriorly along the back of the lens, which can often be seen as a line moving against the red reflex (Figure 5.3). As this occurs the lens is displaced

a)

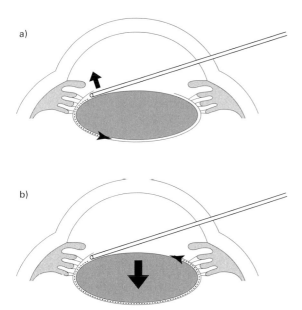

b)

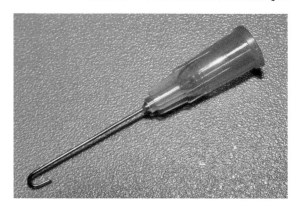

Figure 5.4 J-shaped Pearce hydrodissection cannula (BD Ophthalmic Systems) for accessing the subincisional capsular bag.

Figure 5.2 Steps in hydrodissection. (a) The cannula is advanced through the main incision and under the rhexis, and the capsule is tented anteriorly as fluid is injected. (b) The lens is pushed posteriorly to propagate the fluid wave and prevent anterior lens dislocation.

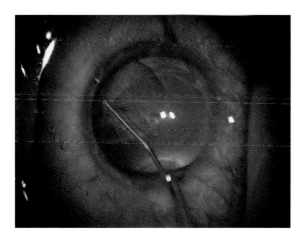

Figure 5.3 The hydrodissection fluid wave is seen passing between the posterior lens and capsule. Note that the cannula is perpendicular to the rhexis edge.

forward and may threaten to be dislocated into the anterior chamber. The cannula should therefore be used to push the lens posteriorly (Figure 5.2b). This serves to propagate the fluid wave across the back of the lens, improving the hydrodissection and decompressing the capsular bag. It is usually necessary to hydrodissect at several sites. The same technique is used, with the cannula placed perpendicular to the rhexis edge (this ensures that the fluid is directed posteriorly).

After hydrodissection the lens should be rotated using the hydrodissection cannula. If this fails then hydrodissection should be repeated. The majority of hydrodissection can be performed using the main incision to access the capsular bag; however, the second instrument paracentesis can be used to approach the subincisional rhexis edge. Alternatively, a J-shaped cannula, inserted through the main wound, can be used to hydrodissect this area (Figure 5.4). In practice rotation of the lens can usually be achieved without resorting to such manoeuvres.

Hydrodelamination is usually performed after hydrodissection by inserting the same cannula into the body of the lens. When it has been advanced 1–2 mm or as resistance is met, fluid is injected (Figure 5.5a). To propagate the fluid wave and prevent anterior displacement of the nucleus, it may be necessary to apply pressure over the central lens with the cannula (Figure 5.5b). Where a good red reflex exists, the injected fluid is visible

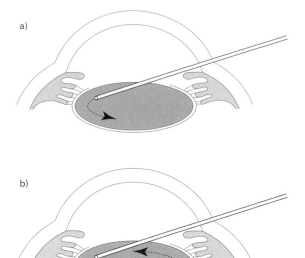

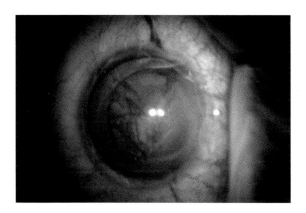

Figure 5.5 Steps in hydrodelamination (a) The cannula is advanced into the body of the lens. (b) Fluid is injected to separate the nucleus from the epinucleus.

Figure 5.6 The "golden ring" appearance after hydrodelamination.

as a "golden ring" demarcating the nucleus, but with denser lenses this is often not apparent (Figure 5.6). Usually, hydrodelamination need only be performed once and multiple injections may cause delamination at several levels, which can hinder segment extraction after chopping.

Complications: avoidance and management

Over-vigorous hydrodissection can cause capsule and zonule damage. The hydrostatic force generated during hydrodissection varies with the size of the syringe and the diameter of the cannula used. A surgeon using an unfamiliar cannula for the first time should therefore be cautious when performing hydrodissection.

The risks associated with hydrodissection are particularly relevant where zonule weakness exists already, for example in eyes with pseudoexfoliation or long axial lengths.[4] During hydrodissection in these cases, only gentle hydrostatic pressure should be applied to the lens and over-inflation of the capsular bag avoided. This is also important with large brunescent cataracts in which hydrodissection brings the rhexis and the anterior lens into close contact. The resulting capsular block[5] and high hydrostatic pressures can cause a posterior capsule tear and a dropped nucleus. Sudden deepening of the anterior chamber accompanied by pupil constriction during hydrodissection ("the pupil snap sign") may suggest that a posterior capsule tear has occurred.[6] A similar risk has been reported with posterior capsular cataracts, in which a weakness in the posterior capsule may pre-exist. Reducing hydrostatic pressure may be achieved by hydrodissecting at multiple sites and using gentle posterior pressure on the lens to decompress injected fluid.

As already mentioned, before commencing phaco the lens (nucleus–epinucleus complex) should rotate with ease. If zonule damage is a recognised problem then the lens should be rotated with care. A bimanual technique, for example using both the phaco probe and a second instrument, minimises stress on the zonules (see Chapter 10).

Nuclear disassembly strategies

Many methods have been described for removal of the lens nucleus, but they fall into two broad categories:

- Sculpting techniques, in which phacoemulsification is used to sculpt the nucleus in order to reduce its bulk, and to create trenches or gutters along which the nucleus may be fractured; the nuclear fragments so liberated are then emulsified[7-14]

- Chopping techniques, in which a sharpened, hooked, or angulated second instrument is drawn through the nucleus to divide and fracture it into smaller fragments; these can then be disengaged from the main body of the nucleus and emulsified.[15,16]

Each has its advantages and disadvantages. Sculpting techniques, such as "divide and conquer",[5] are safe and technically relatively easy to perform because there is plenty of room in the capsular bag to manipulate the nucleus. Chopping techniques, such as Nagahara's "phaco chop",[15] require a greater degree of bimanual dexterity and there is a risk of capsule and zonule damage from both the chopping instrument and from the high vacuum required to disengage nuclear fragments. However, sculpting techniques take longer to perform than chopping, and use more ultrasound energy with consequently greater endothelial cell loss.[17-20] Other techniques have been devised to reduce the risk to the capsule[21,22] and endothelium.[23-26] Nuclear disassembly methods that combine elements of fracturing and chopping techniques have been developed in an attempt to balance the advantages and disadvantages.[27-30]

There are a great number of variations on the above themes, often given eponyms, and readers are encouraged to try as many as they can find descriptions of until the technique that works best for them, under whatever circumstances, is identified and employed routinely. It is certainly true to say that no single technique should be employed in every case. The learning phaco surgeon should be prepared to learn a number of these techniques and become flexible enough to utilise the different methods in different situations.

Sculpting techniques

Divide and conquer (a basic "fail-safe" technique)

As with a great many surgical procedures, having a thoroughly well practised default method provides the surgeon first with a platform on which to build more advanced techniques and second, and perhaps more importantly, a method to fall back upon when complications are encountered. A good example of such a method is divide and conquer phacoemulsification, which, although employed to great effect by the learning phaco surgeon, is also of great value, for example with a small pupil when chopping can present difficulties. Most experienced surgeons will admit that their preferred default technique is a combination of different elements that have survived over the course of their learning curves. Other nuances having been tried and discarded in this evolutionary process. The basic concept of divide and conquer, outlined in Chapter 1, is to separate the nucleus into quadrants of equal size that are freely mobile and can safely be phacoemulsified in the "safe central zone" within the capsular bag (Figure 1.5).

Troubleshooting with Divide and conquer

Lens density A consideration in relation to nuclear division, which is also discussed in Chapter 1, is assessment of nuclear hardness. Surgeons commencing phacoemulsification should choose nuclei of only moderate hardness. This might mean selecting patients with mild to moderate nuclear sclerosis rather than those with posterior subcapsular cataracts or dense brunescence. A useful guide is visual acuity, in that patients with visual acuity between 6/18 and 6/60 are likely to have nuclear sclerosis that should be within the "range" of the learning phaco surgeon. These nuclei are relatively easy to sculpt, there is a good red reflex to aid capsulorhexis, and even if the grooves are not of ideal depth or length (i.e. too shallow and too short) they divide readily. Soft nuclei require a different method (see the section on "bowl technique", below) and greater experience, as do dense brunescent nuclei.

Sculpting the lens Having ensured that the nuclear complex (nucleus and epinucleus with or without the cortex) will rotate in the capsular bag, two grooves are sculpted within the nucleus. It is important to sculpt the grooves with a relatively high degree of precision so that they have almost parallel sides and are more or less at right angles to each other. This will then make it much easier to divide the nucleus into four.

When sculpting, the flow and vacuum settings can be low because little flow is required to aspirate the fine ultrasound generated particles and vacuum is not needed to hold or grip the nucleus (Table 5.1). In reality the flow setting is usually at a baseline of 20 ml/min and, although vacuum can be as little as 0 mmHg, in practical terms it is usually set at approximately 30–40 mmHg. The power used (usually in the range 50–70%) is selected on the basis of the apparent hardness of the nucleus; usually, this is readily apparent after the first few sculpting "passes".

The objective is to produce a groove that follows the "lens-shaped" profile of the posterior capsule (i.e. down, across, and then up to create a large "fault line" in the nucleus; (Figure 5.7). This is created initially by a "down-sculpting" pass of the phaco probe commencing nearest to the main wound (the subincisional area), just beyond the proximal limit of the rhexis (i.e. avoiding the edge of the rhexis closest to the surgeon). By down-sculpting, more tissue is removed from the central nucleus before up-sculpting distally. Care should be taken when phacoemulsifying the distal part of the groove because the tip of the probe can rapidly approach the posterior capsule. Similarly, care should be taken on the upstroke not to damage the anterior capsule. In order to sculpt more deeply it is necessary to widen the superficial part of the groove to admit the metal phaco tip

Table 5.1 Typical basic machine settings for a "Divide and conquer" technique

	Maximum vacuum (mmHg)	Apiration rate (ml/min)	Maximum power (%)	Mode setting
Sculpting	30–40	15–20	50–70	Linear
Quadrant Removal	70–150	20–25	50–70	Pulsed

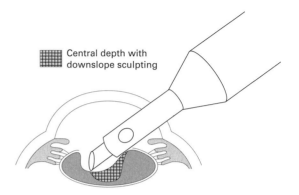

Central depth with downslope sculpting

Figure 5.7 Profile of "Divide and conquer" groove. Note the region of "down-sculpting", which achieves central depth.

plus the surrounding irrigation sleeve, and therefore several passes are required in slightly different lateral locations so that the groove becomes approximately 1·5 times the diameter of the phaco needle (Figure 5.8). This factor is particularly important in dense nuclei.

During formation of the first groove it may be helpful to stabilise the lens–nucleus complex with a second instrument (usually a "micro-finger" or "manipulator"; Figure 5.9), which is then in position to rotate the nucleus. Having created part of the first groove the nuclear complex is then rotated 90° and the process is repeated to initiate the second groove. If the lens–nucleus complex does not rotate with ease, a bimanual technique can be tried (see Chapter 10) or hydrodissection repeated.

After another 90° rotation the phaco tip can now be used to down-sculpt and meet the initial groove, completing the symmetry of the fault line. At this stage the initial groove

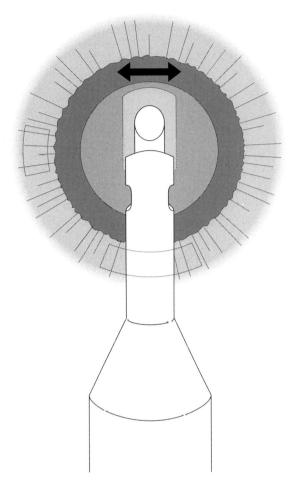

Figure 5.8 Increasing width of groove accommodates the irrigation sleeve.

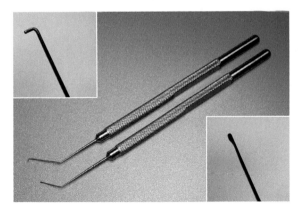

Figure 5.9 Typical second instruments. Hara nucleus divider (top) and Drysdale rotator (bottom; both Duckworth and Kent). Note the corresponding close-ups of instrument.

accommodates the irrigation sleeve of the phaco tip and allows deep central sculpting. A further 90° rotation completes the symmetry of the second groove but it will almost certainly be necessary to repeat the whole process until both grooves are deep and long enough to permit division into freely mobile quadrants.

Assessment of the required depth and length of each groove comes with experience but there are some signs to aid judgement. The most helpful guide to depth is probably the increase in the red reflex centrally as the posterior capsule is approached. Some surgeons consider the 1 mm diameter of the phaco tip to be a useful gauge or measure and will cease to sculpt when the groove is approximately 3 mm, or three tip diameters, in depth. In any event, it is quite understandable that the most common problem facing learning phaco surgeons is their reluctance to sculpt deeply enough. Once this problem has been overcome (with practice), division of the nucleus becomes straightforward. With a 5–6 mm diameter rhexis there is usually little need to lengthen the grooves beyond the dimensions of the rhexis. If the grooves are extended beneath the anterior capsule then the epinucleus here should not be phacoemulsified. This prevents any risk of anterior capsule damage and usually does not diminish the view of the groove. Although hydrodelamination is not usually necessary with a divide and conquer technique, it generates a golden ring appearance that outlines the nucleus. This may provide a useful guide to the extent that the phaco probe can be safely advanced during sculpting. Phacoemulsification beyond the golden ring introduces a significant risk of capsule damage. Here the soft epinucleus can suddenly be aspirated because it has little resistance to the advancing phaco probe.

Phaco tip selection The importance of the design of the phaco tip is discussed in Chapter 4. To sculpt effectively it is desirable to have a tip that is shaped or angled in such a way as to act like a spade or a shovel (Figure 4.6), and the greatest mechanical advantage is perhaps with a 60° phaco tip. However, later in the procedure (i.e. during quadrant removal) it is more important to be able to occlude the phaco tip with a nuclear fragment, and a 0° tip would be more effective. In practice a compromise is sought, and the most commonly used phaco tips have a 30–45° angle, which combines effective sculpting and quadrant holding functions. Newer tip designs, for example the Kelman microtip and the flared tip, have distinct advantages over standard phaco hand piece tips when dealing with harder nuclei. Once the phaco surgeon has mastered the basic techniques it is essential that they then "experiment" with different tips to assess for themselves whether those tips confer any significant benefit over and above their current experience.

Dividing the nucleus into quadrants

Having sculpted two grooves at right angles to each other that are of adequate depth and length, the whole structure must be divided, or cracked into four pieces. To achieve this it is important to produce a "separation force" in the very deepest parts of each groove (Figure 5.10). Two instruments are usually required, typically the tip of the phaco hand piece and the second instrument. By positioning both instruments deep within the groove the greatest mechanical advantage is achieved, and the two halves can be separated relatively easily in a controlled manner. The importance of the relatively smooth vertical sides of each groove becomes apparent at this stage because partially formed or irregular grooves do not provide easy purchase for the instruments. The groove width is also important because the irrigating sleeve can prevent the phaco tip from reaching the bottom of the groove. When the phaco tip and the second instrument are deep within one groove, they are then separated either away from each other (Figure 1.5h) or in a "cross action" manner (Figure 5.11) to push (or pull) the two halves apart. It is usually evident that the two halves of

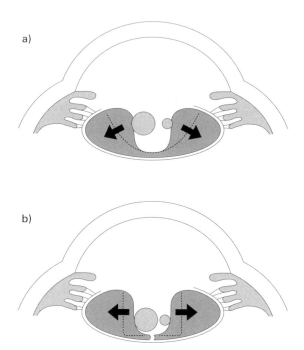

Figure 5.10 "Divide and conquer": instrument depth and separating the nucleus. (a) Incorrect: insufficient depth – separation force causes hinging and not cracking. (b) Correct: deep position – separation force causes cracking.

the lens are free from each other because a clear red reflex becomes instantly visible between the fragments. If this is not achieved then the process is repeated and several attempts may have to be made. To improve the mechanical advantage of the two instruments, the groove may be rotated to lie equidistant between the two instruments (i.e. if the main incision and paracentesis are 90° apart then the groove is placed at 45° from each (Figure 5.12). The nuclear complex is then rotated 90° once again and the separation process is repeated within the second groove. The nucleus has now been divided into four separate pieces (quadrants), each of which can be phacoemulsified relatively easily.

Although the phaco probe and second instrument are used in a bimanual technique to crack the lens, instruments are available that allow the lens to be cracked single-handedly. A

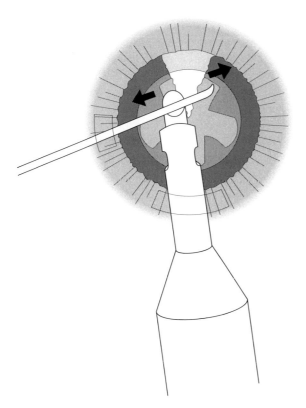

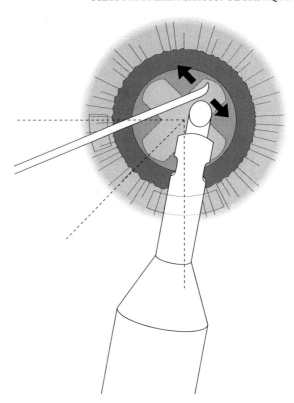

Figure 5.11   Cracking of the nucleus by crossing the instruments (compare with Figure 1.5h).

Figure 5.12   Improving the mechanical advantage during cracking by positioning the groove between the main incision and the second instrument paracentesis.

similar effect can be obtained by gently opening a capsule forceps while its tips are located deep within the groove. This of course first requires the phaco probe to be removed from the eye and the anterior chamber to be filled with a viscoelastic.

Quadrant removal During quadrant removal it is usual to increase the flow settings (by increasing the speed of the pump) to aid movement of the quadrants toward the phaco tip. To improve the holding or gripping power of the phaco tip the maximum vacuum is increased to 70–150 mmHg, depending upon the machine used, the phaco hand piece/tip design, and surgeon preference (Table 5.1).

Removal of the first quadrant is most difficult because there is an inevitable jigsaw or interlocking effect between it and the other three quadrants. It is often necessary to "dislocate" one of the quadrants using the second

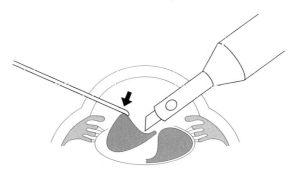

Figure 5.13   Dislocating a quadrant forward to allow removal (arrow indicates direction in which second instrument is used).

instrument. By pressing peripherally and slightly backward on the centre of a quadrant, the deep central tip of the quadrant will usually move forward (Figure 5.13). The phaco tip can then be advanced over this exposed part of the quadrant, which then occludes its lumen. A short burst of phaco power is often required to promote a tight seal, allowing the vacuum to build up. The quadrant can then be gripped and drawn into the central safe zone to be emulsified. The procedure is then repeated for the three remaining quadrants.

If a standard linear phaco mode is used during quadrant removal, particularly if the nucleus is relatively hard, then the quadrant will tend to "chatter" on the phaco tip. This is because the quadrant moves back and forth with the vibrating phaco needle, which breaks vacuum and can allow the fragment to leave the tip completely. Use of a pulsed phaco mode allows vacuum to be maintained and this problem can usually be prevented. Because of the increased efficiency of the process the total energy required is also reduced. It is possible to mimic this pulsing effect by rapid depression and elevation of the foot pedal between positions 2 and 3, avoiding the need to switch formally to pulsed mode.

During removal of the last quadrant, the capsular bag is virtually empty and it is often safer to lower the maximium vacuum and flow rate settings to prevent inadvertent damage to

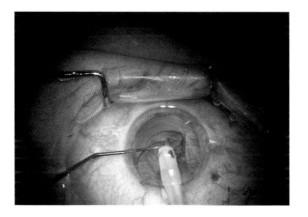

Figure 5.14   Protecting the posterior capsule using a second instrument.

the posterior capsule. Only low vacuum is required to grip the freely mobile quadrant, which can then be gently supported from behind by the second instrument. Ensuring that the second instrument is always below the quadrant and phaco probe at this stage protects the posterior capsule from accidental aspiration (Figure 5.14).

Management of the soft nucleus (the "Bowl technique")

With minimal cataract or cataract that is not of the nuclear sclerotic type, such as a posterior subcapsular cataract, the nucleus may be only partially formed and relatively soft. In these cases it is often impossible to use a default divide and conquer technique. Any attempt to rotate the lens or use two instruments to separate the nucleus impales the soft tissue on the instruments themselves. The "shape" of the grooves is quickly lost and it becomes impossible to divide, let alone conquer.

A different strategy is called for. First, even more attention must be paid to hydrodissection than normal, and hydrodissection from several different entry sites might be necessary to ensure excellent rotation of the nuclear complex. Even after extensive hydrodissection it might still be difficult to rotate these soft lenses within the capsular bag. The next step is to use medium aspiration rate and vacuum settings to phaco aspirate the bulk of the central portion of the nucleus–lens complex (Figure 5.15a). A Bowl of lens remains that will then separate from the capsule and fold on itself (Figure 5.15b). Very little phaco power is required, and the bowl technique is the best example of phaco assisted lens aspiration. High vacuum levels with newer machines (which reduce the risk of postocclusion surge) make the Bowl technique safe and efficient. Despite this, the removal of the bowl can be difficult and techniques such as those used in the management of the epinucleus may be useful (see below).

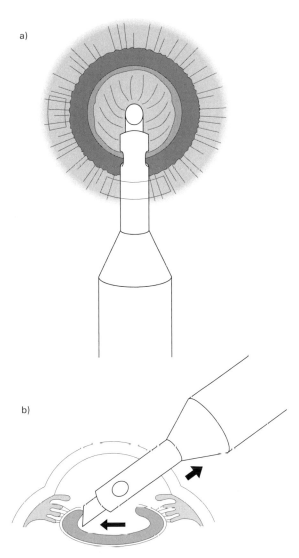

Figure 5.15 The "Bowl technique". (a) Debulking the nucleus to create a bowl. (b) Removal of the bowl.

Chopping techniques

"Nagahara chop" (horizontal chopping)

Nagahara[15] was the first to report nuclear disassembly using chopping and described a technique that does not require sculpting. This is therefore also known as "non-stop chop" or "pure chop". Because the chopper passes from the periphery toward the centre of the lens, it is

classified as a type of horizontal chopping technique. Good hydrodissection is required and, like for most chopping techniques, hydrodelamination is beneficial.

Nagahara chop employs a 0–15° phaco tip and high vacuum. A short burst of ultrasound is first used to impale and grip the nucleus (Figure 5.16a). The lens is then drawn slightly toward the surgeon as the chopper is inserted under the rhexis edge and around the periphery of the nucleus. The chopper is next pulled through the lens toward the phaco tip (Figure 5.16b). Just before contact between the two instruments is made, they are slightly separated to propagate a fracture through the entire lens (Figure 5.16c). The lens–nucleus complex is next rotated approximately 30° (clockwise in the case of a surgeon holding the phaco hand piece in his right hand), reimpaled by the phaco probe, and chopped in the same manner (Figure 5.16d). A small wedge-shaped segment of nucleus held by the phaco probe is thus broken off the main nucleus. By maintaining high vacuum this is then moved into the central safe zone of the capsular bag, where it is phacoemulsified (Figure 5.16e). The process is then repeated (Figure 5.16f) until the entire nucleus is removed.

"Quick chop" (vertical chopping)

This differs from the technique described by Nagahara by using a modified chopper to penetrate the nucleus vertically while it is held by the phaco probe (Figure 5.17a). Upward force simultaneously applied to the lens by the probe results in shearing forces that create a fracture (Figure 5.17b). This fracture is further propagated by also slightly separating the two instruments. The method has the advantage that the chopper is not placed under the capsule at the periphery of the nucleus, but is positioned within the capsular rhexis adjacent to the buried phaco probe. This is particularly advantageous where little epinucleus exists, in which case placement of the Nagahara chopper may cause

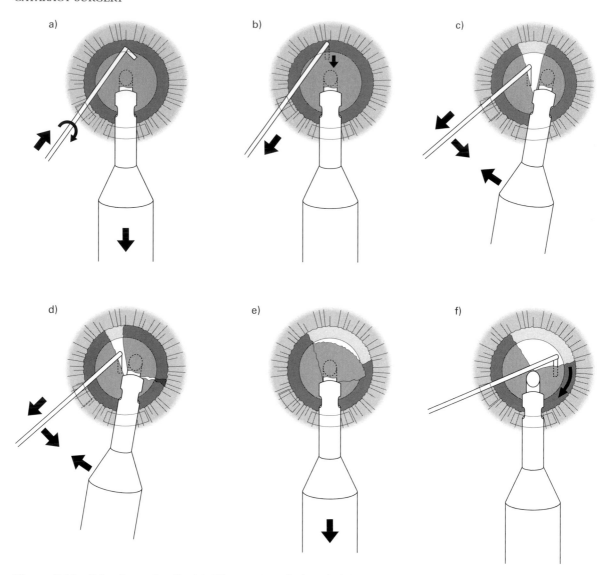

Figure 5.16 "Nagahara chop". (a) The nucleus is impaled by the phaco probe, held with vacuum, and withdrawn to facilitate positioning the chopper (tilted to go beneath the rhexis). (b) The chopper is drawn alongside the phaco tip. (c) Separating the chopper and phaco tip propagates the first fracture. (d) After rotating, the chopping process is repeated to generate a second fracture. (e) The liberated fragment, which continues to be held with vacuum, is drawn into the central rhexis area and emulsified. (f) The remaining nucleus is again rotated to position the nucleus for the next chop.

capsule damage. However, quick chop does rely on brittle, relatively hard lenses for the fracture to propagate, and may be difficult to perform in eyes with deep anterior chambers or with a small capsulorhexis.

Although vertical and horizontal chopping techniques can be employed as distinct entities (Table 5.2), elements of each are often combined. For example, as the chopper approaches the tip of the phaco probe using a Nagahara Chop technique, the fracture may best be propagated by separating the instruments, and elevating the impaled lens and pressing posteriorly with the chopper.

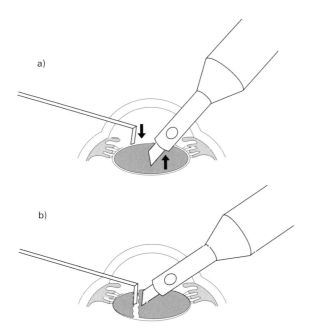

Figure 5.17 "Vertical chop". (a) The nucleus is stabilised by the impaled phaco probe, and as the chopper vertically penetrates the nucleus a vertical separation force is applied. (b) A fracture is created through the nucleus.

Table 5.2 Relative indications for horizontal and vertical chopping techniques

Horizontal chopping (for example, "Nagahara chop")	Vertical chop (for example, "Quick chop")
Deep anterior chamber	Difficulty visualising rhexis edge
Moderately dense nuclei	Dense brittle nuclei
Small rhexis	Little epinucleus

"Stop and chop"

This method is a variation of the Nagahara chop that provides space within the capsular bag for nuclear manipulation and aids removal of the first lens fragment. Although hydrodissection is essential, stop and chop may be performed without hydrodelamination. In this technique, described by Dr Paul Koch,[27] a central trench is first sculpted and the nucleus is cracked into two halves, or heminuclei (Figure 5.18a). The surgeon next "stops" sculpting and starts "chopping".

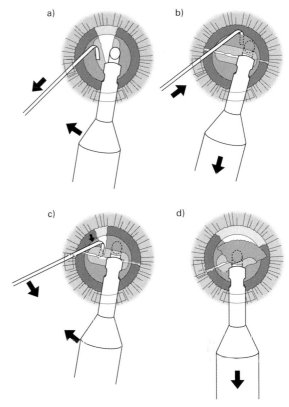

Figure 5.18 "Stop and chop". (a) Cracking the lens along the single groove to create two heminuclei. (b) Gripping the distal heminucleus after the lens–nucleus complex has been rotated and drawing it into the "central safe zone" of the capsular bag while the chopper is positioned. (c) Performing the chop. (d) Phacoemulsifying the chopped lens fragment.

After dividing the nucleus, the fractured nuclear complex is rotated through 90° and the vacuum is increased to approximately 100 mmHg. The phaco tip is then engaged into the heminucleus at about half depth, using a short burst of ultrasound (Figure 5.18b). The vacuum is maintained, and this allows the gripped heminucleus to be drawn centrally and upward into the rhexis plane. The chopping second instrument is passed out to the lens periphery, around the nucleus, and is then drawn toward the phaco tip (Figure 5.18c). Separating the two instruments liberates a fragment from the main body of the lens, which is easily phacoemulsified

(Figure 5.18d). The process is repeated and continued until the first heminucleus is removed. The remaining half is rotated and the same technique is applied.

"Phaco slice"

Another variation of chopping was described by David Gartry of Moorfields Eye Hospital (Video presentation, Royal College of Ophthalmologists Annual Congress, 2000). This uses a very safe horizontal slicing action with a blunt second instrument and reduces the risk of rhexis or capsule damage. The first part of the procedure is exactly as for stop and chop. Once the two heminuclei are completely separated, relatively high vacuum is used to engage and then pull the distal end of a heminucleus out of the bag and into the plane of the rhexis/pupil (Figure 5.19a). The second instrument (either a manipulator of an iris repositor) is next directed in a horizontal plane across the anterior chamber, slicing a fragment from the heminucleus (Figure 5.19b). This is then phacoemulsified and the process repeated.

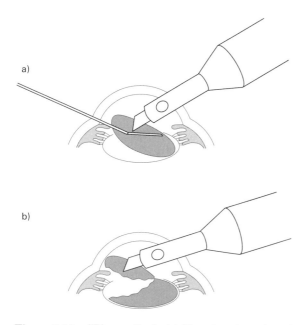

Figure 5.19 "Phaco slice". (a) Drawing the gripped heminucleus up into the plane of the rhexis. (b) Slicing with the second instrument.

Learning chopping techniques

Many of the principles of learning phacoemulsification discussed in Chapter 1 are also relevant when making the transition from techniques such as divide and conquer to those that involve chopping. Patient selection is particularly important, and the features that make a case ideal for learning phacoemulsification (Table 1.4) also apply to developing chopping skills. Although hard nuclei are usually more efficiently dealt with using a chopping technique, these lenses are nonetheless difficult to chop and are not suitable when learning.

A structured approach to learning chopping is necessary, and where possible relevant courses and practical sessions should be attended. A proficient divide and conquer technique is the ideal starting point for learning to chop. In the first instance it is possible to practice chopping once the lens has been divided in quadrants using a divide and conquer technique. Early in the learning phase chopping is best tried after one quadrant has already been removed in the standard manner and the second quadrant can easily be drawn into the central safe zone of the capsular bag. The anxiety experienced when a sharp and hooked chopper (Figure 5.9) is first inserted into the eye may be avoided by using the second instrument to chop the quadrant in a method similar to "phaco slice". This helps to develop the bimanual skills and confidence to proceed to more complex techniques using chopping instruments. At all times the divide and conquer method can safely be returned to in order to complete the procedure. The next step is to perform a stop and chop or phaco slice technique, in which reverting to divide and conquer" is still relatively straightforward. Once these techniques are mastered, progressing to Nagahara chop or quick chop is then possible, provided the case is favourable.

Troubleshooting when chopping

Gripping the nucleus Maintaining sufficient grip on the nucleus is essential to performing an

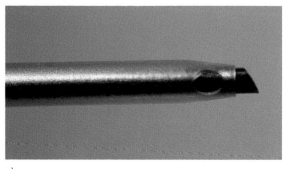

a)

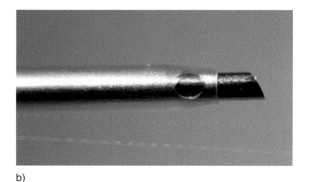

b)

Figure 5.20 Position of the irrigating sleeve. (a) Sculpting techniques. (b) Chopping techniques.

efficient chop. Adequate vacuum settings should be used and these will vary between machines. Initially, a setting similar to that used during the quadrant removal stage of a divide and conquer technique will usually be sufficient, but with experience higher levels may be used (Table 5.1). Exposing more of the phaco needle by moving the irrigation sleeve up the hand piece ensures that the probe can be driven deeper into the nucleus and provides a better hold on the lens (Figure 5.20b). Grip can also be improved by using a burst phaco mode and a phaco tip with a narrow angle (< 30°), which is more easily occluded.

During the early stages of most chopping techniques it is possible to displace the impaled lens from the phaco tip while positioning the chopper. Learning this manoeuvre is particularly difficult because of the need to maintain high vacuum with the foot pedal and keep the dominant hand stationary while manipulating the chopper with the non-dominant hand. Placing the chopper in position before impaling the lens on the phaco probe is much easier and has the added advantage that it then stabilises the lens while the phaco probe is driven into the nucleus.

Avoiding capsule damage The primary concern during the learning phase of chopping is the risk of damaging the anterior capsule with the chopper. If a technique such as stop and chop is used, then chopping predominantly takes place in the central capsular bag and reduces this risk. When sufficient epinucleus exists, placing the chopper out to the equatorial aspect of the nucleus is relatively safe and the vertical portion of the chopper can easily be seen as it passes through the peripheral lens. In contrast, with large dense nuclei, in which little epinucleus is present, placement of the chopper can be difficult. The vertical portion of the chopper must be rotated to lie horizontally as it is introduced under the rhexis. If the chopper is thought to be anterior to the capsule then the rhexis should be examined as the instrument is gently moved. The rhexis should not move if the chopper is correctly placed. In circumstances in which the red reflex is poor the use of a capsule stain (see Chapter 3) greatly improves visualisation of the capsule and helps with safe positioning of the chopper.

Although most choppers have protected tips and pose relatively little risk to the posterior capsule in the initial phases of chopping, some may become sharp after contact with other instruments. During the learning curve, eyes with small pupils should be avoided because the tip of the chopping instrument may not easily be visualised at the peripheral edge of the lens. With experience, however, chopping can be performed despite a reduced view. The period of highest risk of damage to the posterior capsule is during the removal of the final pieces of the lens.

Sudden postocclusion surge may bring the capsule into contact with the chopper, and replacing it with a blunt second instrument at this stage may be advisable. This instrument can then be placed under the final fragment as it is emulsified to prevent accidental aspiration of the capsule into the phaco probe (Figure 5.14). It is then also in position for removal of the epinucleus.

Failure to chop When using a Nagahara chopping technique a common mistake is to enter the lens with the phaco probe at the centre of the rhexis. This causes the buried tip to lie in the relative periphery of the lens and chopping does not occur at the central nucleus (Figure 5.21a). The entry of the phaco probe into the lens should therefore be initiated as close as possible to the subincisional aspect of the rhexis, ensuring that the phaco tip then becomes located close to the centre of the lens (Figure 5.21b).

As previously mentioned, a combination of vertical and horizontal movements with the chopper may be required to propagate a fracture within the nucleus, and these may have to be repeated.

Fracturing advanced brunescent lenses may be particularly difficult unless they are brittle. The optimal chopping technique to use in these circumstances is open to debate. The main problem is failure to crack the central posterior region of the lens. As the instruments are separated, lens fibre bridges may be visible against the red reflex in the posterior aspect of the fracture. Advancing the chopper into the crack may allow these to be individually cut, but there is a risk of posterior capsule damage and the surgeon should proceed with care. In some cases a dense posterior plate of lens may remain, and replacing the phaco probe with a second chopper or similar instrument allows this to be chopped with a bimanual technique. Viscoelastic injected under the plate also helps to manoeuvre the plate so that it can be either broken up or directly phacoemulsified.

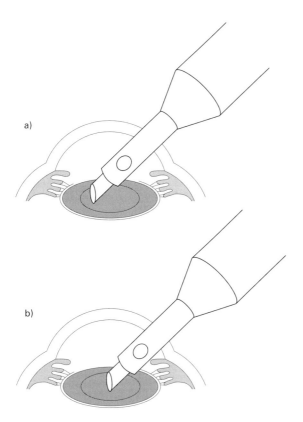

Figure 5.21 Positioning the phaco probe during "Nagahara chop". (a) Incorrect: phaco tip in the peripheral lens. (b) Correct: phaco tip in the central nucleus.

Removing the first segment The difficulty in "unlocking" the first segment or fragment chopped from the nucleus when using a Nagahara Chopping technique led to development of methods in which space was first created (such as Stop and chop). However, when the nucleus is efficiently chopped, removing a segment should be possible assuming adequate vacuum is used. If, after the initial two chops, the first segment cannot be extracted, then after rotating the lens a further chop can be made in an attempt to liberate an adjacent segment. If this also fails then the lens can again be rotated and the procedure repeated until a fragment is extracted and emulsified. Alternatively, the chopper can be used to help dislocate a fragment centrally. Once one fragment is removed the space created allows the others to follow easily.

When chopping hard lenses, creating small segments may make it easier to liberate the fragments. To further facilitate segment removal, and minimise the ultrasound power used, the extracted segment can be chopped again and forced (or "stuffed") into the aspiration port of the phaco probe.[28]

Removing the epinucleus Hydrodelamination produces an epinuclear layer that maintains a protective barrier between the instruments and the capsule while the nucleus is chopped and phacoemulsified. The surgeon is then faced with removing the epinucleus, which, even when soft, can be time consuming if it is removed as part of the lens cortex aspiration. This has similarities to removing the soft peripheral lens when using a bowl technique (Figure 5.15). In most circumstances the phaco probe, with its large aspiration port, is used but little or no ultrasound is required. The epinucleus is first engaged using moderately high vacuum in the region of the peripheral anterior capsule opposite the main incision. It is then drawn centrally and, using a bimanual technique, the epinucleus located over the posterior capsule is swept away from the incision using a second instrument. Simultaneously, the vacuum is increased using the foot pedal and the epinucleus is aspirated. Hence the epinucleus is fed back on itself and removed in one piece. Debulking the epinucleus may facilitate this manoeuvre but an adequate peripheral piece of epinucleus should be retained to allow it to be aspirated and initiate the manoeuvre. If a plate of posterior epinucleus is difficult to remove, then viscoelastic placed behind it will move it anteriorly and allow safe aspiration.

Cortex aspiration

Following successful phacoemulsification, and despite cortical cleaving hydrodissection, remnants of cortical lens (soft lens matter) almost invariably remain. Thorough removal of

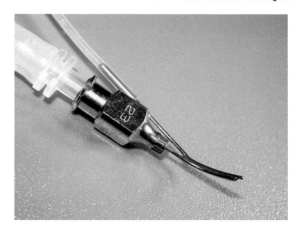

Figure 5.22 Manual syringe system for cortex aspiration (Simcoe).

the lens cortex ("cortical clean up") reduces the risk of postoperative lens related inflammation and the incidence of posterior capsule opacification.[2] It may be removed using either manual or automated systems, both of which simultaneously maintain the anterior chamber by gravity-fed fluid infusion and permit aspiration of soft lens matter. Manual systems use a hand held syringe to generate vacuum (Figure 5.22) whereas an automated system produces vacuum that is controlled by the foot pedal. All manual systems and most automatic systems use a coaxial irrigation and asiration cannula or hand piece.

Technique

By aspirating under the anterior lens capsule cortical lens matter is engaged, and this is then drawn centripetally and aspirated (Figure 5.23). It is important that aspiration is not commenced until the port is placed into the periphery of the capsular bag. This ensures that the port is fully occluded and the cortex is gripped. Care has to be taken, however, to ensure that the capsule is not engaged. If this is suspected then the aspiration should be reversed. An advantage of a manual syringe system is that this can be done very quickly. Automatic systems regurgitate

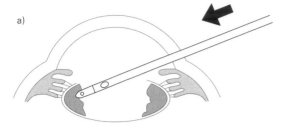

a)

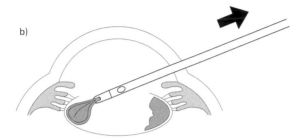

b)

Figure 5.23 Cortex aspiration technique. (a) Engaging cortex in the peripheral capsular bag. (b) Stripping and aspirating cortex.

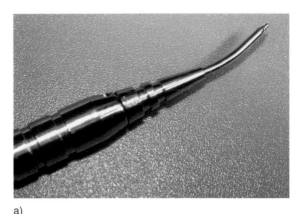

a)

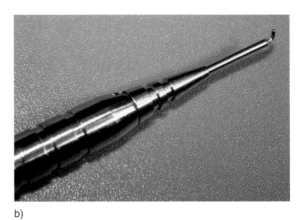

b)

Figure 5.24 Automated hand piece instruments (Allergan). (a) 145° tip. (b) 90° tip.

aspirated fluid by reversing the pump, which is controlled by a switch on the foot pedal.

Assuming only cortex is engaged the process of aspiration is repeated around the circumference of the capsular bag. Using the main incision it is relatively easy to access the majority of the bag with either a straight, curved, or 145° angled (Figure 5.24a) instrument. However, the subincisional cortex is more difficult to remove because the instrument disorts the cornea in this area. Many phaco systems with automatic aspiration have an interchangeable 90° angled tip (or "hockey stick"; Figure 5.24b) that can be used to remove the cortex in this region.[31] An alternative is to enlarge the existing second instrument paracentesis (Figure 5.25) or to create a second paracentesis to accommodate the irrigation and aspiration instrument.[32] To avoid this additional surgical step, the second paracentesis may be deliberately oversized at the beginning of surgery. Unfortunately, this may

lead to leakage of irrigation fluid around the second instrument during phacoemulsification (a particular problem if a shallow anterior chamber already exists). Using the second instrument paracentesis also usually necessitates using the irrigation and aspiration instrument in the non-dominant hand. A bimanual technique with separate infusion and aspiration cannulas allows improved access to the subincisional cortex without enlarging the second instrument paracentesis (Figure 5.26).[33] The two instruments also stabilise the globe and, if necessary, enable the iris to be retracted, improving visualisation of the capsular bag (Box 5.1). If both instruments have the same external diameter and one is used through the main incision, then substantial leakage of

a)

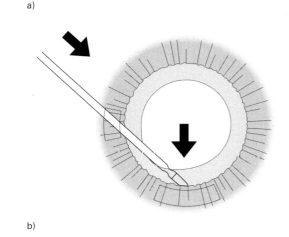

b)

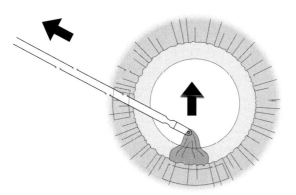

Figure 5.25 Using the paracentesis to access the subincisional cortex. (a) Cortex is engaged in the peripheral capsular bag. (b) Cortex is stripped and aspirated in the "central safe zone".

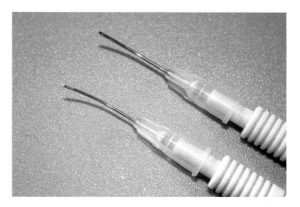

Figure 5.26 Bimanual irrigation and aspiration instruments (BD Ophthalmic Systems).

Box 5.1 Advantages of bimanual irrigation and aspiration

- Entire capsular bag accessible
- Easy access to subincisional cortex
- Simultaneous retraction of iris possible
- Stabilisation of globe
- Capsule polishing without additional instrumentation
- Residual nuclear fragments easily broken up and aspirated

---

irrigation fluid may occur. An additional paracentesis is therefore recommended for the second cannula, and this allows each instrument to be used in either hand.

Small fragments of nucleus that have not been phacoemulsified may be discovered during cortical aspiration. Using a manual system these cannot usually be aspirated and the phaco tip should be reintroduced into the eye. A coaxial automated system allows a second instrument to be placed into the anterior chamber, which can then be used to break up the fragment against the aspiration port. When a bimanual technique is used the irrigation instrument can be used against the aspiration instrument in a similar manner.

The irrigation and aspiration equipment can also be used to remove or "polish" lens epithelial cells from the anterior capsule using low levels of vacuum. This capsule polishing may prevent anterior capsule opacity or phimosis, which is associated with, for example, silicone plate haptic lenses.[34] Posterior capsule plaques should be approached with care because it is possible to cause vitreous loss. During capsule polishing, aspiration is often unnecessary and several single lumen cannulas are available that can be attached to the gravity-fed infusion (Figure 5.27). The external surface of these cannulas are textured or have a soft flexible sleeve to allow the plaque to be gently abraded. The aspiration cannulas of some bimanual systems are similarly treated so further instrumentation is unnecessary. Bimanual

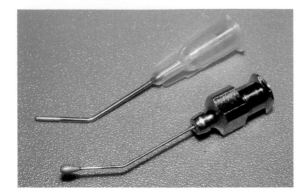

Figure 5.27 Capsule polishing cannulas (BD Ophthalmic Systems).

systems also have the advantage that all of the capsular bag can be accessed easily.

Complications: avoidance and management

The process of cortical clean up can cause both capsule rupture and zonule dehiscence. If the cortex seems particularly adherent, it is important to be patient. With time the cortical matter hydrates and should become easier to remove. Inserting the intraocular lens and rotating it can help to liberate cortex but the haptics, like a capsular tension ring, may also trap cortical matter in the equatorial capsular bag and make it difficult to aspirate.

Most concern during irrigation and aspiration centres on removal of the subincisional cortex. When using a 90° tip, the instrument should be held as close to vertical as is possible without distorting the cornea (Figure 5.28a). Once the tip is within the capsular bag, rotating the instrument swings the aspiration port under the rhexis toward the peripheral subincisional capsular bag (Figure 5.28b). The aspiration port thus remains in view and aspiration can then be commenced to engage the cortex. Once vacuum has built up the instrument is gently rotated back to its original position, stripping cortex. This piece of cortex can then be fully aspirated in the safe central zone (Figure 5.28c). If a 90°

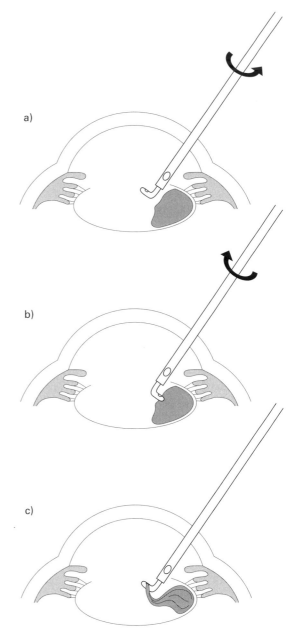

a)

b)

c)

Figure 5.28 Using the 90° tip. (a) Near vertical position of the hand piece within the eye. (b) Accessing the subincisional capsular bag by rotating the tip under the rhexis. (c) Aspiration of stripped cortex after rotating tip back to "central safe zone".

angle tip is found to distort the view of the anterior segment, then this problem may be reduced in the future by altering the construction and length of the incision (see

Chapter 2). Alternatively, a bimanual system can be used or a separate paracentesis employed.

In eyes with known zonule damage cortex aspiration needs to proceed with caution (see Chapter 10). It should commence in areas of normal zonule support and initially avoid areas of dialysis. Stripping of aspirated cortex should employ tangential rather than radial movements, and where possible it should be directed toward the areas of weakness.

References

1 Fine IH. Cortical cleaving hydrodissection. *J Cataract Refract Surg* 1992;**18**:508–12.

2 Peng Q, Apple DJ, Visessook N, *et al*. Surgical prevention of posterior capsule opacification. Part 2: enhancement of cortical cleanup by focusing on hydrodissection. *J Cataract Refract Surg* 2000;**26**: 188–97.

3 Gimbel HV. Hydrodissection and hydrodelineation. *Int Ophthalmol Clin* 1994;**34**:73–90.

4 Ota I, Miyake S, Miyake K. Dislocation of the lens nucleus into the vitreous cavity after standard hydrodissection. *Am J Ophthalmol* 1996;**121**:706–8.

5 Miyake K, Ota I, Ichihashi S, Miyake K, Tanaka Y, Terasaki H. New classification of capsular block syndrome. *J Cataract Refract Surg* 1998;**24**:1230–4.

6 Yeoh R. The "pupil snap" sign of posterior capsule rupture with hydrodissection in phacoemulsification [letter]. *Br J Ophthalmol* 1996;**80**:486.

7 Shepherd JR. In situ fracture. *J Cataract Refract Surg* 1990;**16**:436–40.

8 Davison JA. Hybrid nuclear dissection technique for capsular bag phacoemulsification. *J Cataract Refract Surg* 1990;**16**:441–450.

9 Gimbel HV. Divide and conquer nucleofractis phacoemulsification: development and variations. *J Cataract Refract Surg* 1991;**17**:281–91.

10 Pacifico RL. Divide and conquer phacoemulsification: one-handed variant. *J Cataract Refract Surg* 1992; **18**:513–7.

11 Johnson SH. Split and lift: nuclear quadrant management for phacoemulsification. *J Cataract Refract Surg* 1993;**19**:420–4.

12 Fine IH, Maloney WF, Dillman DM. Crack and flip phacoemulsification technique. *J Cataract Refract Surg* 1993;**19**:797–802.

13 Gimbel HV, Chin PK. Phaco-sweep. *J Cataract Refract Surg* 1995;**21**:493–6.

14 Corydon L, Krag S, Thim K. One-handed phacoemulsification with low settings. *J Cataract Refract Surg* 1997;**23**:1143–8.

15 Nagahara K. Phaco-chop technique eliminates central sculpting and allows faster, safer phaco. *Ocular Surgery News* 1993;**October**:12–3.

16 Arshinoff SA. Phaco-slice and separate. *J Cataract Refract Surg* 1999;**25**:474–8.

17 Hayashi K, Nakao F, Hayashi F. Corneal endothelial cell loss after phacoemulsification using nuclear cracking procedures. *J Cataract Refract Surg* 1994;**20**:44–7.

18 Pirazzoli G, D'Eliseo D, Ziosi M, Acciari R. Effects of phacoemulsification time on the corneal endothelium using phacofracture and phaco-chop techniques. *J Cataract Refract Surg* 1996;**22**:967–9.

19 DeBry P, Olson RJ, Crandall AS. Comparison of energy required for phaco-chop and divide and conquer phacoemulsification. *J Cataract Refract Surg* 1998; **24**:689–92.

20 Ram J, Wesendahl TA, Auffarth GU, Apple DJ. Evaluation of in situ fracture versus phaco-chop techniques. *J Cataract Refract Surg* 1998;**24**:1464–8.

21 Maloney WF, Dillman DM, Nichamin LD. Supracapsular phacoemulsification: a capsule-free posterior chamber approach. *J Cataract Refract Surg* 1997;**23**:323–8.

22 Ayoub MI. Three phase phacoemulsification. *J Cataract Refract Surg* 1998;**24**:592–4.

23 Hara T, Hara T. Endocapsular phacoemulsification and aspiration (ECPEA): recent surgical technique and clinical results. *Ophthalmic Surg* 1989;**20**:469–75.

24 Anis AY. Hydrosonic intercapsular piecemeal phacoemulsification or the "HIPP" technique. *Int Ophthalmol* 1994;**18**:37–42.

25 Joo C-K, Kim YH. Phacoemulsification with a bevel-down phaco tip: phaco-drill. *J Cataract Refract Surg* 1997;**23**:1149–52.

26 Kohlhaas M, Klemm M, Kammann J, Richard G. Endothelial cell loss secondary to two different phacoemulsification techniques. *Ophthalmic Surg Lasers* 1998;**29**:890–95.

27 Koch PS, Katzen LE. Stop and chop phacoemulsification. *J Cataract Refract Surg* 1994;**20**:566–70.

28 Vasavada AR, Desai JP. Stop, chop, chop and stuff. *J Cataract Refract Surg* 1996;**22**:526–9.

29 Dada T, Sharma N, Dada VK, Vajpayee RB. Modified phacoemulsification in situ. *J Cataract Refract Surg* 1998;**24**:1027–9.

30 Dada T, Sharma N, Dada VK. Petalloid phacoemulsification. *Ophthalmic Surg Lasers* 2000;**31**: 170–2.

31 Hagan JC III. Irrigation/aspiration handpiece with changeable tip for cortex removal in small incision phacoemulsification. *J Cataract Refract Surg* 1992;**18**: 318–20.

32 Hagan JC III. A new cannula for removal of 12 o'clock cortex through a sideport corneal incision. *Ophthalmic Surg* 1992;**23**:62–3.

33 Colvard DM. Bimanual technique to manage subincisional cortical material. *J Cataract Refract Surg* 1997;**23**:707–9.

34 Joo CK, Shin JA, Kim JH. Capsular opening contraction after continuous curvilinear capsulorhexis and intraocular lens implantation. *J Cataract Refract Surg* 1996;**22**:585–90.

6 Biometry and lens implant power calculation

Improvements in surgical techniques have provided an added impetus to improve the precision of lens implant power calculation. Determination of the lens implant power to give any desired postoperative refraction requires measurement of two key variables:

- The anterior corneal curvature in two orthogonal meridia
- The axial length of the eye.

These measurements are then entered into an appropriate formula.

Anterior corneal curvature measurement

The cornea acts as a mirror reflecting the images of luminous objects, and it is the curvature of the "mirror" that is measured when using a keratometer. The anterior cornea is not uniformly curved but in most individuals progressively flattens in the periphery.[1] The corneal apex is also slightly decentred. Keratometers measure anterior corneal curvature over a small annular zone and assume that this is spherical. The size of this zone varies with corneal curvature but generally lies between 2 and 4 mm in diameter.[2] Contact lenses should be removed at least 48 hours before keratometry because their long-term use can induce a reversible corneal flattening (~0·05 mm). If the contact lens fit is tight then this distortion or warpage may be

more pronounced, especially with rigid polymethylmethacrylate (PMMA) lenses. In such circumstances removal of the contact lenses 6 weeks before biometry is ideal although rarely practical for most individuals.

Keratometry "setup"

The room lighting should be adjusted to avoid stray reflections on the cornea. The keratometer's telescopic eyepiece should be focused for the examiner's eye, before the examination begins, using the in-built graticule designed for this purpose. Failure to focus the eyepiece in certain instruments could lead to errors in measurement of corneal radius of curvature of the order of 0·05 mm and as great as 0·15 mm in some instruments.[3] Individuals are usually examined in a seated position with their chin on a rest and their forehead placed against a band. If the patient's upper eyelid drops to within a few millimetres of the corneal apex then it may be necessary for the examiner to raise the eyelid, carefully avoiding indentation of the globe and artefactually steepening the cornea.

Manual keratometers

A central fixation target within the instrument is provided and must be viewed by the patient. If the individual is unable to see the fixation light, then it is vital to fixate the fellow eye. Internally illuminated targets (the mires) are mounted on a viewing telescope and their reflections on the cornea, viewed through the keratometer's telescopic system, are then centred in the field of view by the examiner. In order to overcome any eye movements by individuals undergoing examination, doubling devices such as prisms are incorporated into the viewing telescope. The instrument is set to read the corneal curvature when two halves of a mire image just touch or when two identical mire images are superimposed. While the examiner adjusts the mire image separation with one hand, the focus of the mire reflections should be monitored continuously and adjusted by altering the separation between the telescope and the patient's eye using a joystick controlled with the other hand. The corneal image size of the mires is related to corneal curvature by Newton's magnification equation, but for accuracy instruments are calibrated against steel spheres of known curvature. Some instruments measure to 0·05 mm and others to 0·01 mm. Reproducibility of measurements is within 0·05 mm.[4] Some instruments require the telescope to be rotated through 90° to take an orthogonal reading of corneal curvature (two-position keratometer), whereas others permit two orthogonal readings to be taken with the telescope stationary (one-position keratometer).

Instruments generally have two scales, one giving the corneal radius of curvature in millimeters and the other giving corneal power in dioptres (D). Currently, most but not all instruments use a hypothetical corneal refractive index of 1·3375 to calculate corneal power that takes into account the small minus power of the posterior corneal surface. Gullstrand, however, has shown that a refractive index of 1·333 produces a more accurate estimate of corneal power, and some practitioners elect to use this value in lens implant power formulae. Corneal power can be calculated from Equation A in Appendix I.

The angles at which keratometer readings are taken should be noted because surgeons may decide intentionally to induce corneal flattening in a meridian to reduce corneal astigmatism. Flattening in the steep meridian is associated with some steepening in the orthogonal meridian (known as coupling), although the flattening exceeds the steepening.[5] Arcuate keratotomy therefore induces a hyperopic shift dependent upon the degree of corneal coupling (typically 0·25 times the intended correction). In practice, approximately 0·25 D should be subtracted from the average preoperative corneal power for each 1 D of astigmatism to be corrected (otherwise there is a risk of residual hypermetropia).

Automatic keratometers

Automatic keratometers have the advantage of virtually eliminating operator subjectivity. However, it is very important to confirm that the patient is fixating correctly, and in some automatic keratometers it is difficult to view the eye directly. The mires of automated keratometers are generally light emitting diodes and the corneal image positions of the mires are detected using solid state detectors. The fast response of such detectors overcomes problems associated with eye movement, thus negating the need for doubling devices.

Hand-held keratometers

Portable hand-held keratometers can be used with patients in seated, standing, or supine positions, and therefore are ideal for use on infants, individuals with restricted physical mobility, or those supine under general anaesthesia. Highly accurate hand-held automatic keratometers are now commercially available. However, care must be taken to hold the instrument parallel to the plane of the face, and to check that the eye is fixating correctly and that the eyelids do not obscure the cornea.

Difficult and complex keratometry

Poor fixation

The examiner should ensure that the patient is fixating on the target light by observing the patient's eye and the reflections of ocular structures viewed both directly and through the keratometer eyepiece. The radius of curvature of the cornea increases in the periphery by approximately 0·5 mm at 3 mm nasal to the corneal apex and 0·4 mm at 3 mm temporal to the apex.[6] If measurements are taken when the patient is not fixating correctly then large errors will be encountered. When fixation is not possible a target for the fellow eye should be used. Poor fixation by the patient is the major source of keratometry error.

Poor tear film

If the tear film constantly breaks up then it may be necessary to insert a drop of normal saline to clear the film for the few seconds required for a measurement to be taken. More viscous substances such as methylcellulose should be avoided because they produce random curvature readings.

Nystagmus

The keratometer should be roughly aligned and then the patient should be asked to close their eyes for 10 seconds. The nystagmus is generally reduced on initial opening of the eyes, which allows fine adjustment of the mire separation.

Combined corneal graft and cataract surgery

In eyes that are to be treated with combined cataract extraction and keratoplasty, some surgeons assume an average postoperative anterior corneal curvature of 7·60 mm on the basis that successful grafts tend to have a steeper rather than a flatter curvature. Other surgeons assume an average keratometry value of 7·80 mm. If keratometry is possible then some surgeons use these measured values in the lens implant power calculation and try to maintain the corneal curvature. Keratometry readings from the fellow eye are also sometimes used and amended according to the corneal donor button

size. Binder[7] suggests that a corneal donor button 0·25 mm larger than the recipient trephine reduces the chance of corneal flattening, whereas 0·5 mm larger induces steepening associated with a 1–2 D myopic shift postoperatively. Less postoperative steepening is associated with larger grafts (7·5–8·0 mm).

Following refractive surgery

It has been reported that keratometric measurements following refractive surgery show a significantly smaller refractive change than the optometric refraction.[8-11] Consequently, the use of postkeratotomy keratometric readings in lens implant formulae may lead to large postoperative refractive errors. Some surgeons use corneal topography (see below) and select a smoothing algorithm over the pupillary zone to determine an effective corneal power. Two other methods for determining the true effective corneal power following refractive surgery have been suggested:[9]

- The known refractive history method
- The contact lens method.

In the known refractive history method (Box 6.1), the level of myopia or hypermetropia surgically corrected is first converted from the spectacle plane to the corneal plane (see Equation B in Appendix I). This value is then subtracted from the prerefractive surgery average corneal power (keratometry).

In the contact lens method (Box 6.2), refraction is performed and its spherical equivalent (SE) at the corneal plane is calculated. After keratometry, a rigid contact lens (CL) of known power (preferably plano) and known base curve is inserted. The base curve is selected using the flatter keratometry reading (typically 40, 35, or 30 D). A further refraction is performed and again the SE at the corneal plane is calculated. The effective corneal power for use in a lens implant formula is given by the formula (base curve CL) + (CL power) +

Box 6.1 Example of effective corneal power calculation following refractive surgery using the known refractive history method

- If the prerefractive surgery average corneal power is 40 D
- And 2 D of myopia was corrected
- Then the average effective corneal power for use in lens implant formula is 40 D − 2 D = 38 D

D, dioptres

Box 6.2 Example of effective corneal power calculation following refractive surgery using the contact lens method

- CL base curve is 40 D (use refractive index 1·3375 to convert a base curve from mm to D if necessary)
- CL power is 0 D (plano)
- SE at corneal plane with CL is −4 D
- SE at corneal plane with CL is −2 D
- Then the average effective corneal power is [40 + 0 + (−4) − (−2)] = 38 D

CL, contact lens; SE, spherical equivalent

(SE corneal plane with CL) − (SE corneal plane without CL).

Both techniques can conveniently be performed using commercially marketed intraocular lens (IOL) software programs. In some instances there is an incomplete refractive history. For example, the pretreatment keratometry or corneal topography may not be available. In other cases, such as in those with poor visual acuity, the contact lens technique may be unsuitable. In these situations, providing the pretreatment and six month post-treatment refractions are available, published data defining corneal flattening versus corrected myopia or hyperopia may be used to predict the original keratometry for use in the refractive history formula.

Irregular astigmatism

The keratometer mire reflections viewed by the examiner are distorted in eyes with irregular astigmatism, such as those with corneal disease or those after corneal surgery. In these cases corneal topography may be useful. The corneal topographer uses a large number (typically 20) of illuminated concentric rings that are reflected by the anterior corneal surface. A digital video

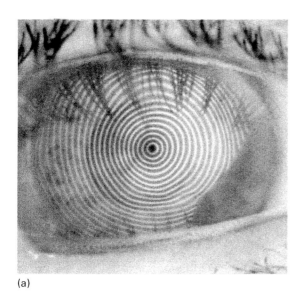

(a)

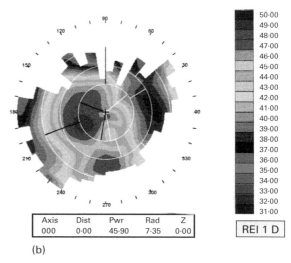

Axis	Dist	Pwr	Rad	Z
000	0·00	45·90	7·35	0·00

REI 1 D

(b)

Figure 6.1 Corneal topography maps: post-photorefractive keratectomy for hypermetropia. (a) Rings suggest the central cornea is regular. (b) Colour scale image of same eye shows treatment zone is decentred by 1·3 mm.

camera linked to a computer enables the reflected corneal rings to be simultaneously sampled at several thousand points. Once processed, these data provide a detailed three-dimensional corneal shape map. Such corneal mapping (Figure 6.1) is useful for measuring the corneal curvature of eyes in which keratometry is difficult, particularly those with irregular astigmatism. The averaging of a large number of data points makes topography more accurate than keratometry in such situations, although only the central readings should be used. A study has shown that a corneal topography system, an automated keratometer, and a hand-held keratometer are as accurate as the "gold standard" manual Javal-Schiotz keratometer.[12]

If neither keratometry nor topography is possible, then a best estimate of anterior corneal curvature must be used. The options in these circumstances are as follows:

- Directly view the cornea in profile and estimate curvature

- Estimate curvature using ultrasound B-mode images (see below) in two orthogonal planes

- Use measurements obtained from the fellow eye

- Assume an average value (7·80 mm).

Axial length measurement

Axial length of the eye is measured from the corneal vertex to the fovea. This visual axis measurement is made using either A-mode ultrasound, on occasions aided by B-mode ultrasound, or an optical interferometric technique.

A-mode ultrasound

Preparation

Anaesthetic drops are first instilled into the eye. In infants or sensitive (non-pregnant) adults, Proxymetacaine is the local anaesthetic of choice because it does not sting. Alternatively,

Oxybuprocaine 0·4% may be used. The patient is usually seated at a slit-lamp assembly with their chin on a rest and their forehead against a band. The ultrasound probe is commonly housed in a spring-loaded assembly, such as a tonometer (set at ≤10 mmHg). This avoids indenting the globe on contact, a source of error that produces a short axial length measurement. If preferred, the ultrasound probe can be hand held, and this is often useful if a patient has restricted physical mobility. Not all hand-held probes are housed in a spring-loaded sleeve and care must be exercised to avoid globe indentation.

Ideally, the transducer contains a central light on which the patient fixates and aids visual axis alignment. The patient should be asked specifically whether they can see the transducer light; if they are unable to do so then it is vital to encourage the fellow eye to fixate (see below). As the probe is brought into direct contact with the anaesthetised cornea, the patient is asked to look into the centre of the transducer light and the operator should use the corneal reflex of the fixation light as an aid to alignment. The tear film should provide sufficient "couplant" to allow efficient transmission of ultrasound pulses into the eye.

Technique

The A-mode transducer is commonly 5 mm in diameter and emits short pulses of weakly focused ultrasound with a nominal frequency of 10 MHz. In the intervals between these emissions, echoes are received by the same transducer, converted to electrical signals, and plotted as spikes on a display. The height of a spike on the y-axis indicates the amplitude of an echo. The position of a spike along the x-axis of the display is dependent upon the arrival time of an echo at the transducer face (Figure 6.2). Most systems presuppose a higher velocity of sound in the cataractous lens than in the aqueous and vitreous (which are assumed to have equal velocities). Table 6.1 gives a list of some of the velocities used in commercially available systems. Most use

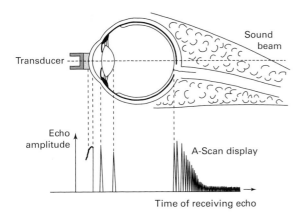

Figure 6.2   A-mode ultrasound trace.

Table 6.1 Calibrated sound velocities in some commercially available A-mode systems

Tissue/material	Calibrated sound velocity (m/s at 37°C)
Aqueous	1532
Vitreous	1532
Cataractous lens	1640
Intumescent cataract	1590
Phakic eye (mean velocity)	1550–1555
Aphakic eye (mean velocity)	1533
Pseudophakic eye (mean velocity)	1553
Lens implant PMMA	2381–2720
Lens implant silicone	980–1000

Note that some systems allow the user to input a specific velocity. PMMA, polymethylmethacrylate.

in-built pattern recognition criteria to determine a "good" trace. Typically, these are three echoes, greater than a predetermined amplitude, which occur within ranges (or gates) predicted for the anterior lens interface, posterior lens interface, and vitreo–retinal interface. No system can determine the origin of the echoes, and it is up to the operator to determine whether the trace is acceptable. It is therefore advantageous if the system indicates which echoes have been selected for a measurement.

Axial length measurement is given as a digital read-out alongside the A-mode trace. The accuracy to which systems will measure a calibrated distance depends upon a number of factors and is typically 0·03 mm (if full wave

rectification of the radiofrequency echo signal should be used to produce the echo "spike" on the display, and measurements taken on the leading edge of the echo). The accuracy of measurements from a skilled operator in a regularly shaped eye is generally within 0·1 mm. Visual axis A-mode traces are shown in Figure 6.3a–f,h. The major source of error in the measurement of axial length is due to misalignment of the transducer with respect to the eye. Misalignment errors can be extremely large (Figure 6.3g) and typically overestimate the axial length measurement.

Avoiding misalignment errors

Corneal illumination and pupil size   The eye should be illuminated and/or the room light adjusted so that it can be seen clearly without stray corneal reflections. If the eye is directly illuminated, then care must be taken not to bleach the patient's retina and impair their ability to fixate. Accurate alignment of the probe with respect to the visual axis is easier with a constricted pupil. However, if the selected formula for lens implant power calculation requires an anterior chamber depth, then it is theoretically better to dilate the eye before measurement. This prevents accommodation, which may cause anterior chamber shallowing and the lens thickness to increase. A 0·7 mm increase in lens thickness during accommodation has been reported,[13] but even in such an extreme case the overall axial length measurement would be increased by only 0·04 mm.

Echo appearance   As previously mentioned, A-mode axial length measurement depends on the echo characteristics of three key interfaces. The anterior lens interface arises after the echolucent anterior chamber. The cataractous lens is often echogenic but the posterior lens interface is the last echo before the echolucent vitreous cavity (although an artefactual echo, a reflection from the internal lens, may be seen after the posterior lens interface echo, or echoes

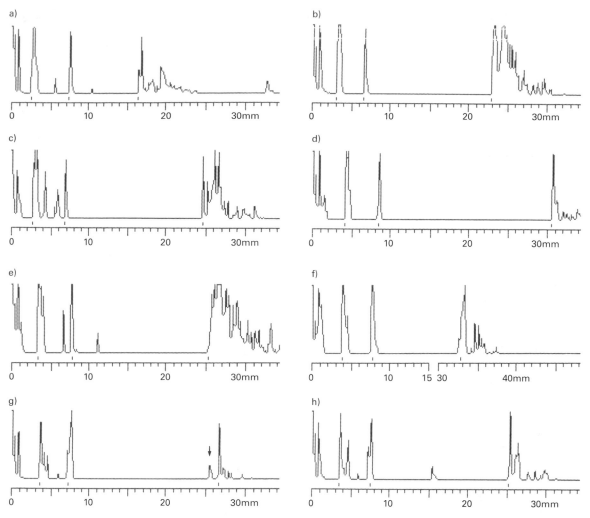

Figure 6.3   A-mode traces: cursors directly above horizontal axis indicate echoes accepted by machine in measurement. (a) Nanophthalmic eye (visual axis). (b) Average length eye (visual axis). (c) Dense cataract with multiple internal lens echoes (visual axis). (d) Highly myopic eye (visual axis). (e) Posterior staphyloma: note the gradual slope of vitreo–retinal interface (visual axis). (f) Highly myopic eye with posterior staphyloma: note the gradual slope of vitreo–retinal echo (visual axis). (g) Non-visual axis A-mode trace: system ignores vitreo–retinal interface echo (arrow) as amplitude too low and accepts echo from a more posterior structure; measurement 1·4 mm too long. (h) Same eye as (g) but with visual axis alignment.

may arise from vitreous opacities). The next echo is from the vitreo–retinal interface. If the pulses of ultrasound strike the lens and vitreo–retinal interfaces perpendicularly then the echoes arising from those interfaces will be higher in amplitude, more steeply rising from the baseline, and shorter in duration (narrower). These features are not observed if the transducer is misaligned obliquely.

Eye fixation   If the individual cannot see the transducer fixation light then the fellow eye should used to fixate on a separate target. In all cases, the reflection of the transducer fixation light on the cornea as it is placed on the eye, and the position of the transducer tip, should be observed carefully. The machine should be positioned so that it is easy to observe the display and the patient's eye at the same time.

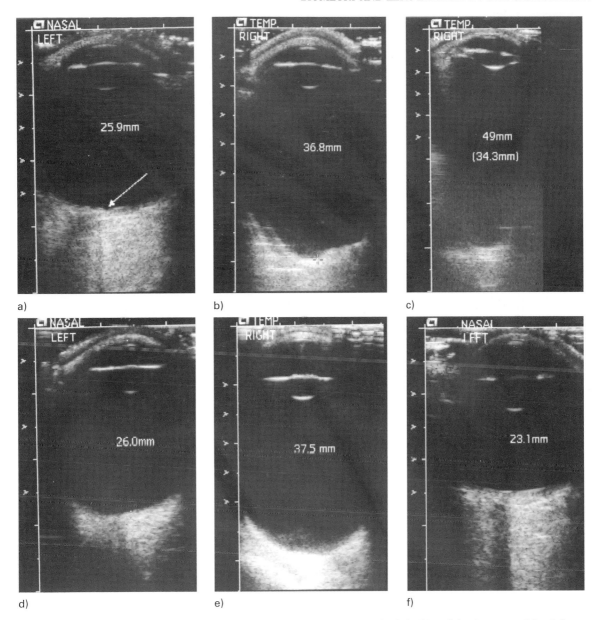

Figure 6.4 B-mode sections (for right eyes the temporal globe is on the left side of the image and for left eyes on the right side of the image). (a) Long eye (25·9 mm): foveal dip (arrow). (b) Very long eye (36·8 mm): massive posterior pole staphyloma. (c) Silicone oil filled vitreous cavity: eye measures 49 mm on B-scan, but actual axial length is 34·3 mm. (d) Long eye (26·0 mm): posterior staphyloma centred nasal to disc. (e) Buphthalmic globe: very long eye (37·5 mm): deep anterior chamber. (f) Megalocornea: average length eye (23·1 mm): deep anterior chamber (5·2 mm).

Gain control To confirm the acquisition of a "good" A-mode trace, the gain (or sensitivity) setting should be varied to alter the echo amplification. The gain should be increased to check whether an echo is present before the presumed vitreo–retinal interface echo. If an

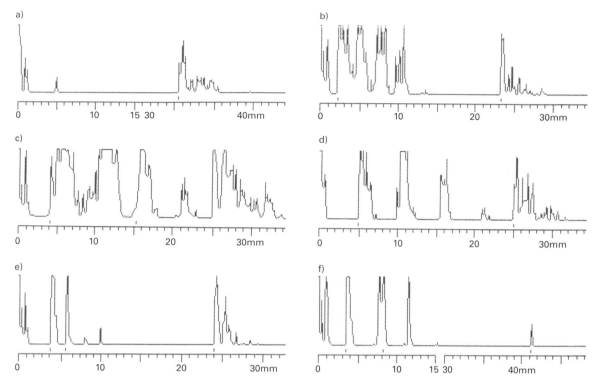

Figure 6.5 A-mode traces. (a) Aphakic, myopic eye. (b) Anterior chamber polymethylmethacrylate (PMMA) implant in situ: note the multiple reflection echoes from implant displayed in vitreous cavity. (c) Posterior chamber PMMA implant in situ: multiple reflections from implants displayed in vitreous cavity; machine accepts multiple reflection as the vitreo–retinal interface and measures globe inaccurately as 15·3 mm. (d) Same eye as (c): manual gates used to indicate to system which echo to accept; correct axial length 25·0 mm. (e) Silicone implant in situ (thickness 1·4 mm). (f) Silicone oil filled vitreous cavity: low amplitude echo from vitreo–retinal interface and multiple reflection artefact at approximately 12·0–15·0 mm, which the system may mistake for the vitreo–retinal interface; system measures axial length as 41·2 mm using manual gates (corrected axial length 29·4 mm, obtained by scaling vitreal length by × 0·64).

echo does appear then the transducer alignment is probably poor (Figure 6.3g). Should ultrasonic pulses strike the vitreo–retinal interface very obliquely and the gain is set to a low value, then the interface echo may not be displayed. The instrument then measures from the anterior cornea to a structure beyond the vitreo–retinal interface. This trace appearance also occurs in eyes with a dense nuclear cataract, in which an internal lens echo is mistaken by the instrument for the posterior lens interface.

The gain should be reduced to prevent echo saturation. Echo saturation is seen as flattening at the top of the amplitude spikes when the display maximum is reached on the y-axis scale. These amplitudes cannot be compared because they all appear to be the same height.

Ultrasound B-mode

This technique uses pulses of ultrasound to produce cross-sectional images of the globe. Patients are usually examined seated. The probe is smeared with a coupling gel and placed horizontally on the centre of the closed upper eyelid. Pulses of sound are sent from the transducer probe, through the eyelid, and into the eye. Echoes from the ocular structures are received by the same transducer and plotted as brightness modulated spots on the display. A bright spot indicates a high amplitude echo and a dim spot a low amplitude echo.

The images shown here were taken using a Sequoia 512 whole body scanner (Acuson). The probe consists of an array of 128 transducer elements, which are fired electronically in overlapping batches to simulate a single moving transducer. For each probe position, a cross-sectional B-mode image is produced and refreshed at a rate of 25 B Scans per second, so that any eye movement is clearly resolved on the image. Positional and angular adjustment of the probe allows the central horizontal section of the globe to be displayed. Figure 6.4 shows B Scans taken on eyes of various dimensions. Appearing echolucent internally, the anterior and posterior surfaces of the cornea are clearly resolved. With less sophisticated scanners, 3 mm thick solid gel pads can be used as a "stand-off" to improve resolution of the anterior chamber. It is sometimes possible to see the foveal dip (Figure 6.4a) and posterior staphyloma are easily imaged. In patients with poor fixation or a posterior staphyloma, B-mode measurement of vitreal length is likely to be considerably more accurate than A-mode. In contrast, aphakic eyes (Figure 6.5a) are generally easy to measure using A-mode examination because there is no attenuation of the sound by the lens.

Complex and difficult axial length measurements

Dense cataracts

A dense cataract can attenuate sound pulses strongly and reduce the amplitude from the vitreo–retinal interface echoes. Alignment is more difficult if the patient is unable to fixate and the corneal reflex of the transducer light is more difficult to see on the background of a white or brown cataract. In these circumstances it may be worthwhile crosschecking measurements using the B-mode technique.

Posterior staphyloma/irregularity of eye shape

Myopic eyes may be difficult to measure in the presence of a posterior pole staphyloma. In such cases the foveal interface presents obliquely to the incoming pulses of ultrasound and the criteria of a steeply rising vitreo–retinal interface echo is not met (Figure 6.3e,f). It is worthwhile crosschecking measurements in such eyes using the B-mode technique or by optical interferometry.

Vitreal echoes

Vitreal echoes arise in pseudophakic eyes from multiple reflections between the implant and the transducer face (Figure 6.5b–d). Vitreous opacities such as asteroid hyalosis also generate high amplitude echoes. Such echoes may be accepted by the A-mode system as the vitreo–retinal interface (Figure 6.5c) If so, manual gate selection should be used to aid the machine in locating the true vitreo–retinal interface echo.

The B-mode appearances of the pseudophakic eye (implanted with one IOL) are shown in Figures 6.6 and 6.7a. It is possible to distinguish the material from which an implant is made and to estimate lens implant power using B mode. Most implants are made from PMMA, acrylic, or silicone. Of these materials PMMA scatters ultrasound waves the most, and silicone does so the least. Thus, PMMA generates the highest amplitude echoes from the implant surfaces and appears brightest on B mode, producing stronger multiple reflections. The refractive index of PMMA is highest (1·49) and that of silicone is lowest (1·41). PMMA lens implants therefore appear much thinner than do silicone implants of the same power (for example, a 18 D PMMA implant measures 0·90 mm centrally).

Silicone oil/heavy liquid in vitreous

The presence of silicone oil or heavy liquid in the vitreous has a dramatic affect on the

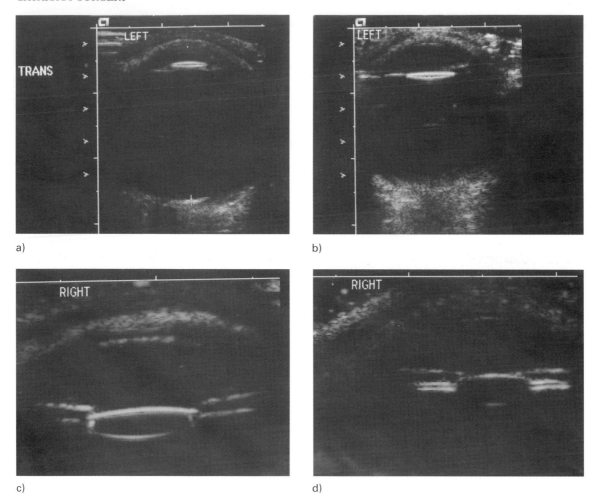

a) b)

c) d)

Figure 6.6 Transverse B-mode images: pseudophakic eyes. (a) Anterior chamber polymethylmethacrylate (PMMA) implant in situ. (b) Posterior chamber PMMA implant in situ. (c) Posterior chamber Acrysoft™ implant in situ. (d) Posterior chamber 21D silicone implant plate haptic (C11UB; Bausch and Lomb) in situ (measures 2·2 mm thick on B-scan scale; 1·4 mm when corrected for velocity in silicone as compared with system velocity of B-scanner).

appearance of both the A-mode trace (Figure 6.5f) and the B-mode (Figure 6.4c) image. The velocity of ultrasound in these liquids is very low in comparison with that in biological tissues (for example, velocity in 1000 cS silicone oil is 982 m/s). Because the A-mode system assumes a velocity of 1532 m/s in the vitreous and the B-mode system assumes an average velocity in tissue of either 1540 m/s or 1550 m/s, the imaged eye may appear considerably elongated (Figures 6.4c and 6.5f). To determine the actual vitreal length, the measured vitreal length should be multiplied by the ratio of the sound velocity in silicone oil to that in vitreous (a factor of 0·64). Further confusion occurs because the acoustic properties of silicone oil and heavy liquid differ so much from vitreous that the echo from the posterior lens interface is increased and multiple reflections commonly occur. This may cause a high amplitude echo at twice the expected distance from the transducer face, typically arising at around 12–15 mm (Figure 6·5f), which then fools the instrument (and some examiners) to record that the eye is very short. Oil also attenuates the sound strongly, resulting in a reduction in amplitude of the echo

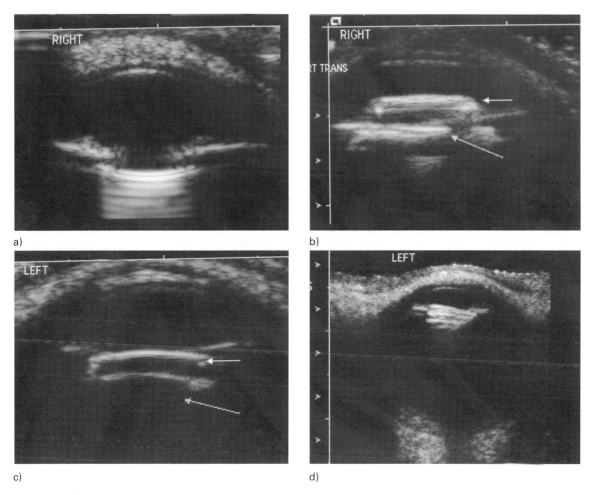

a)

b)

c)

d)

Figure 6.7 Transverse B-mode images: pseudophakic eyes (unusual situations). (a) Anterior globe: posterior chamber polymethylmethacrylate (PMMA) negative power implant (minus 3 D) in situ; note the multiple reflections from implant displayed in vitreous. (b) Anterior globe: anterior chamber PMMA implant (short arrow) and posterior chamber PMMA implant long arrow) in situ. (c) Anterior globe: two silicone "piggy back" implants in bag; anterior implant is of lower power (10 D) and therefore thinner than the posteriorly positioned implant (26 D). (d) Nanophthalmic eye (15·6 mm): three PMMA "piggyback" implants in the bag; note that attenuation of sound by implants gives rise to shadowing in the orbital fat pad.

from the vitreo–retinal interface (Figure 6.4c and 6.5f).

Usually, silicone oil is removed at the time of lens implantation, but if oil is to be retained it has been recommended that convex–plano (plano posterior) implants be used.[13] Silicone lens implants should not be used in conjunction with silicone oil (see Chapter 7). If biconvex lenses are used then the loss of refracting power of the implant in oil has been calculated as 67·4/r, where r is the back radius of the IOL in millimetres.[14] This is negative for a biconvex lens and positive for a meniscus lens. In contrast, for a convex–plano implant r is infinity and 67·4/r is therefore equal to 0. It has also been suggested that the IOL power should be calculated to allow for the refractive index of silicone oil (1·4034). This requires the addition of a constant that is dependent on the axial length of the eye and is calculated as 67·4/[(0·708 × Axial length in millimetres) + 2·93]. For example, IOL power would be + 3·5 D for an axial length of 23·0 mm and + 2·8 D for an axial length of 30·0 mm (if using convex–plano implants).

Optical interferometry

An optical interferometer specifically designed for lens implant power calculation is commercially available (IOL Master; Carl Zeiss). This system can be used for optical measurement of the axial length, keratometry, and optical measurement of anterior chamber depth. In-built formulae (Haigis, Hoffer Q, SRK T, and Holladay 1) allow calculation of lens implant power. It can be used for measuring axial length in eyes in which visual acuity is 6/18 or better but dense cataract, corneal opacification, or vitreous opacities preclude measurement. The system is a non-contact one and is therefore ideal in terms of patient comfort and compliance. The patient sits with their chin on a rest and forehead against a band and is asked to fixate on a target light. The operator merely has to use the joystick to focus the instrument and to press a button to record the axial length. A measure of trace quality is given in a signal: noise ratio, which must be greater than 2·0 to be accepted by the machine. The system is ideal for use in those eyes that are difficult to measure using ultrasound, for example eyes in which there are posterior staphylomata (especially if eccentric) or eyes with nystagmus.

The system uses a low coherence Doppler interferometer to measure axial length.[15] A collimated beam of near infrared (780 nm) from a multimode laser diode is transmitted to the globe via a Michelson interferometer. Light is partially reflected at the ocular interfaces. Moving one of the interferometer mirrors varies the optical path difference between the two arms of the interferometer. When the path difference corresponds to the axial length of the eye, concentric interference fringes are generated. The intensity of these fringes are plotted as a function of the position of the mirror. The position of the mirror is converted to an axial length measurement by assuming an average refractive index along the beam path from prior calibration. Experimental studies on chick eyes suggest that the first peak seen on the interferometer display arises at the retinal inner limiting membrane and the second at Bruch's membrane.[16]

The traces represent a plot of intensity of fringes converted to a voltage versus axial length. Figure 6.8 shows a series of traces from the IOL Master interferometer taken in phakic eyes, an aphakic eye, pseudophakic eyes, and a highly myopic eye with silicone oil filled vitreous. The system has proved to be highly accurate and simple to use in a variety of difficult measurement situations.

Intraocular lens calculation formulae

Fedorov and Kolinko[17] introduced the first lens implant formula. This was a "theoretical" formula based on geometrical optics using axial length, average keratometry measurements, the predicted postoperative anterior chamber depth, and the refractive index of aqueous and vitreous (see Equation C in Appendix I). Several inherent errors occur using a theoretical formula:

- Postoperative anterior chamber depth cannot be predicted from preoperative anterior chamber depth alone

- The corneal refractive index used to convert the anterior corneal curvature readings (mm) to corneal power (D) is hypothetical

- The axial length measured is to the vitreo–retinal interface and not to the sensory retina

- Corneal flattening and shortening of the eye may be induced surgically.

Subsequently, many authors have introduced or amended correction factors to improve the

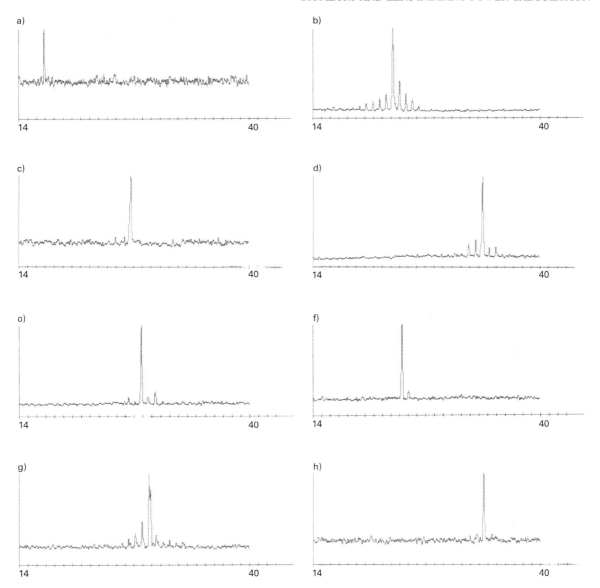

Figure 6.8 Optical interferometry traces (IOL Master, Carl Zeiss). (a) Nanophthalmic eye. (b) Average length eye. (c) Myopic eye. (d) Aphakic, highly myopic eye. (e) Pseudophakic (polymethylmethacrylate implant), highly myopic eye. (f) Pseudophakic eye [acrylic (Acrysof; Alcon) implant]. (g) Pseudophakic eye (silicone implant). (h) Highly myopic eye (34·2 mm) with silicone filled vitreous.

formulae for IOL power calculation.[18–23] To increase the accuracy of predicted postoperative anterior chamber depth, Binkhorst[19] adjusted the preoperative anterior chamber depth according to axial length. In contrast, Holladay and Olsen use a corneal height formula (the distance between the iris plane and the optical

plane of the implant). This is referred to as "the surgeon factor" in the Holladay formula[21] and "the offset" by Olsen.[23]

In the 1980s, while many authors continued to improve and refine theoretical formulae, Sanders, Retzlaff and Kraff produced the SRK I regression formula.[24,25] This formula used an empirically determined A constant that is specific to the lens implant style, and showed a linear relationship between lens implant power and both axial length and corneal power. The A constant encompassed the predicted anterior chamber depth and could be individualised by the surgeon. This formula evolved to SRK ll, in which the A constant was adjusted in a stepwise manner according to whether the axial length was short, average, or long. In 1990 the SRK T formula was introduced.[26,27] This is a theoretical formula with a regression methodology optimising the postoperative anterior chamber depth, corneal refractive index, and retinal thickness corrections. It also uses the A constant, which some authors have correlated with theoretical anterior chamber depth determinations.[22,28] Because axial length determined by ultrasound is only measured to the vitreo–retinal interface and not to the sensory retina, the SRK T formula is adjusted by adding a figure derived from the measured axial length ($0.65696 - 0.02029 \times$ axial length in millimeters). The Holladay formula simply adds 0.2 mm to the axial length of the eye.

Software has been introduced by several authors for use on personal computers. This software allows a surgeon to calculate lens implant powers using a variety of formulae and to input their own refractive outcomes into a database. These results can then be used to further refine their lens power calculations. Alternatively, surgeons can share refractive postoperative data by adding it to a large database that is available on the internet. These data can then be used to improve the accuracy of lens implant calculations.

Formula(e) choice in complex cases

Extremes of axial length

Hoffer[29] suggests that different formulae perform optimally according to the axial length of the eye (Table 6.2). For average length eyes ($22.0-24.5$ mm), an average of the powers calculated using the Holladay, Hoffer Q, and

Table 6.2   Choice of formulae according to the axial length

Axial length (mm)	Proportion of eyes in population	Recommended formula(e)
< 22·0	8%	Hoffer Q
22·0–24·5	72%	Average Holladay, Hoffer Q, and SRK T
24·5–26·0	15%	Holladay
> 26·0	5%	SRK T

SRK T formulae is recommended. For shorter eyes (< 22·0 mm) the Hoffer Q formula is recommended. For eyes with axial lengths in the range 24·5–26·0 mm, the Holladay formula is best and for eyes longer than 26·0 mm, the SRK T formula is optimal. Olsen's Catefract formula, the Haigis formula, and the Holladay 2 formula require the input of the measured preoperative anterior chamber depth. These formulae are therefore particularly suited to eyes with shallow or deep anterior chambers (Figure 6.4e,f).

Extremes of corneal curvature

The Holladay 2 formula may be inaccurate for calculating implant power in eyes with extremely flat corneas and a single implant. For example, in an eye with average keratometry of 11·36 mm (29·7 D) and an axial length of 28·7 mm, Holladay 2 overestimates the lens implant power by 4 D as compared with Holladay 1 (which accurately predicts the correct lens implant power). Conversely, the SRK T formula may fail with very steep corneas. For example, in an eye with an average keratometry of 6·45 mm (52·3 D) and an axial length of 22·5 mm, SRK T predicts a lens implant power that is 4 D too high, as compared with the Holladay 1 and Hoffer Q formulae (which both predict lens implant power correctly).

Piggyback lenses

Modern third generation formulae do not accurately predict the strength of piggyback implants, and it has been shown that the use of such formulae may result in an average of 5 D postoperative absolute refractive error.[30] As a result it has been suggested that personalised constants be adjusted to force the mean predicted errors to zero (for the Holladay formula + 2·1 D and for the SRK T formula + 4·5 D).

The Holladay 2 formula uses the horizontal white to white corneal diameter, anterior chamber depth, and crystalline lens thickness to predict better the position of the implant in the eye and to determine whether an eye is short overall or just has a short vitreal length. As such this formula is able to predict accurately the optimum piggyback lens implant powers for use in extremely short eyes. Surgeons can elect whether to use two lens implants of the same power, or to set the anteriorly or posteriorly positioned implant to a power of choice (depending on the availability of implants or surgeon preference). B-mode images of a variety of piggyback lens implant configurations are shown in Figure 6.7b–d. Figure 6.7b shows combined anterior chamber and posterior chamber implants. In the nanophthalmic eye shown in Figure 6.7d, three rather than two implants were used to provide a total power +58 D.

Postoperative biometry errors

In the event of a significant difference between the calculated and achieved postoperative refraction, the axial length and keratometry measurements should be repeated (Box 6.3). Additionally, the postoperative anterior chamber depth should be measured and compared with the formula prediction (an anterior chamber depth greater than that predicted corresponds to a hypermetropic shift in postoperative refractive error, and vice versa).[31] It is also worthwhile performing a B-mode examination to determine any irregularity in shape of the posterior globe, for example a posterior staphyloma. The thickness of the implant as measured on both A and B modes

---

Box 6.3 Outcome of corneal curvature or axial length measurement error

- + 0·1 mm error in radius of corneal curvature = + 0·2 D postoperative refraction error
- + 1·0 mm error in axial length = + 2·3 D postoperative refraction error

---

should be noted. This thickness should be consistent with the lens implant power claimed to have been implanted. Implantation of the wrong lens implant by the surgeon or mislabelling of an implant by the manufacturer should also be considered as possibilities.

Correction of biometry errors

Lens exchange

If a lens exchange is planned, then in addition to remeasurement of the axial length, keratometry, and anterior chamber depth, a calculation should be performed using the postoperative refraction to determine the power of the new implant. A simple way to do this is to decide whether the error originated in determining true corneal power (for example, an eye post-photorefractive keratectomy with a poor refractive history) or, as is more commonly the case, in the axial length measurement. A trial and error method is then used in the chosen formula, inserting, for example, the measured corneal curvature but a guessed axial length, along with the actual postoperative refraction as the desired target outcome. The axial length guess is then adjusted until the implant power recommended coincides with that which was implanted. This axial length is then used in the formula as the "true" axial length and the real target refraction set to calculate the exchange lens implant power. This lens implant power is the best prediction of lens exchange power because it is based on the postoperative refraction in that individual. Ideally, the exchange lens implant power calculated in this way should be the same as that calculated using the new measurements of axial length, anterior chamber depth, and keratometry. If they differ, then the exchange lens power calculated from the postoperative refraction should be used (assuming the implant thickness measured on A or B mode is consistent with the IOL power claimed to have been implanted).

For medicolegal purposes, the removed lens implant should have its central thickness measured using an electronic calliper and it should be returned to the manufacturers to have the power checked and a labelling error excluded. The central thickness of the implant can be used, with a calibration chart for the lens material, in order to determine its power in the eye (for example, a PMMA implant of power 12 D has a central thickness of 0·64 mm). It should be noted that most hospital focimeters do not have the range to measure lens implant power because the IOL power is 3·2 times greater in air than the labelled power for within the eye (for example, a 15 D IOL has a power of 48 D air).

"Piggyback" lens implant

If a lens implant has been in situ for a considerable period, then lens exchange may be difficult. It may be preferable to correct postoperative refractive error by inserting a second, or piggyback, implant. The measurements of the corneal curvature, axial length, and anterior chamber depth should be repeated and an accurate postoperative refraction obtained. The Holladay R formula should then be used to calculate the required lens implant power to piggyback an IOL either into the capsular bag or the sulcus.

Refractive surgery

An alternative to either lens exchange or piggyback lens implantation is to correct postoperative refractive error using a corneal laser refractive technique. This has the advantage of avoiding a further intraocular procedure. Laser in situ keratomileusis has been reported as effective, predictable, and safe for correcting residual myopia after cataract surgery.[32] To avoid IOL or cataract incision related complications, it should not be performed until 3 months after the initial surgery.

References

1 Guillon M, Lydon DPM, Wilson C. Corneal topography a clinical model. *Ophthalmic Physiol Opt* 1986;**6**:47–56.
2 Lehman SP. Corneal areas used in keratometry. *Optician* 1967;**154**:261–6.
3 Rabbetts RB. Comparative focusing errors of keratometers. *Optician* 1977;**173**:28–9
4 Clark BAJ. Keratometry: a review. *Aus J Optom* 1973;**56**:94–100.
5 Russell JF, Koch DD, Gay CA. A new formula for calculate changes in corneal astigmatism. *Symposium on Cataract, IOL and Refractive Surgery*; Boston, April 1991.
6 Mandell RB. Corneal topography. In: *Contact lens practice, basic and advanced*, 2nd ed. Illinois: Charles C Thomas, 1965.
7 Binder PS. Secondary intraocular lens implantation during or after corneal transplantation. *Am J Ophthalmol* 1985;**99**:515–20.
8 Koch DD, Liu JF, Hyde LL, Rock RL, Emery JM. Refractive complications of cataract surgery following radial keratotomy. *Am J Ophthalmol* 1989:**108**:676–82.
9 Soper JW, Goffman J. Contact lens fitting by retinoscopy. In: Soper JW, ed. *Contact lenses: advances in design, fitting and application.* Miami: Symposia Specialist, 1974.
10 Holladay JT. Intraocular lens calculations following radial keratotomy surgery. *Refract Corneal Surg* 1989;**5**:39.
11 Colliac J-P, Shammas HJ, Bart DJ. Photorefractive keratotomy for correction of myopia and astigmatism. *Am J Ophthalmol* 1994;**117**:369–80.
12 Tennen DG, Keates RH, Montoya CBS. Comparison of three keratometry instruments. *J Cataract Refract Surg* 1995;**21**:407–8.
13 Rabie EP, Steele C, Davies EG. Anterior chamber pachymetry during accommodation in emmetropic and myopic eyes. *Ophthalmic Physiol Opt* 1986;**6**:283–6.
14 Meldrum ML, Aaberg TM, Patel A, Davis J. Cataract extraction after silicone oil repair of retinal retachments due to necrotising retinitis. *Arch Ophthalmol* 1996;**114**:885–92.
15 Hitzenberger CK. Optical measurement of the axial length of the eye by laser doppler interferometry. *Invest Ophthalmol Vis Sci* 1991;**32**:616–24.
16 Schmid GF, Papastergiou GI, Nickla DL, Riva CE, Stone RA, Laties AM. Validation of laser Doppler interferometric measurements in vivo of axial eye length and thickness of fundus layers in chicks. *Curr Eye Res* 1996;**15**:691–6.
17 Fedorov SN, Kolinko AI. A method of calculating the optical power of the intraocular lens. *Vestnik Oftalmologii* 1967;**80**:27–31.

18 Colenbrander MD. Calculation of the power of an iris-clip lens for distance vision. *Br J Ophthalmol* 1973;**57**:735–40.

19 Binkhorst RD. Pitfalls in the determination of intra-ocular lens power without ultrasound. *Ophthalmic Surg* 1976;**7**:69–82.

20 Hoffer KJ. The effect of axial length on posterior chamber lenses and posterior capsule position. *Curr Concepts Ophthalmic Surg* 1984;**1**:20–22.

21 Holladay JT, Prager TC, Chandler TY, Musgrove KH, Lewis JW, Ruiz RS. A three part system for refining intraocular lens power calculations. *J Cataract Refract Surg* 1988;**14**:17–24.

22 Olsen T. Theoretical approach to intraocular lens calculation using Gaussian optics. *J Cataract Refract Surg* 1987;**13**:141–5.

23 Olsen T, Corydon L, Gimbel H. Intra-ocular lens implant power calculation with an improved anterior chamber depth prediction algorithm. *J Cataract Refract Surg* 1995;**21**:313–9.

24 Retzlaff J. A new intraocular lens calculation formula. *J Am Intraocular Implant Soc* 1980;**6**:148–52.

25 Sanders DR, Kraff MC. Improvement of intraocular lens calculation using empirical data. *J Am Intraocular Implant Soc* 1980;**6**:263–7.

26 Retzlaff J, Sanders DR, Kraff MC. Development of the SRK/T lens implant power calculation formula. *J Cataract Refract Surg* 1990;**16**:333–40.

27 Sanders DR, Retzlaff JA, Kraff MC, Gimbel HF, Raanan MG. Comparison of SRK/T formula and other theoretical formulas. *J Cataract Refract Surg* 1990;**16**:341–346.

28 McEwan JR. Algorithms for determining equivalent A-constants and Surgeon's factors. *J Cataract Refract Surg* 1996;**22**:123–34.

29 Hoffer K. The Hoffer Q formula: a comparison of theoretical and regression formulas. *J Cataract Refract Surg* 1993;**19**:700–12.

30 Holladay JT. Achieving emmetropia in extremely short eyes with two piggy-back posterior chamber intra-ocular lenses. *Ophthalmology* 1996;**103**:118–22.

31 Haigis W. Meaurement and prediction of the post-operative anterior chamber depth for intraocular lenses of different shape and material. In: Cennamo G, Rosa N, eds. *Proceedings of the 15th bi-annual meeting of SIDUO (Societas Internationalis pro Diagnostica Ultrasonica in Ophthalmologica)*. Boston: Dordect, 1996.

32 Ayala MJ, Perez-Santonja JJ, Artola A, Claramonte P, Alio JL. Laser in situ keratomileusis to correct residual myopia after cataract surgery. *J Refract Surg* 2001;**17**:12–6.

Appendix I: equations

Equation A: corneal power

$$F_c = (n_c - n_a)/r_m = 337 \cdot 5/r_{mm}$$

Where:

F_c = corneal power (D)

n_c = hypothetical corneal refractive index (1·3375)

n_a = refractive index of air (1·0000)

r_m = radius of anterior corneal curvature (m)

r_{mm} = radius of anterior corneal curvature (mm)

Equation B: conversion of refraction from the spectacle to the corneal plane

$$R_c = Rs/(1 - 0 \cdot 012\ Rs)$$

Where:

R_c = refraction at corneal plane

Rs = refraction at spectacle plane (12 mm back vertex distance)

Equation C: theoretical intraocular lens formula

$$P = n/(l - a) - nk/(n - ka)$$

Where:

P = IOL power for emmetropia (D)

n = refractive index of aqueous and vitreous

l = axial length (mm)

a = predicted post-operative anterior chamber depth (mm)

k = average keratometry reading (D)

7 Foldable intraocular lenses and viscoelastics

Foldable intraocular lenses

Since 1949, when Harold Ridley implanted the first intraocular lens (IOL),[1] polymethylmethacrylate (PMMA) has been the favoured lens material, and the "gold standard" by which others are judged. Using a rigid material, such as PMMA, the minimum optic diameter is 5 mm and hence the wound needs to be of a similar dimension. To preserve the advantages of a small phacoemulsification incision, various materials have been developed that enable the IOL to be folded.

Designs and materials

There are a number of features and variables by which a lens material and design are judged. Of these, capsule opacification and need for laser capsulotomy is considered particularly important. This is the main postoperative complication of IOL implantation and as such is discussed in Chapter 12. Other relevant aspects of lens performance that influence the choice of implant include the following:

- Ease and technique of implantation
- IOL stability after implantation
- Biocompatibility
- Lens interaction with silicone oil.

Three foldable materials are in widespread use: silicone, acrylic, and hydrogel. Acrylic and hydrogel are both acrylate/methacrylate polymers but differ in refractive index, water content, and hydrophobicity (Table 7.1).

Table 7.1   Comparison of foldable materials

Comparison	Silicone elastomers	Acrylate/methacrylate polymers	
		Acrylic	Hydrogel
Typical components	Dimethylsiloxane	2-Phenylethylmethacrylate	6-Hydroxyhexylmethacrylate
	Dimethlydiphenylsiloxane	2-Phenylethylacrylate	2-Hydroxyethylmethacrylate
Refractive index	1·41 (1st generation)	1·55	1·47
	1·47 (2nd generation)		
Hydrophobicity	Hydrophilic	Hydrophobic	Hydrophilic
Biocompatibility			
Foreign body reaction	High (1st generation)	Low	Very low
	Low (2nd generation)		
LEC growth (?related to PCO)	Low	Low	High
Silicone oil coating	High	Moderate/low	Low

LEC, lens epithelial cell; PCO, posterior capsule opacification.

Table 7.2   Comparison of intraocular lens designs

	Loop haptic	Plate haptic
Implantation method	Manually folded or by injection device	Usually injection device
Vitreous loss/posterior capsule rupture	May be used with careful haptic positioning	Use contraindicated
Anterior capsular tears	May be used with careful haptic positioning	Use contraindicated
Sulcus fixation	Possible depending on overall lens size	Use contraindicated
Post-Nd:YAG	Stable	Early and late subluxation or dislocation recognised
Non-corneal astigmatism	Rare	Recognised

Nd:YAG, neodymium: yttrium aluminium garnet.

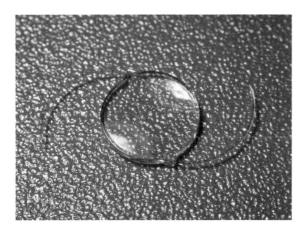

Figure 7.1   A typical foldable silicone three-piece loop haptic intraocular lens (Allergan). Note that the haptics are posteriorly angulated.

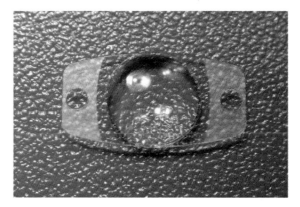

Figure 7.2   A typical foldable silicone plate haptic lens with large haptic dial holes (Staar Surgical).

Silicone lenses have been extensively used with millions implanted worldwide,[2] although acrylic lenses have become increasingly popular.[3] The first hydrogel IOL was implanted in 1977, but only more recently have these lenses been developed further. Subtle differences exist between the optical performances of these lens materials,[4–6] but these are not thought to be clinically significant.

IOL haptic configuration is broadly divided into loop or plate haptic designs (Table 7.2). Loop haptic lenses are constructed either as one piece (optic and haptic made of the same material) or three pieces (optic and haptic made of different materials). The majority of foldable loop haptic lenses are of a three piece design (Figure 7.1), with haptics typically made of either PMMA or polypropylene. Plate haptic lenses are constructed of one material (Figure 7.2).

Implantation

Foldable IOLs are inserted into the capsular bag with either implantation forceps or an injection device. Injection devices simplify IOL implantation and allow the lens to be inserted through a smaller wound,[7] while minimising potential lens contamination. Foldable plate haptic silicone lenses were among the first to be implanted using an injection device; they have been widely used and are available in a broad range of lens powers. An advantage of plate

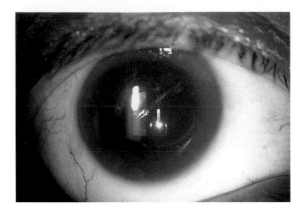

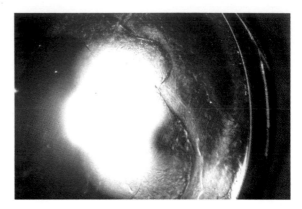

Figure 7.4   Lens epithelial growth on the surface of a hydrogel lens.

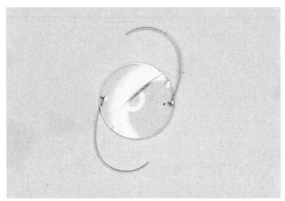

Figure 7.3   A damaged acrylic lens optic following folding and implantation. (a) Intraocular lens in situ. (b) Explanted intraocular lens.

haptic lenses is that they can easily be loaded into an injection device and reliably implanted directly into the capsular bag. However, because these lenses have a relatively short overall length (10·5 mm typically) they are not suitable for sulcus placement. Acrylic IOLs are more fragile than other foldable materials and they may be scratched or marked during folding (Figure 7.3). Although explantation has been reported for a cracked acrylic optic,[8] usually the optical quality of the IOL is not affected unless extreme manipulations are applied during folding or implantation.[9,10] Both hydrogel and acrylic lenses are easily handled when wet. In contrast silicone lenses are best kept dry until they are placed into the eye.

Stability

Studies comparing decentration and tilt of lenses of differing materials and haptic design have emphasised the importance of precise IOL placement into the capsular bag with an intact capsulorhexis.[11,12] Subluxation and decentration of plate haptic lenses have been attributed to asymmetrical capsule contraction from capsule tears.[13] It is also recognised that the unfolding of a silicone lens may extend any pre-existing capsule tear. For these reasons, the implantation of injectable silicone plate haptic lenses is contraindicated unless the rhexis and capsular bag are intact.[14] In contrast, a loop haptic foldable lens can often be successfully inserted by careful positioning of the haptics despite a capsule tear.[15] Although plate haptic lenses may rotate within the capsular bag immediately after implantation, they show long-term rotational stability compared with loop haptic lenses.[16] This may make them more suitable for use as a toric lens implant to correct astigmatism.

In the presence of an intact capsule, contraction of the capsular bag and phimosis may cause compression and flexing of a plate haptic lens, resulting in refractive change[17] or non-corneal astigmatism.[18] This lens compression is also a contributing factor to the phenomenon of silicone and hydrogel plate haptic lens subluxation or dislocation following neodymium:

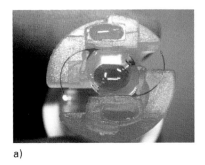
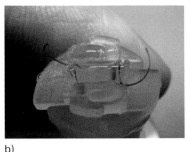

a)   b)

Figure 7.5   Packaging that folds the lens implant (Hydroview; Bausch and Lomb). (a) Unfolded lens seated in the lens carrier. (b) Squeezing the lens carrier folds the optic to allow transfer to implantation forceps.

yttrium aluminium garnet (Nd:YAG) laser capsulotomy (see Chapter 12). Plate haptic lenses are therefore not the IOL of choice in patients who are at risk of capsule contraction, for example those with weakened zonules.

Biocompatibility

This is the local tissue response to an implanted biomaterial. It consists of two patterns of cellular response to an IOL: lens epithelial cell (LEC) growth and a macrophage derived foreign body reaction. LEC growth is relevant in the development of capsule opacification (see Chapter 12). In patients who are at higher risk of cell reactions, such as those who have had previous ocular surgery or have glaucoma, uveitis or diabetes, biocompatibility may influence IOL selection. Compared with silicone and PMMA, hydrogel IOLs are associated with a reduced inflammatory cell reaction but have more LEC growth on their anterior surface (Figure 7.4).[19] Inflammatory deposits are greater on first generation silicone plate IOLs than on acrylic or second generation silicone IOLs.[20] LEC growth was found to be lowest on an acrylic lens, but in the same study a second generation silicone lens had the least incidence of cell growth overall.[21]

Silicone oil

Silicone oil can cover and adhere to lens materials causing loss of transparency. This interaction of silicone oil with the IOL optic has implications for vitreo–retinal surgery following cataract surgery[22] and governs the choice of IOL in patients undergoing cataract surgery in which silicone oil has been or may be used for retinal tamponade. Silicone lenses are particularly vulnerable to silicone oil coverage and should be avoided in patients with oil in situ or who may require oil tamponade.[23] Hydrogel and non-surface modified PMMA lenses show lower levels of oil coating as compared with acrylic lenses.[24]

Intraocular lens implantation techniques

Forceps folding

Depending on the optic–haptic configuration, a loop haptic lens may either be folded along its 12 to 6 o'clock axis or its 3 to 9 o'clock axis. It is important that the lens manufacturer's directions are followed because lens damage may occur if incorrect forceps are used[25] or if non-recommended folding configurations are employed.[10] The anterior chamber and capsular bag should first be filled with viscoelastic and the incision enlarged if necessary (see Chapter 2). The AcrySof (Alcon) and Hydroview (Bausch and Lomb) lenses should be folded on the 6 to 12 o'clock axis.[10,26] Acrylic lens implantation is made easier by warming the lens before insertion, protecting the optic with viscoelastic before grasping it with insertion

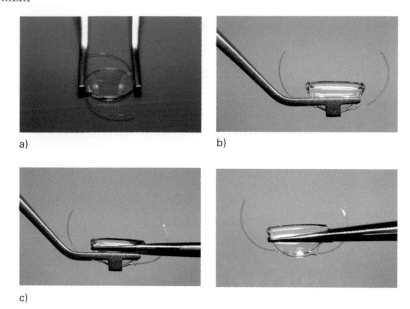

a)

b)

c)

Figure 7.6 "6 to 12 o'clock" forceps folding technique. (a) The intraocular lens optic edge (Allergan) is grasped with folding forceps (Altomed) at the 3 and 9 o'clock positions. (b) The optic is folded symmetrically with gentle closure of the folding forceps. (c) The folded optic is grasped with implantation forceps (Altomed), ensuring it is gripped away from but parallel to the fold. (d) The folded intraocular lens ready to be inserted, haptic first.

forceps, and using a second instrument through the side port during lens rotation and unfolding.[27] Folding some lens types may be achieved using a lens specific folding device that may be part of the packaging rather than using forceps (Figure 7.5). Three piece lenses with polypropylene haptics require particular care because these haptics are easily deformed, which may result in asymmetrical distortion and subsequent decentration. Not tucking the haptics within the folded optic may reduce this problem.[28,29]

"6 to 12 o'clock" folding and implantation technique *(Figure 7.6):* Usually the lens is removed from its packaging using smooth plain forceps and placed on a flat surface. Using folding forceps, the lens optic edge is grasped at the 3 and 9 o'clock positions. With less flexible optic materials, smooth forceps may be used to help initiate the fold. The optic should fold symmetrically with gentle closure of the folding forceps. The folded optic is then grasped with implantation forceps, ensuring that it is gripped away from, but parallel to, the fold. Ideally, the

lens should only be folded immediately before implantation.

During implantation the leading haptic is slowly guided into the enlarged incision, through the rhexis, and into the capsular bag. The optic should follow with minimal force. Slight posterior pressure helps to guide the optic through the internal valve of the incision, and it may be helpful to stabilise the globe with toothed forceps. If optic implantation requires force then it is likely that the incision is of inadequate width. Once the folded optic is within the anterior chamber the forceps are rotated and gently opened to release the optic. Care should be exercised while closing and removing the implantation forceps because the trailing haptic may be damaged. This haptic may then be dialled or placed into the capsular bag and lens centration confirmed.

"3 to 9 o'clock" folding and implantation technique *(Figure 7.7):* The optic is grasped at the 12 to 6 o'clock positions with folding forceps. Once folded, the lens is transferred to implantation forceps in a manner similar to that

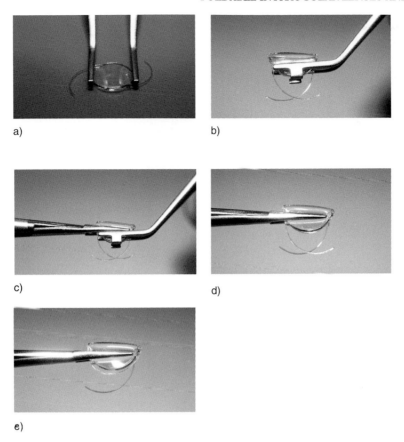

Figure 7.7 "3 to 9 o'clock" forceps folding technique. (a) The intraocular lens optic (Allergan) is grasped with folding forceps (Altomed) at the 12 to 6 o'clock positions. (b) The optic is folded symmetrically with gentle closure of the folding forceps. (c) The folded optic is grasped with implantation forceps (Altomed), ensuring it is gripped away from but parallel to the fold. (d) The haptic end located near the tip of the implantation forceps is at risk of damage during implantation. (e) With the leading haptic tucked into the folded optic, the intraocular lens is ready to be inserted.

described above. The haptics lie overlapped, unlike the 6 to 12 o'clock fold, which produces a leading and trailing haptic. The haptic end located near the tip of the implantation forceps is tucked either into the folded optic or alongside the optic and forceps blade. This ensures the haptic enters the eye without damage. Once the lens is within the eye the implantation forceps are rotated so that both the haptic loops enter the capsular bag. As the forceps are opened gentle posterior pressure ensures that the optic is also implanted directly into the capsular bag.

Injection devices

Each injection device is usually specific to a lens type and the manufacturer's instructions should be followed carefully. Injection devices use viscoelastic and balanced salt solution (BSS) to fill dead space within the device, preventing injection of air bubbles, and to act as a lubricant. Again, the manufacturer's recommendation of type of viscoelastic and dwell time (the time the lens lies within the injector cartridge) should be closely followed.[30] Plate haptic lenses, with their relatively simple construction and lack of posterior vaulting, are

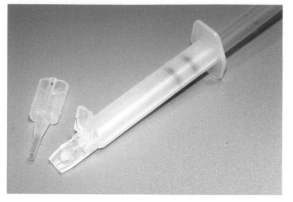

a)

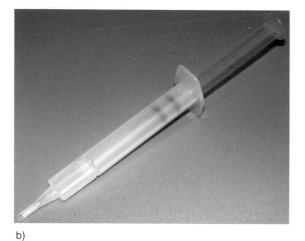

b)

Figure 7.8 Loading technique for a plate haptic lens injection device (Staar Surgical). (a) The intraocular lens is placed in the loading area and the plunger located over the trailing haptic. The injection cannula is filled with a viscoelastic and balance salt solution. (b) The hinged loading area door is closed, the injection cannula is attached, and the plunger is advanced to move the intraocular lens into the distal cannula.

easy to load into and insert using an injection device (Figure 7.8). Loading a loop haptic lens into an injector cartridge or device is generally more complicated because the haptics must be orientated correctly. Most loop haptic lenses are designed to be posteriorly vaulted and must be placed in the capsular bag with the correct anteroposterior orientation. Injection devices that roll the lens may deliver the lens back to front during unfolding. If this should occur

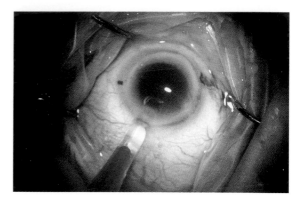

Figure 7.9 Modified injection technique with the injector cannula held in, rather than through, the wound.

then the lens should be repositioned (see below).

Some injection devices are of a syringe type and allow one handed operation, the free hand is then available to stabilise the globe with toothed forceps if required. When advancing the injection plunger it is important to ensure correct contact is made between it and the IOL, and care should be taken to check that the lens advances smoothly until it is located within the distal aspect of the injection cannula. The lens should be injected soon after the lens has been advanced down the cannula. Its tip should be placed bevel down into the incision. The cannula is gently advanced through the wound so that the tip is positioned within the anterior chamber in the plane of the rhexis. The IOL is then gently advanced and unfolds into the capsular bag (note that during unfolding some injection devices require the barrel to be rotated). The trailing haptic of loop haptic lenses usually requires dialling or placing into the bag. With some injection systems it is possible to hold the injector tip within the wound and inject the lens (Figure 7.9).[31] Although the lens is delivered only partly into the capsular bag, implantation can usually be completed using the irrigation and aspiration cannula, which is then in position to remove viscoelastic.

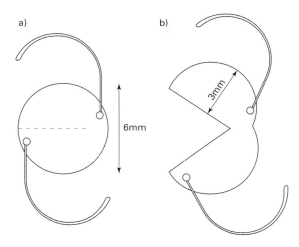

Figure 7.10 Loop haptic intraocular lens explantation without incision enlargement. (a) A partial cut is made through two thirds of the optic via a paracentesis. (b) The optic is hinged to allow explantation through the main wound (for example, if the optic diameter is 6 mm then the cut lens will pass through a 3 mm incision).

Intraoperative implantation complications

Inserting the lens back to front ("antero-posterior malposition" or "IOL flip") is usually a result of incorrect IOL unfolding. IOL haptic or optic damage may occur to both folding and rigid lenses during insertion, although the need to fold the optic and the soft materials may make foldable lenses more vulnerable. Postoperative IOL related complications are discussed in Chapter 12.

Intraocular lens anteroposterior malposition

Anteroposterior malposition may occur intraoperatively using either forceps or an injection device with loop haptic lenses.[32] Failure to correct this may result in a myopic postoperative refractive outcome, pupil block glaucoma, and an increased rate of posterior capsule opacification.

The lens can be rotated or tumbled within the capsular bag to reposition it. The anterior chamber and capsular bag should be fully filled with a viscoelastic. A bimanual technique is employed using either a pair of second instruments, one through the main incision and another through the side port, or an instrument through the side port and forceps to manipulate the trailing haptic. The optic is initially pushed posteriorly and then rotated along its long axis.

Intraocular lens optic or haptic damage

IOL explantation may be required intraoperatively because of inadvertent lens optic or haptic damage sustained during folding or implantation. It is preferable to avoid enlarging the existing main incision during explantation, and a number of techniques have been described. The lens optic may be bisected using Vannas scissors[33] or using a specialised lens bisector,[34] and the IOL halves then extracted. Partially bisecting the optic may be sufficient to reduce the maximum diameter of the optic to match the incision width (Figure 7.10)[35] or in some cases the lens may simply be manipulated through the existing wound.[36] An alternative is to refold the IOL within the anterior chamber.[37] In this technique, a side port is constructed opposite the main incision and haptic loop is pulled through the main incision. A second instrument is then introduced through the side port and under the lens optic. This applies counter force as the lens is folded using implantation forceps inserted through the main incision. Once the lens is folded, the forceps are rotated clockwise and withdrawn. Following IOL removal, a new folding IOL can be inserted through the same incision that then does not require suturing.

Intraocular lens selection in special circumstances

Lens implant selection in patients with uveitis, diabetes, glaucoma, and zonular instability is discussed in Chapter 10. In the presence of vitreous loss it is normally possible to implant an

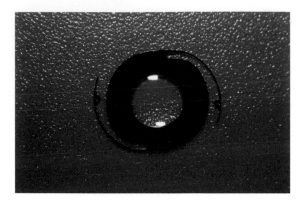

Figure 7.11   Aniridic intraocular lens (Morcher).

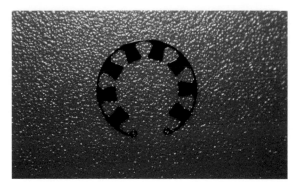

Figure 7.12   Aniridic ring (Morcher).

IOL, but it may be necessary to use a different lens (see Chapter 11).

Iris defects

Complete or partial iris defects often coexist with cataract, and lens implants with opaque segments have been developed to simulate the iris following cataract extraction. The most widely used "aniridic IOL" is a sulcus placed posterior chamber lens with an opaque peripheral segment constructed of rigid black PMMA (Figure 7.11).[38,39] Its minimum diameter is 10 mm and implantation requires a large incision. Traumatic iris defects often present in conjunction with severe anterior segment disruption, including corneal scaring, and congenital aniridia is associated with corneal opacity. Cataract extraction and IOL implantation in these circumstances is often combined with penetrating keratoplasty. The large diameter aniridic IOL can then usually be inserted through the corneal trephine opening.[38] In the absence of combined penetrating keratoplasty, it is possible to avoid the need for a large incision by using phacoemulsification with a folding IOL followed by implantation of two modified capsule tension rings (Figure 7.12). The castellated (rampart-like) ring shape allows them to flex as they are implanted through the main incision and placed into the capsular bag. Once in place, one ring is rotated relative to the other so that the castellations overlap and create a circular diaphragm.

Postoperative glaucoma is a common problem in many aniridic patients. It has been suggested that the large PMMA sulcus lens may be partly responsible. In fact, in the absence of iris tissue, the supporting haptics are often located not in the sulcus but rather in the anterior chamber angle.[38] The use of two rings and an IOL placed within the capsular bag may therefore have some advantage.

High hyperopia

If emmetropia is desired following cataract surgery in a hyperopic eye, then a high implant power will usually be required. In the past IOL powers in excess of +30 dioptres (D) were not readily available, and the concept of inserting multiple lenses into the capsular bag was developed, termed poly-pseudophakia or piggyback lens implantation.[40] The availability of high power folding lenses remains limited, and employing piggyback lenses in patients with short axial lengths reduces optical aberrations.[41]

Acrylic folding lenses have been advocated for multiple lens implantation because they are thinner than other foldable materials.[42] A flattened contact zone has been observed between the optics of such acrylic lenses, which may induce multifocality.[43] A more significant complication, often requiring acrylic lens explantation, is the formation of interlenticular

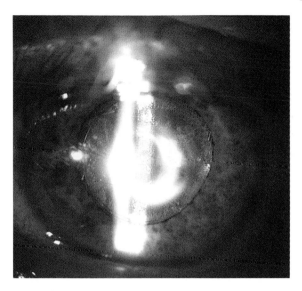

Figure 7.13 Interlenticular opacity between two piggyback acrylic lens implants in a hyperopic eye.

a)

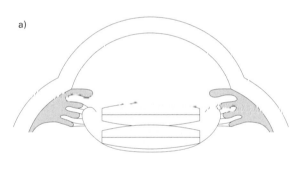

b)

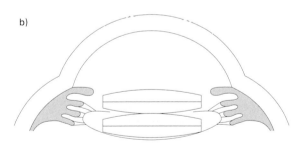

Figure 7.14 Piggyback lenses: methods of preventing interlenticular opacification. (a) Capsular rhexis diameter larger than lens optic diameter, both lenses in the capsular bag. (b) Capsular rhexis diameter less than the lens optic diameter, one lens in the capsular bag and the other in the sulcus.

opacification (Figure 7.13). This is either a membrane[44] or Elschnig's pearls[45] caused by proliferating LECs between the IOL optics trapped within the capsular bag.[46] This complication has also been reported following implantation of multiple silicone plate haptic lenses.[45] To prevent this problem the capsulorhexis should be larger than the lens optic (Figure 7.14a). Alternatively, one IOL should be placed within the capsular bag (with a rhexis size less than the optic diameter) and the other lens is placed in the sulcus, thus preventing LEC access to the interlenticular area (Figure 7.14b).[44]

Intraocular lenses and presbyopia

The majority of patients undergoing cataract surgery are presbyopic and use glasses for near tasks. The power of an implanted monofocal IOL is usually selected to provide distant focus emmetropia (or a low level of myopia to avoid an unexpected hyperopic outcome), and the resulting dependence on reading glasses is not usually regarded as a problem, except in the pre-presbyopic age group. A number of options reduce the need for reading glasses and allow a compromise between near and distance vision.

Monovision relies on the dominant eye becoming emmetropic for distance, and the contralateral eye is then made deliberately myopic (−1·50 to −1·75 D). Unfortunately, stereopsis is reduced and some patients may feel unbalanced even with low levels of anisometropia. It is also essential that the dominant eye is correctly identified. Pre-existing cataract can make this difficult and monovision is therefore usually reserved for refractive procedures in which its effect can be demonstrated first to the patient using contact lenses. Huber's myopic astigmatism is an alternative method that attempts to "solve" presbyopia by deliberately creating a final refraction of, for example, −0·75/ + 0·50 × 090. This level of myopic "with the rule" astigmatism produces two blur foci for near and distant vision so that 6/9 and N6 can be achieved unaided.[47] Despite this, patients often remain dependant on spectacles for some visual tasks.

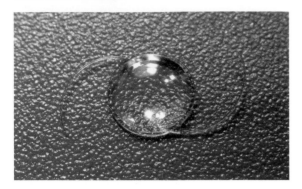

Figure 7.15 Multifocal silicone Array intraocular lens (Allergan).

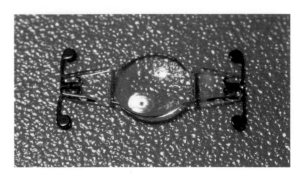

Figure 7.16 Accommodative silicone model AT-45 hinged plate intraocular lens (C&C Vision).

Two types of multifocal lens implants have been designed to overcome presbyopia: diffractive and refractive. The diffractive type achieves multifocality with a modified phase plate that creates constructive interference, directing light rays to near or far foci. As a result most diffractive IOLs are bifocal with no intermediate foci, and a percentage of light is unfocused or lost by destructive interference. This causes a loss of contrast sensitivity, and glare may be a problem. The refractive IOL uses a change in optical refractive power in different areas of the optic to create a range of foci, directing light for distant, intermediate, and near vision. The refractive Array® lens, (Allergan) has a foldable silicone optic that can be inserted through a small incision (Figure 7.15). Good results for both unaided distance and near vision have been reported with this lens.[48] Although there may be some loss of low level contrast sensitivity and glare or halos may occur, patient satisfaction is high and their spectacle dependance is low.[48,49] Irrespective of the type of multifocal IOL used, patient selection and refractive outcome are key. To function effectively, accurate biometry to achieve emmetropia is essential and postoperative astigmatism must be minimal (<1·0 D see Chapters 2 and 6).

In an attempt to avoid the optical compromises of multifocal IOLs, attempts have been made to produce lens implants that accommodate. These are designed to move along the visual axis in response to ciliary muscle contraction and pressure changes in the vitreous and anterior chamber. A recent clinical trial of a flexible plate accommodating IOL (Figure 7.16) reported a good range of near, intermediate, and distance acuities in an uncontrolled group of patients.[50] However, as discussed in Chapter 14, the future of accommodating IOL technology perhaps lies in capsular bag refilling, which may more closely mimic the physiological properties of the natural lens.

Viscoelastics

Viscoelastic materials or devices are an integral part of many aspects of cataract surgery. An essential feature is that they behave as a fluid during injection and removal, but in their static state they act as a semisolid within the eye. Viscoelastics are then able to maintain and compartmentalise intraocular space allowing instrumentation, as well as coat and protect structures such as the endothelium.

Molecular components

Viscoelastics are sophisticated biopolymers that are transparent, isotonic, pH balanced, non-toxic and non-inflammatory. Their physical properties are determined by the charge, molecular weight, concentration, and chain length of their molecular components. The most

Table 7.3   Comparison of physical properties of some viscoelastics

Comparison	Cohesive			Dispersive	
	Healon GV*	Provisc†	Healon*	Viscoat‡	Ocucoat‡
Zero shear (or resting) viscosity (mPas)	2 000 000	4 800 000	280 000	41 000	4 000
Content(s) %	Na HA 1·4	Na HA 1·0	Na HA 1·0	Na HA 3·0 CDS 4·0	HPMC 2·0
Molecular weight (Da)	5 000 000	7 900 000	4 000 000	500 000 25 000	86 000

Manufacturers are *Pharmacia Ophthalmology, †Alcon, and ‡Bausch and Lomb. CDS, chondroitin sulphate; Da, daltons; HPMC, hydroxypropylmethyl cellulose; mPas, millipascal-seconds; Na HA, sodium hyaluronate.

common constituents are glycosaminoglycans (GAGs) and hydroxpropylmethyl cellulose (HPMC).

Glycosaminoglycans

GAGs are polysaccharides composed of repeating disaccharide units, each of which is a hexosamine (either galactosamine or glucosamine) that is glycosidically linked to uronic acid or galactose. Unlike those used as viscoelastics, GAGs do not usually occur in vivo as free polymers and are covalently linked to a protein to form a proteoglycan. These occur naturally in many animal connective tissues where they interact with collagen fibrils. Two types of GAG are commonly used as viscoelastic agents:

• Sodium hyaluronate

• Chondroitin sulphate.

Sodium hyaluronate has a high molecular weight and a single negative charge. Hyaluronic acid is found within both the vitreous and aqueous, and the endothelial surface has sites that specifically bind sodium hyaluronate. The sodium hyaluronate found in viscoelastics is either extracted from rooster combs or produced by bacterial fermentation. After surgery it is metabolized in the aqueous, where it has a half-life of approximately 24 hours.

Chondroitin sulphate is similar to sodium hyaluronate but has a sulfphated group and a double negative charge. It is typically derived from shark's fins.

Hydroxypropylmethyl cellulose

Cellulose is a plant-derived structural carbohydrate found in plant cell walls and is not present in animals. It is extracted from wood pulp and modified by the addition of hydroxypropyl and methyl groups to form HPMC. This is a negatively charged molecule that binds to some intraocular tissues. Within the anterior chamber HPMC is not metabolised but is eliminated with the aqueous.

Physical properties

The electrical charge of the molecular components of a viscoelastic primarily affects the type and extent of bonds between other molecules and adjacent intraocular structures. Chain length determines the degree of tangling between molecules and, together with electric charge, it influences cohesion within the material and hence its viscosity. The intraocular behaviour of viscoelastic materials in different circumstances has been used to subdivide them broadly, based on their on cohesiveness, into either highly cohesive or dispersive agents (low cohesiveness; Table 7.3).[51]

Viscosity, elasticity, and pseudoplasticity

Numerous terms are used to describe the properties of viscoelastics. Viscosity is the

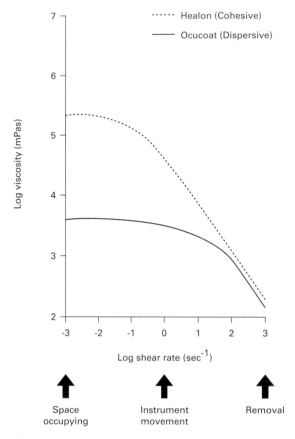

Figure 7.17 Pseudoelasticity curve of cohesive and dispersive viscoelastics compared. (Modified from Arshinoff[51])

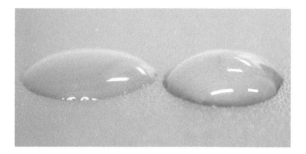

Figure 7.18 Comparison of Coatel (Chauvin Opsia SA), a dispersive viscoelastic (left), and Healon (Pharmacia Ophthalmology), a cohesive viscoelastic (right), both placed on a flat surface (at room temperature).

resistance that a material or fluid has to flow, whereas elasticity is the ability of a material to resume its previous distribution after compression or distortion. The viscosity of a viscoelastic material varies as energy is transmitted to it. This allows it to be injected into the eye and to remain in situ during the instrument movement necessary to perform, for example, capsulorhexis, but permits its removal at the end of the procedure. This change in behaviour is known as pseudoplasticity, which is measured at different shear rates (s⁻¹). Viscosity is measured in mPas (millipascal-seconds), and pseudoplasticity is assessed by comparing the log viscosity with log shear rate (Figure 7.17). Resting or stationary viscosity, which represents the ability of a viscoelastic to occupy a space, is

at zero shear (10^{-3} log s⁻¹). Zero shear viscosity also tends to correspond to the elasticity a material possesses. Mid-shear rates ($10^0 - 10^1$ log s⁻¹) are said to be equivalent to normal instrument movement during surgery, and the viscosity of a material in this state is related to the concentration of its constituent polymer(s). Higher shear rates (10^3 log s⁻¹) are representative of the resistance to flow during injection of viscoelastic into, or aspiration out of, an eye.

Less viscous materials are better at coating surfaces and this is particularly apparent when different viscoelastics are placed on the anterior cornea or a flat surface (Figure 7.18). The stationary or zero shear viscosity of a viscoelastic determines this phenomenon, termed the "contact angle". It is also related to a material's surface tension, where those with a lower surface tension have a lower contact angle.

Cohesive (high viscosity) viscoelastics

Cohesive viscoelastics have a zero shear of greater than 100 000 mPas and typically contain sodium hyaluronate with a high level of non-covalently linked entangled long chains. These substances are highly viscous and effectively create or maintain space, allowing complex surgical maneouvres. Because the material is cohesive and remains localised in one site, it is easily removed by irrigation and aspiration. Unfortunately, the same attribute allows a cohesive viscoelastic to be aspirated during phacoemulsification, potentially reducing endothelial protection.

Dispersive (low viscosity) viscoelastics

Dispersive viscoelastics have lower viscosity, with a zero shear typically of less than 100 000 mPas. Most commonly they are composed of HPMC, which has shorter, less entangled chains and reduced cohesion. This allows the molecules to disperse, coat, and protect tissues such as the endothelium. The negatively charged molecules can bind to these structures and are less easily removed with irrigation. They can therefore be used to partition space during surgery, for example during vitreous loss, when irrigation may disturb a cohesive viscoelastic. A disadvantage is that an interface may form between the viscoelastic and fluid, which can be visually distracting. Also bubbles may become trapped within the material and reduce the view.

Surgical uses

The uses of viscoelastic agents in cataract surgery are summarised in Table 7.4.

Intraocular

The most important of intraocular uses is the protection of the endothelium. During surgery

Table 7.4 Uses of viscoelastic agents in cataract surgery

Site of use	Examples
Intraocular	Coat and protect endothelium Maintain anterior chamber (for example, during capsulorhexis or phaco tip insertion) Open capsular bag for intraocular lens implantation Viscodissection/Viscoexpression Mobilisation of lens fragments Compartmentalisation of surgical field (for example, during vitreous loss)
Extraocular	Coat anterior corneal epithelium to prevent drying and improve anterior segment view To fill dead space within intraocular lens injection devices

several mechanisms may lead to endothelial injury, including direct trauma from instruments, lens fragments, or air bubbles (from the infusion or the phaco probe). Ultrasound energy from phacoemulsification and irrigation fluid turbulence can also damage the endothelium. An ideal viscoelastic therefore coats and protects the endothelium while maintaining space to allow instrumentation. To date no one viscoelastic has demonstrated unequivocal superiority. As discussed, dispersive viscoelastics are thought to protect the endothelium most effectively and are less easily removed from the

Table 7.5 Cohesive and dispersive viscoelastics relative advantages and disadvantages

	Cohesive	Dispersive
Zero shear (mPas)	>100 000	<100 000
Typical content	Sodium hyaluronate	Hydroxypropylmethyl cellulose
Advantages	Create space allowing complex manoeuvres (for example, IOL implantation) High elasticity (for example, fattens anterior capsule, allowing capsulorhexis) Easy to remove (all in one site)	Coats endothelium Used to partition space (for example, during vitreous loss)
Disadvantages	May be aspirated accidentally, with loss of endothelial protection	May form an interface with fluid Resistant to removal Traps air bubbles

mPas, millipascal-seconds; IOL, intraocular lens.

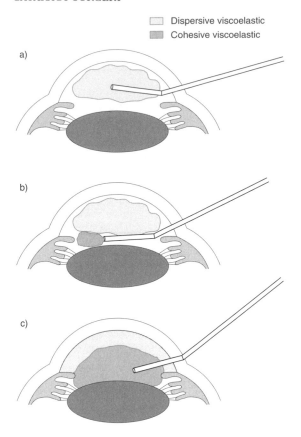

Dispersive viscoelastic
Cohesive viscoelastic

a)

b)

c)

Figure 7.19   The "soft shell" technique. (a) Injection of dispersive viscoelastic. (b) Injection of cohesive viscoelastic beneath the dispersive viscoelastic. (c) Dispersive viscoelastic in close contact with the endothelium and cohesive viscoelastic occupying the central anterior chamber.

eye, but they do not maintain intraocular space well. In contrast, cohesive viscoelastics are excellent at maintaining space, but coat surfaces poorly and can be accidentally removed by aspiration (Table 7.5).

To maximise the benefit of each type of viscoelastic it has been suggested that a dispersive and cohesive agent should used together. In the "soft shell" technique, the dispersive viscoelastic is first injected followed by the cohesive one (Figure 7.19).[52] This second injection take places under the first, ensuring that the dispersive agent is positioned in an even layer over the endothelium. The viscous cohesive agent then fills the anterior chamber and its elastic properties flatten the lens capsule, facilitating capsulorhexis. Although the cohesive viscoelastic may be aspirated during phacoemulsification and cortex aspiration, the dispersive agent is retained and maintains endothelial protection.

Viscoelastics are employed routinely during capsulorhexis and before incision enlargement (if required) and IOL implantation. It may also be helpful to inject additional viscoelastic after completing the rhexis to aid insertion of the phaco hand piece. A further important role for viscoelastics is as a surgical tool in the management of difficult cases or complications. During surgery viscoelastics can be used to mobilise the lens or lens fragments either by viscodissection (i.e. injecting viscoelastic between the lens and the capsule) or by viscoexpression (i.e. moving the lens or lens fragment out of the eye with viscoelastic injected behind them), assuming that the incision is sufficiently large.[53] Alternatively, viscoelastic may be simply placed under a lens fragment to protect the posterior capsule and allow phacoemulsification. Dispersive viscoelastics are most effective at partitioning spaces, particularly when irrigation may disturb a cohesive viscoelastic. This may be relevant, for example, following zonular dialysis where vitreous is present in the anterior chamber. Here a dispersive agent may be used to isolate that area while cortex is aspirated from the rest of the capsular bag. Similarly, if a small posterior capsule tear is identified then viscoelastic can be used to tamponade the vitreous and minimise its movement into the anterior segment.

Extraocular

In addition to their intraocular uses, viscoelastics are commonly used to fill the dead space within foldable IOL injection devices. This prevents injection of air bubbles into the anterior chamber during IOL delivery. The use of high viscosity agents has been implicated in the failure of injection devices and cracking of the injection cannula or cartridge.[54] Although these problems

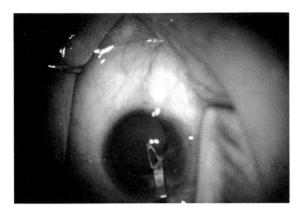

Figure 7.20 Removing viscoelastic by placing the irrigation and aspiration cannula behind the lens optic.

may in fact be related to technique and the design of injection devices, some manufacturers either specify a type of viscoelastic or suggest that balanced salt solution should also be used.[55]

A further extraocular use for low viscosity viscoelastics is on the corneal surface. When placed on the corneal epithelium they reduce corneal drying and smooth corneal surface irregularities. This removes the need to frequently wet the corneal surface with balanced salt solution during surgery and can improve the view of the anterior segment.

Viscoelastic removal

Following lens implantation the viscoelastic is removed from the anterior segment using the same instrument used for cortex aspiration. This reduces postoperative intraocular pressure peaks caused by viscoelastic blocking the trabecular meshwork. Ideally, the viscoelastic should also be removed from behind the IOL optic. This can be achieved by moving the lens optic from side to side, within the capsular bag, using the aspiration hand piece. Alternatively, the tip of the instrument can be placed with care behind the lens optic (Figure 7.20). A second instrument, used to tilt the lens optic, aids this manoeuvre when using a coaxial irrigation and aspiration hand piece. It is easier to use bimanual irrigation and aspiration instruments because the irrigation cannula can then be used to tilt the lens while the relatively narrow diameter aspiration cannula passes behind the optic. If viscoelastic remains behind the optic it may become trapped, causing a form of capsular block, which distends the capsular bag.[56] This can result in a myopic shift of refraction, raised intraocular pressure, or acute angle closure. Although this can usually be treated with Nd:YAG capsulotomy,[57] it can be avoided by thorough removal of the viscoelastic from behind the lens. It may be that this complication is more prevalent with acrylic lens implants that are strongly adherent to the capsule.[58] Careful removal of viscoelastic behind the lens optic may therefore be more important in this group of lens implants.

To some extent the ease of viscoelastic removal depends on whether it has predominately cohesive or dispersive properties. Because cohesive materials tend to remain localised in one site, they are more easily removed by irrigation and aspiration, and in theory this reduces the risk of a postoperative increase in intraocular pressure. In contrast, dispersive agents are difficult to aspirate from the anterior segment, and may therefore be more likely to be associated with a postoperative pressure rise. Although neither animal[59] nor human[60] trials have demonstrated that dispersive viscoelastics are more associated with a rise in intraocular pressure (assuming the majority of the viscoelastic is aspirated), the additional time required to remove these agents could cause endothelial damage.[61] In these circumstances it is preferable to leave some viscoelastic in the anterior chamber after surgery. This is cleared via the trabecular meshwork within 24 hours, but in some individuals it may cause a substantial, albeit transient, rise in intraocular pressure. The use of topical or oral prophylaxis to lower the IOL in the immediate postoperative period should therefore be considered, particularly in patients with compromised optic discs.[62]

References

1 Ridley H. Intraocular acrylic lenses. *Trans Ophthalmol Soc UK* 1952;71:617–21.

2 Kohnen T. The variety of foldable intraocular lens materials. *J Cataract Refract Surg* 1996;22(suppl 2):1255–8.

3 Leaming DV. Practice styles and preferences of ASCRS members: 2000 survey. *J Cataract Refract Surg* 2001;27:948–55.

4 Kulnig W, Skorpik C. Optical resolution of foldable intraocular lenses. *J Cataract Refract Surg* 1990;16:211–6.

5 Knorz MC, Lang A, Hsia TC, Poepel B, Seiberth V, Liesenhoff H. Comparison of the optical and visual quality of polymethyl methacrylate and silicone intraocular lenses. *J Cataract Refract Surg* 1993;19:766–71.

6 Weghaupt H, Menapace R, Wedrich A. Functional vision with hydrogel versus PMMA lens implants. *Graefes Arch Clin Exp Ophthalmol* 1993;231:449–52.

7 Kohnen T, Koch DD. Experimental and clinical evaluation of incision size and shape following forceps and injector implantation of a three-piece high-refractive-index silicone intraocular lens. *Graefes Arch Clin Exp Ophthalmol* 1998;236:922–8.

8 Lee GA. Cracked acrylic intraocular lens requiring explantation. *Aust N Z J Ophthalmol* 1997;25:71–3.

9 Oshika T, Shiokawa Y. Effect of folding on the optical quality of soft acrylic intraocular lenses. *J Cataract Refract Surg* 1996;22(suppl 2):1360–4.

10 Milazzo S, Turut P, Blin H. Alterations to the AcrySof intraocular lens during folding. *J Cataract Refract Surg* 1996;22(suppl 2):1351–4.

11 Hayashi K, Harada M, Hayashi H, Nakao F, Hayashi F. Decentration and tilt of polymethyl methacrylate, silicone, and acrylic soft intraocular lenses. *Ophthalmology* 1997;104:793–8.

12 Ram J, Apple DJ, Peng Q, *et al.* Update on fixation of rigid and foldable posterior chamber intraocular lenses. Part I: elimination of fixation-induced decentration to achieve precise optical correction and visual rehabilitation. *Ophthalmology* 1999;106:883–90.

13 Schneiderman TE, Johnson MW, Smiddy WE, Flynn HW Jr. Bennett SR, Cantrill HL. Surgical management of posteriorly dislocated silicone plate haptic intraocular lenses. *Am J Ophthalmol* 1997;123:629–35.

14 Cumming JS. Surgical complications and visual acuity results in 536 cases of plate haptic silicone lens implantation. *J Cataract Refract Surg* 1993;19:275–7.

15 Haigh PM, Lloyd IC, Lavin MJ. Implantation of foldable intraocular lenses in the presence of anterior capsular tears. *Eye* 1995;9:442–5.

16 Patel CK, Ormonde S, Rosen PH, Bron AJ. Postoperative intraocular lens rotation: a randomized comparison of plate and loop haptic implants. *Ophthalmology* 1999;106:2190–5.

17 Spiegel D. Widmann A. Koll R. Noncorneal astigmatism related to polymethyl methacrylate and plate-haptic silicone intraocular lenses. *J Cataract Refract Surg* 1997;23:1376–9.

18 Shammas HJ. Relaxing the fibrosed capsulorhexis rim to correct induced hyperopia after phacoemulsification. *J Cataract Refract Surg* 1995;21:228–9.

19 Hollick EJ, Spalton DJ, Ursell PG, Pande MV. Lens epithelial cell regression on the posterior capsule with different intraocular lens materials. *Br J Ophthalmol* 1998;82:1182–1188.

20 Samuelson TW, Chu YR, Kreiger RA. Evaluation of giant-cell deposits on foldable intraocular lenses after combined cataract and glaucoma surgery. *J Cataract Refract Surg* 2000;26:817–23.

21 Mullner-Eidenbock A, Amon M, Schauersberger J, *et al.* Cellular reaction on the anterior surface of 4 types of intraocular lenses. *J Cataract Refract Surg* 2001;27:734–40.

22 Kusaka S, Kodama T, Ohashi Y. Condensation of silicone oil on the posterior surface of a silicone intraocular lens during vitrectomy. *Am J Ophthalmol* 1996;121:574–5.

23 Apple DJ, Federman JL, Krolicki TJ, *et al.* Irreversible silicone oil adhesion to silicone intraocular lenses. A clinicopathologic analysis. *Ophthalmology* 1996;103:1555–61.

24 Apple DJ, Isaacs RT, Kent DG, *et al.* Silicone oil adhesion to intraocular lenses: an experimental study comparing various biomaterials. *J Cataract Refract Surg* 1997;23:536–44.

25 Carlson KH, Johnson DW. Cracking of acrylic intraocular leness during capsular bag insertion. *Ophthalmic Surg Lasers* 1995;26:572–3.

26 Dada T, Sharma N, Dada VK. Folding angle critical with hydrogel lens. *Ophthalmic Surg Lasers* 1999;30:244.

27 Shugar JK. Implantation of AcrySof acrylic intraocular lenses. *J Cataract Refract Surg* 1996;22(suppl 2):1355–9.

28 Oh KT, Oh KT. Simplified insertion technique for the SI-26NB intraocular lens. *J Cataract Refract Surg* 1992;18:619–22.

29 Davison JA. Modified insertion technique for the SI-18NB intraocular lens. *J Cataract Refract Surg* 1991;17:849–53.

30 Singh AD, Fang T, Rath R. Cartridge cracks during foldable intraocular lens insertion. *J Cataract Refract Surg* 1998;24:1220–2.

31 Coombes AGA, Sheard R, Gartry DS, Allan BDS. Plate haptic lens injection without prior incision enlargement. *J Cataract Refract Surg* 2001;27:1542–4.

32 Patel CK, Rosen PH. Per-operative malposition of foldable implants (IOL flip). *Eye* 1999;13:255–8.

33 Koo EY, Lindsey PS. Bisecting a foldable acrylic intraocular lens for explantation. *J Cataract Refract Surg* 1996;22(suppl 2):1381–2.

34 Koch HR. Lens bisector for silicone intraocular lens removal. *J Cataract Refract Surg* 1996;22(suppl 2):1379–80.

35 Batlan SJ, Dodick JM. Explantation of a foldable silicone intraocular lens. *Am J Ophthalmol* 1996;122:270–2.

36 Geggel HS. Simplified technique for acrylic intraocular lens explantation. *Ophthalmic Surg Lasers* 2000;31:506–7.

37 Neuhann TH. Intraocular folding of an acrylic lens for explantation through a small incision cataract wound. *J Cataract Refract Surg* 1996;22(suppl 2):1383–6.

38 Thompson CG, Fawzy K, Bryce IG, Noble BA. Implantation of a black diaphragm intraocular lens for traumatic aniridia. *J Cataract Refract Surg* 1999;25:808–13.

39 Reinhard T, Engelhardt S, Sundmacher R. Black diaphragm aniridia intraocular lens for congenital aniridia: long-term follow-up. *J Cataract Refract Surg* 2000;26:375–81.

40 Gayton JL, Sanders VN. Implanting two posterior chamber intraocular lenses in a case of microphthalmos. *J Cataract Refract Surg* 1993;**19**:776–7.

41 Hull CC, Liu CSC, Sciscio A. Image quality in polypseudophakia for extremely short eyes. *Br J Ophthalmol* 1999;**83**:656–63.

42 Shugar JK, Lewis C, Lee A. Implantation of multiple foldable acrylic posterior chamber lenses in the capsular bag for high hyperopia. *J Cataract Refract Surg* 1996;**22**(suppl 2):1368–72.

43 Findl O, Menapace R, Rainer G, Georgopoulos M. Contact zone of piggyback acrylic intraocular lenses. *J Cataract Refract Surg* 1999;**25**:860–2.

44 Gayton JL, Apple DJ, Peng Q, et al. Interlenticular opacification: clinicopathological correlation of a complication of posterior chamber piggyback intraocular lenses. *J Cataract Refract Surg* 2000;**26**:330–6.

45 Shugar JK, Schwartz T. Interpseudophakos Elschnig pearls associated with late hyperopic shift: a complication of piggyback posterior chamber intraocular lens implantation. *J Cataract Refract Surg* 1999;**25**:863–7.

46 Eleftheriadis H, Marcantonio J, Duncan G, Liu C. Interlenticular opacification in piggyback AcrySof intraocular lenses: explanation technique and laboratory investigations. *Br J Ophthalmol* 2001;**85**:830–6.

47 Bradbury JA, Hillman JS, Cassells-Brown A. Optimal postoperative refraction for good unaided near and distance vision with monofocal intraocular lenses. *Br J Ophthalmol* 1992;**76**:300–2.

48 Steinert RF, Aker BL, Trentacost DJ, Smith PJ, Tarantino N. A prospective comparative study of the AMO ARRAY zonal-progressive multifocal silicone intraocular lens and a monofocal intraocular lens. *Ophthalmology* 1999;**106**.1243–55.

49 Javitt JC, Wang F, Trentacost DJ, Rowe M, Tarantino N. Outcomes of cataract extraction with multifocal intraocular lens implantation: functional status and quality of life. *Ophthalmology* 1997;**104**:589–99.

50 Cumming JS, Slade SG, Chayet A. Clinical evaluation of the model AT-45 silicone accommodating intraocular lens: results of feasibility and the initial phase of a Food and Drug Administration clinical trial. *Ophthalmology* 2001;**108**:2005–9.

51 Arshinoff SA. Dispersive and cohesive viscoelastic material in phacoemulsification. *Ophthalmic Pract* 1995;**13**:98–104.

52 Arshinoff SA. Dispersive-cohesive viscoelastic soft shell technique. *J Cataract Refract Surg* 1999;**25**:167–173.

53 Corydon L, Thim K. Continuous circular capsulorhexis and nucleus delivery in planned extracapsular cataract extraction. *J Cataract Refract Surg* 1991;**17**:628–32.

54 Singh AD, Fang T, Rath R. Cartridge cracks during foldable intraocular lens insertion. *J Cataract Refract Surg* 1998;**24**:1220–1222.

55 Dick HB, Schwenn O, Fabian E, Neuhann T, Eisenmann D. Cartridge cracks with different viscoelastics. *J Cataract Refract Surg* 1998;**25**:463–465.

56 Miyake K, Ota I, Ichihashi S, Miyake S, Tanaka Y, Terasaki H. New classification of capsular block syndrome. *J Cataract Refract Surg* 1998;**24**:1230–4.

57 Masket S. Postoperative complications of capsulorhexis. *J Cataract Refract Surg* 1993;**19**:721–4.

58 Oshika T, Nagata T, Ishii Y. Adhesion of lens capsule to intraocular lenses of polymethyl methacrylate, silicone, and acrylic foldable materials: an experimental study. *Br J Ophthalmol* 1998;**82**:549–53.

59 Dua HS, Benedetto DA, Azuara-Blanco A. Protection of corneal endothelium from irrigation damage: a comparison of sodium hyaluronate and hydroxypropylmethylcellulose. *Eye* 2000;**14**:88–92.

60 Henry JC, Olander K. Comparison of the effect of four viscoelastic agents on early postoperative intraocular pressure. *J Cataract Refract Surg* 1996;**22**:960–6.

61 Holzer MP, Tetz MR Auffarth GU, Welt R, Volcker HE. Effect of Healon5 and 4 other viscoelastic substances on intraocular pressure and endothelium after cataract surgery. *J Cataract Refract Surg* 2001;**27**:213–8.

62 Rainer G, Menapace R, Findl O, et al. Intraocular pressure rise after small incision cataract surgery: a randomised intraindividual comparison of two dispersive viscoelastic agents. *Br J Ophthalmol* 2001;**85**:139–42.

8 Non-phacoemulsification cataract surgery

Before the widespread acceptance of extracapsular techniques, the majority of cataract surgery involved removal of the cataractous lens, including its capsule, using the intracapsular technique (Figure 8.1a). Experience of extracapsular cataract extraction (ECCE) had shown that if the posterior lens capsule was preserved then it was likely to become opaque, necessitating further surgery to restore vision. However, correction of the high degree of hypermetropia induced by intracapsular cataract extraction (ICCE) was not entirely satisfactory[1] because of the optical properties of aphakic spectacles and difficulties with contact lens usage in the age group prone to cataract. The development of the intraocular lens (IOL) made it possible to circumvent these problems, but anterior chamber (Figure 8.2) or iris fixated (Figures 8.2b and 8.3) lenses implanted during intracapsular surgery were associated with some ocular morbidity.[2]

Attention then became focused on refining the extracapsular technique to permit more physiological lens implantation in the posterior chamber. At about the same time, the introduction of the neodymium : yttrium aluminium garnet (Nd:YAG) laser permitted outpatient management of posterior capsule opacification. The improved extracapsular technique (Figure 8.1b) permitted cataract surgery to be timed according to patients' visual needs, unlike the intracapsular approach, in which surgery was often deferred until visual loss was marked and the physical properties of the cataract were favourable to cryoextraction. As a consequence, the extracapsular technique became established as the principal means of cataract extraction in the developed world. However, advances in phacoemulsification surgery and then foldable IOL technology have provided more rapid visual rehabilitation and fewer wound related complications. More recently, this has resulted in a shift away from use of the traditional extracapsular technique, which has come to occupy a more circumscribed role. Intracapsular extraction is now usually reserved for unstable subluxed lenses in which neither phacoemulsification or extracapsular surgery is possible. An alternative to ICCE for these cases is lensectomy (Figure 8.1c), in which cataract surgery is combined with pars plana vitrectomy.

Extracapsular cataract extraction

Indications for extracapsular technique

Although phacoemulsification is regarded as the technique of choice for the bulk of cataract surgical procedures, there are nonetheless certain clinical contexts in which the extracapsular approach may be preferred (Table 8.1). These include significant corneal opacity that may preclude safe capsulorhexis or phacoemulsification; marked endothelial cell loss, in which postoperative corneal decompensation

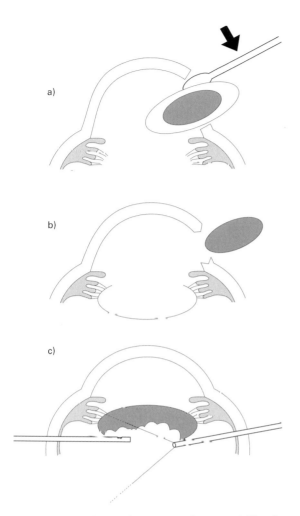

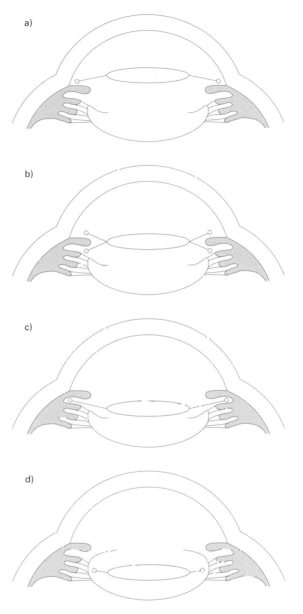

Figure 8.1 The various non-phacoemulsification techniques for cataract extraction. (a) Intracapsular cataract extraction: the entire lens, including the capsule, is removed with a cryoprobe (arrow). (b) Extracapsular cataract extraction: the anterior lens capsule, lens nucleus and cortex are removed, and the posterior lens capsule is left in situ. (c) Lensectomy: during pars plana vitrectomy the lens is removed using either ultrasound (fragmatome) or the vitrector (seen here). Note that the anterior capsule may be partly preserved.

Figure 8.2 Possible locations for an intraocular lens. (a) Anterior chamber. (b) Iris fixated. (c) Sulcus fixated. (d) Capsular bag.

may result; anterior capsular fibrosis preventing capsulorhexis; and white or dark brown lenses, which may be refractory to phacoemulsification. In addition, if capsular complications or corneal decompensation occur during phacoemulsification surgery, then conversion to an extracapsular approach may provide the best means of safely

completing the procedure. For these reasons, the extracapsular technique represents an essential skill for both trainee and trained surgeons.

In addition to these specific clinical indications, there are circumstances in which the extracapsular approach may be used for the

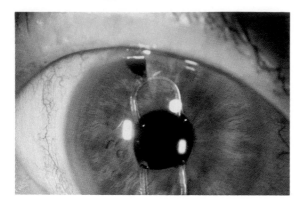

Figure 8.3   Iris clip lens in situ.

Table 8.1   Indications for extracapsular cataract extraction

---

Eyes unfavourable to phacoemulsification:
  Dense white/brown nucleus
  Corneal opacity
  Marked endothelial cell loss
  Anterior capsular fibrosis
Intraoperative complications of phacoemulsification
Phacoemulsification learning curve complications
  unacceptable
Phacoemulsification too expensive
Phacoemulsification logistically impractical

---

majority of cataract surgery. Some surgeons nearing retirement age who have a refined extracapsular technique, may consider the increased potential for surgical complications associated with learning phacoemulsification unjustified.[3] Alternatively, the capital outlay for phacoemulsification equipment or the cost per case of disposable surgical items may exceed resources and prompt the adoption of an extracapsular approach. Finally, in contrast to phacoemulsification, extracapsular surgery can be carried out with simple and portable equipment, requiring little technical support; this is an attractive attribute, especially in the developing world.[4]

Extracapsular technique

The widespread adoption of extracapsular surgery throughout the world is reflected in the diversity of its variations. The following account of the technique therefore emphasises critical phases in the procedure, outlines the approaches that are commonly adopted in each phase, and presents some of the factors that influence the choice of approach, rather than specifying a single technique.

Incision

The incision is made in the cornea, or at the corneoscleral limbus, and is curved to maintain a fixed point of entry into the anterior chamber relative to the iris plane throughout its length. Corneal incisions, being nearer the visual axis, carry a greater risk of astigmatism than do limbal incisions, but the potential for iris trauma may be less. The length of the incision is based on the size of the largest object to pass through it, namely either the nucleus (if large and expressed intact) or the IOL optic (if the nucleus is small or techniques to reduce nuclear size are adopted). Because the wound is curved, its maximum dimension is not its circumferential length but the straight line distance between its ends (i.e. the chord length). The more the wound is extended circumferentially, the less the proportionate increase in chord length, but the greater the potential for wound related complications such as astigmatism (Figure 8.4). It is thus desirable to keep the wound as short as possible. Paradoxically, only a small increase in wound length may permit expression of the nucleus where previously it was not possible. This is because the circumference of the wound aperture increases by up to double the length that the wound is enlarged (Figure 8.5).

The incision is commonly carried out as a two stage procedure. The first is a partial thickness cut in the limbus or cornea along the entire length of the planned incision. At this stage, the eye is firm and this assists accurate wound construction. The small stab incision that follows is sufficiently watertight to help preserve anterior chamber depth during capsulotomy. The second cut, converting the incision to a full thickness wound, is made immediately before

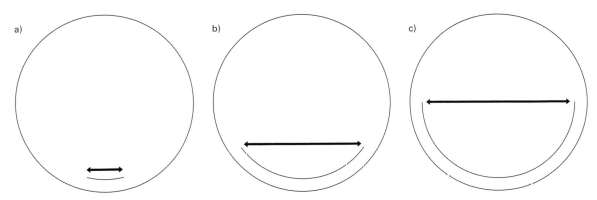

Figure 8.4 The greater the circumferential extension (a–c) of the incision (solid line), the less the proportionate increase in chord length (arrow) and maximum linear wound dimension.

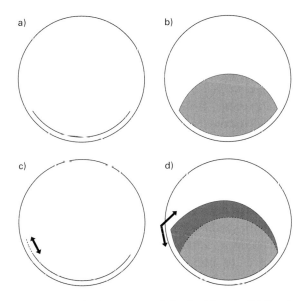

Figure 8.5 Enlargement of the incision (solid line in a) by a given amount (dotted line in c) produces double the increase in wound circumference (b v d).

expression of the nucleus. The resulting incision may be uniplanar, either perpendicular to the cornea (Figure 8.6a) or backward (or reverse) sloping to encourage a watertight seal (Figure 8.6b). Alternatively, the incision may be a biplanar construction, which also improves the accuracy of wound apposition (Figure 8.6c).

Capsulotomy/capsulorhexis

An aperture can be made in the anterior lens capsule by either capsulotomy or capsulorhexis,

commonly using a bent needle. Techniques for capsulorhexis are discussed in Chapter 3. The capsular edge of this type of opening is strong; this property is useful in phacoemulsification surgery, where integrity of the capsular bag is essential for nuclear manipulation and in-the-bag IOL insertion. In extracapsular surgery, however, it may obstruct expression of the nucleus, resulting in delivery of both nucleus and capsule, so-called intracapsular delivery.[5] This creates difficulties in IOL placement and risks vitreous complications. Radial relieving incisions are therefore commonly made in the capsulorhexis edge during extracapsular sugery (Figure 8.7).[6]

Capsulotomy may be performed either using a "can opener" or endocapsular technique. Can opener capsulotomy involves multiple perforations made in a circular pattern in the anterior lens capsule (Figure 8.8a), the centre of which is then torn out (like a car tax disc; Figure 8.8b). This leaves a ragged capsular edge, which presents little resistance to nucleus expression, but may not be sufficient to secure placement of the IOL inside the capsular bag. By contrast, the technique used in endocapsular surgery employs a linear capsulotomy (Figure 8.9), through which the nucleus is expressed, cortex aspirated, and the IOL inserted. Anterior capsulectomy is then performed using either a can opener or capsulorhexis-type approach. The endocapsular

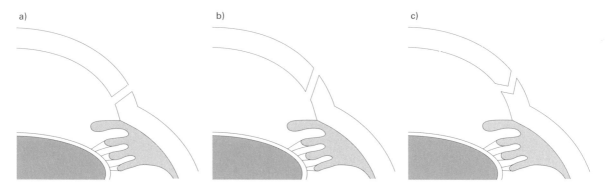

Figure 8.6 Incision profiles. (a) Perpendicular to cornea. (b) Backward (reverse) sloping. (c) Stepped.

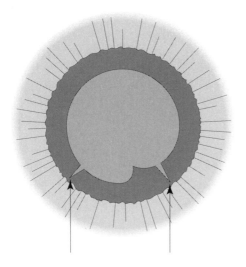

Figure 8.7 Continuous curvilinear capsulorhexis with relieving incisions (arrows) to facilitate nucleus expression and reduce the risk of intracapsular delivery.

technique both protects the corneal endothelium and facilitates placement of the IOL in the capsular bag.

Nucleus manipulation

The separation of the nucleus from lens cortex or capsule may assist its expression. In part, this can be achieved by mechanically dislocating the lens or injecting fluid between capsule and lens (i.e. hydrodissection; see

Chapter 5). At this point the incision may completed and the nucleus expressed. However, given the desirability of minimising the length of the incision, attempts may be made to reduce the size of the lens before expression. The nucleus may be separated from epinucleus by injecting fluid between the two (i.e. hydrodelamination; see Chapter 5) or by mechanical fragmentation of the nucleus (in situ nucleofractis),[7] for example with a wire snare (Figure 8.10) or trisection. Such techniques may permit expression of nuclear fragments through a considerably smaller incision than would be necessary to allow passage of the entire nucleus. Expression is achieved either by application of pressure to the eye, typically behind the completed incision (Figure 8.11a), or by injection of a viscous agent behind the nucleus to expel it under positive pressure (i.e. viscoexpression; Figure 8.11b).

Cortex aspiration

Following successful expression of the nucleus, remnants of cortical lens matter remain. These may be removed by manual or automated systems, both of which simultaneously maintain the anterior chamber by fluid infusion and permit aspiration of soft lens matter. By aspirating under the anterior lens capsule, cortical lens matter is engaged, this is then drawn centripetally and aspirated (see Chapter 5). The process is repeated around the

a)

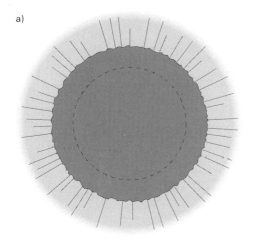

b)

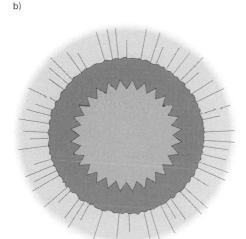

Figure 8.8 "Can opener" capsulotomy. (a) Multiple perforations (dotted circle) are made in the anterior lens capsule with a bent needle. (b) The central portion of the anterior lens capsule is avulsed with a forceps, leaving a serrated edge to the anterior capsular aperture.

circumference of the capsular bag until no lens matter remains. This requires a relatively constant anterior chamber depth, and if this cannot be achieved by appropriate construction of the wound then it may be necessary to insert temporary sutures to appose the wound.

Rigid intraocular lens insertion

To facilitate posterior chamber IOL insertion, the capsular bag and anterior chamber should be inflated with a viscoelastic agent. The incision enables the implantation of a one-piece loop haptic PMMA lens with a large optic diameter (Figure 8.12). It is inserted along its long axis, and once the leading haptic is in place, behind the iris plane and within the capsular bag, the trailing haptic may be rotated (or dialled) into position (Figure 8.2d). Refilling the anterior chamber with viscoelastic may facilitate this. Some lens implants have dial holes drilled into the optic to allow an instrument (for example, a Sinskey hook) to obtain purchase on the IOL; alternatively, the junction of the haptic and optic is engaged. Dialling some polymethylmethacrylate lenses into the capsular bag can be difficult, particularly if there is an intact capsulorhexis. In these cases the trailing haptic may be better placed directly into the bag with forceps and a bimanual technique employed, using a second instrument to apply posterior pressure to the lens optic. It is important to ensure that both haptics are either in the bag or in the sulcus, because if one haptic is in the bag and one in the sulcus then the lens may become decentred.

Wound closure

The wound is closed, commonly with 10/0 monofilament nylon, using either multiple interrupted sutures (Figure 8.13a) or as a single continuous suture (Figure 8.13b). Continuous sutures have the merit that suture tension is distributed evenly along the wound, unlike interrupted sutures, which may differ in tension. There is, however some risk of translational malposition of the wound with continuous sutures, and selective suture removal to counteract astigmatism is not possible (see Chapter 12). Whichever technique is used, knots and suture ends must lie beneath the ocular surface to avoid irritation. This can be achieved by rotating interrupted sutures after they are tied, or by inserting a continuous

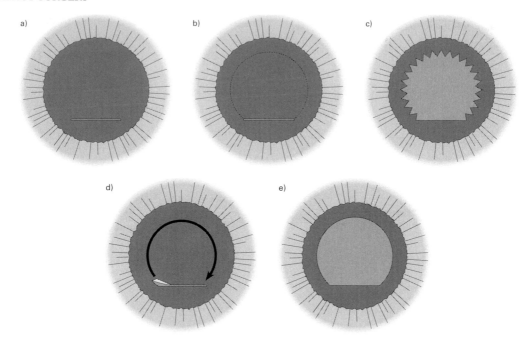

Figure 8.9   Endocapsular capsulotomy. A linear incision (a) is made in the anterior lens capsule with a needle. Through this, nucleus expression, cortex aspiration, and intraocular lens implantation are carried out. The residual anterior capsule may then be removed by can opener (b,c) or capsulorrhexis-type (d,e) technique.

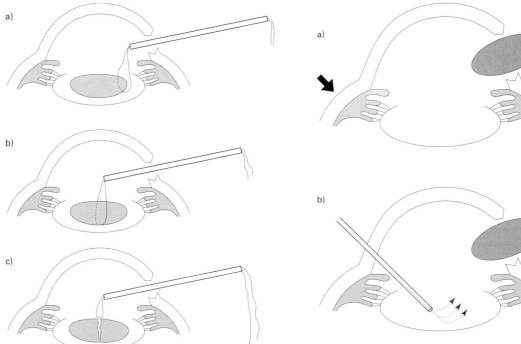

Figure 8.10   In situ mechanical nucleofractis with a wire snare. (a) The snare is introduced into the capsular bag. (b) It is looped around the nucleus. (c) The snare is pulled tight, bisecting the nucleus.

Figure   8.11 Nucleus   delivery.   (a)   Nucleus expression. Delivery is achieved by pressure behind the incision (arrow). (b) Viscoexpression. Delivery is achieved by positive pressure from inferiorly injected viscoelastic agent (dotted arrows).

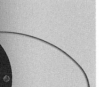

Figure 8.12   Sinskey pattern polymethylmethacrylate posterior chamber lens (Chiron Vision).

Table 8.2   Complications of cataract extraction

	ECCE and ICCE Complications
Incision related ↕ Less incision related	Astigmatism
	Loose suture
	Suture track inflammation
	Suture degradation and breakage
	Wound dehiscence
	Iris prolapse
	Wound leakage
	Suprachoroidal haemorrhage
	Posterior capsule rupture
	Postoperative uveitis
	Endophthalmitis
	Posterior capsule opacification
	Macular oedema
	Retinal detachment

ECCE, extracapsular cataract extraction; ICCE, intracapsular cataract extraction.

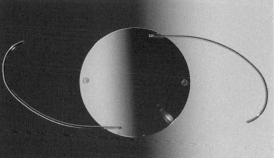

a)

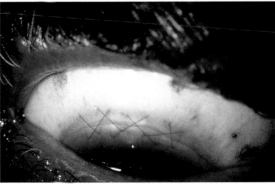

b)

Figure 8.13   Comparison of suture patterns. (a) Interrupted sutures. The sutures have been rotated after tying so that the knots and loose ends lie under the surface. (b) Continuous suture. Suturing starts and ends in the incision so that the knot and suture ends lie beneath the surface.

suture so that the knot is tied within the wound. The viscoelastic agent should be aspirated, because it may produce a postoperative rise in intraocular pressure. The wound is then checked to ensure that it is watertight and additional sutures are inserted as necessary. Finally, antibiotic and steroid may be injected subconjunctivally for prophylaxis against infection and inflammation.

Future developments in extracapsular cataract surgery

Extracapsular surgery is unlikely to be supplanted in the foreseeable future as a means of cataract extraction in eyes in which phacoemulsification would be difficult or has been abandoned because of intraoperative complications. The current shift away from conventional extracapsular surgery toward phacoemulsification is largely driven by the reduced incidence of wound related complications (Table 8.2) and accelerated visual rehabilitation associated with smaller incision size. Techniques such as mechanical nucleofractis, which permit small incision cataract surgery without the need for costly phacoemulsification equipment, are attractive both in the developing world, where financial constraints exist, and in the

Table 8.3 Relative indications and contraindications for lensectomy and intracapsular cataract extraction

	ICCE	Lensectomy
Relative indications	Subluxed unstable hard lens (elderly)	Subluxed unstable soft lens (children/young adults)
	Inadequate resources for ECCE or phacoemulsification	Cataract and need for vitrectomy
		Juvenile idiopathic arthritis
		Proliferative vitreoretinopathy
Relative contraindications	Trauma with capsule rupture	Hard or mature cataract
	Vitreous in anterior chamber	
	High risk of retinal detachment	

ECCE, extracapsular cataract extraction; ICCE, intracapsular cataract extraction.

developed world, where an ageing population places ever-increasing demands on funding for health care.

Intracapsular cataract extraction

Indications for intracapsular technique (Table 8.3)

ICCE, removal of the entire lens and capsule, is commonly employed in the third world, but its disadvantages mean that ECCE with posterior chamber implantation is the preferred technique where resources allow (see Chapter 13).[8] ICCE has the advantage of no posterior capsule opacification, but this precludes capsular or unsutured sulcus IOL placement. Compared with ECCE, there is also a higher risk of vitreous loss and complications such as pupil block glaucoma, cystoid macular oedema, and retinal detachment.[9] ICCE also requires a larger incision and has more potential for wound-related complications (Table 8.2). There is the additional risk of injury to structures such as the cornea or the iris by the cryoprobe.

Where ICCE is not the standard method of cataract extraction, it is usually reserved for hard, subluxed, and unstable cataracts that cannot be removed by either ECCE or phacoemulsification.[10] Lensectomy is an alternative treatment and is preferable in patients with a high risk of retinal detachment, for example those with Marfan's syndrome and high myopia. In children and young adults with

soft unstable lenses, lensectomy is also safer and easier to perform. ICCE should be avoided if the lens capsule has been ruptured or in cases where vitreous is present in the anterior chamber and vitreous traction may occur.

Intracapsular technique

The procedure may be performed under general anaesthesia or local anaesthesia (peribulbar, retrobulbar, or sub-Tenon's). The pupil is dilated preoperatively and a speculum and superior rectus traction suture are inserted. A scleral support ring may be sutured posterior to the limbus in eyes with thin or weak sclera. The principles and considerations of incision construction described in the preceding section on ECCE apply to ICCE (Figures 8.5–8.6), except the wound is longer (12–14 mm or 160–180°). Preplaced 10/0 nylon sutures, inserted before the incision is full thickness, may reduce the risk of translational malposition during wound closure. A 10/0 nylon traction suture, at the mid-point of the anterior wound edge, helps to retract the cornea during lens delivery. A peripheral iridectomy is performed after the incision to prevent pupil block glaucoma and to allow injection of α-chymotrypsin into the posterior chamber. This dissolves the zonules, which should then be irrigated to prevent blockage of the trabecular meshwork. The iris is next dried gently, gently retracted, and the wound opened to allow the cryoprobe access to the anterior lens capsule.

Table 8.4 Choice of intraocular lens (IOL) in eyes without capsular support

	Anterior chamber IOL	Sutured IOL
Relative indications	Old age	Young age
	Patient intolerance of prolonged surgery	Pre-existing glaucoma
Relative contraindications	Risk of corneal decompensation	Ciliary body pathology
	Abnormal angle anatomy	

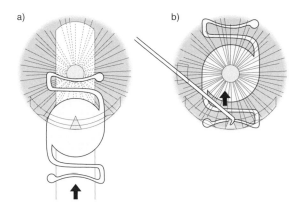

Figure 8.15 Anterior chamber intraocular lens insertion technique. (Note peripheral iridectomy and miosed pupil.) (a) Over a lens glide, the intraocular lens is inserted so that the leading haptic is positioned in the anterior chamber angle. The lens glide is then removed. (b) The trailing haptic is carefully positioned in the subincisional angle. This can be facilitated by using a second instrument through a paracentesis (as shown here).

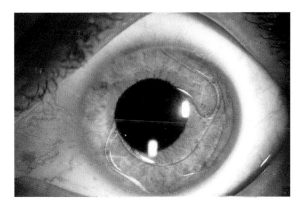

Figure 8.14 An open loop anterior chamber intraocular lens after implantation.

When firmly attached, rotary movement of the probe breaks remaining zonule attachments and the lens can gently be lifted out of the eye. In the event of vitreous loss, an anterior vitrectomy is performed. If an IOL is not to be inserted then the wound is closed in the same manner as an ECCE incision.

Anterior chamber lens insertion

Without capsular support either an anterior chamber lens or posterior chamber sutured IOL may be inserted (Table 8.4). Closed loop anterior chamber IOLs developed a poor reputation, particularly because of corneal endothelial damage and decompensation.[1] Modern open loop anterior chamber IOLs (Figure 8.14) appear to have a lower risk of these complications, and

are less commonly explanted when compared with closed loop lenses.[11] In the absence of glaucoma and with adequate iris support, an open loop anterior chamber IOL may be the lens of choice in an older patient following ICCE.[12] This avoids the risk of vitreous haemorrhage, retinal trauma, and infection associated with sutured lenses (see below).

An anterior chamber lens can usually be successfully inserted without the need for a second procedure.[13] The pupil should first be constricted using acetylcholine (Miochol®; Novartis) and the anterior chamber filled with viscoelastic. A Sheet's glide, placed anterior to the iris, ensures that the IOL does not accidentally enter the posterior chamber or snag peripheral iris (Figure 8.15a). Once the leading haptic is located in the angle, the glide is removed (holding the lens in place). The trailing haptic is then placed into the angle beneath the incision, taking care not to catch the iris. A bimanual technique, using forceps through the main incision and a second instrument through a paracentesis, can facilitate this manoeuvre (Figure 8.18b).

111

Lensectomy

Indications for lensectomy (Table 8.3)

Lensectomy is most frequently performed when cataract surgery is combined with pars plana vitrectomy. It remains the method of choice for removal of cataracts in juvenile idiopathic arthritis related uveitis, in which an anterior or complete vitrectomy is also performed to prevent the development of a cyclitic membrane and hypotony.[15,16] Lensectomy has almost been superseded by phacoemulsification combined with vitrectomy, particularly in other patterns of uveitis. Unlike ECCE, the small phacoemulsification wound is easily closed and is unlikely to leak during vitrectomy, and visualisation of the posterior segment is less often compromised by corneal distortion or pupil miosis. Phacoemulsification, combined with pars plana vitrectomy, allows IOL insertion into the capsular bag and retains the posterior capsule.[16]

However, lensectomy, may be indicated where posterior segment disease exists and placement of an IOL or retention of residual capsule is not desired. This then necessitates either contact lens use or secondary IOL implantation (sutured posterior chamber IOL or an anterior chamber IOL). More typically, lensectomy preserves sufficient capsule to insert a sulcus positioned IOL with lens implantation through a corneal, corneoscleral, or scleral incision at the end of the procedure. Subluxation of the crystalline lens may prevent the use of either an ECCE technique or phacoemulsification. Because ICCE has a high incidence of retinal detachment in patients who are at risk of retinal complications with a subluxed lens, for example those with Marfan's syndrome, lensectomy with vitrectomy is the preferred procedure.[17] Indications for lensectomy also include ocular trauma that necessitates a vitrectomy, particularly in the presence of capsule rupture or a posterior segment intraocular foreign body. In these circumstances, primary IOL implantation is not usually anticipated, particularly because biometry is not likely to be accurate. Lensectomy is also the common form of lens surgery in proliferative vitreoretinopathy, in which the capsule is typically removed and primary IOL implantation avoided.

Lensectomy technique

A standard three-port pars plana approach with an infusion cannula is used. In soft lenses in children and young adults, the vitrector can be used directly to cut and aspirate the lens. In harder lenses, ultrasonic fragmentation is required to emulsify the lens. An MVR blade is used to puncture the lens via the two superior sclerostomies. The fragmatome, set on 10–15% power with up to 300 mmHg suction, is passed through the holes in the capsule and into the lens. If small lens fragments fall posteriorly then these can either be removed with the fragmatome or aspirated using the cutter and then crushed between it and the endoilluminator. The posterior capsule can then be removed using the cutter; although the anterior capsule may be left intact, more usually a central anterior capsulotomy is performed.

The choice and position of lens implant is in part determined by the amount of residual lens capsule available for support. If sufficient capsule support exists, and providing the lens haptic diameter is suitable ($\geq 12\cdot5$ mm), it is possible to insert a sulcus positioned foldable IOL. Although silicone lenses should be avoided in the context of vitrectomy, this allows the patient to benefit from the advantages of small incision surgery. To compensate for the relative anterior position of the IOL when implanting a sulcus placed lens, the optimal posterior chamber IOL power should be reduced by 0·5 dioptres. In the absence of sufficient capsule to support a sulcus placed IOL, either an open loop anterior chamber IOL or a sutured posterior chamber lens can be used. Anterior chamber lenses have the advantages over a sutured lens of simplicity and decreased operating time.[18] However, in young patients or

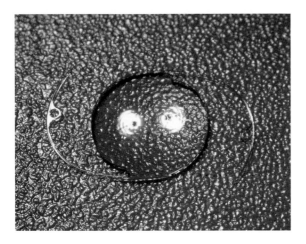

Figure 8.16 Posterior chamber intraocular lens with haptic eyelets to enable attachment of fixation sutures (Alcon).

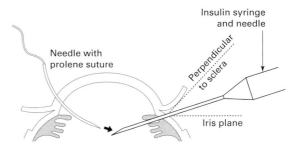

Figure 8.18 Ab externo technique using an insulin syringe to retrieve the prolene suture: the syringe needle is passed into the ciliary sulcus 1·5 mm behind the limbus (at an oblique angle). The prolene suture needle, which has been attached to the intraocular lens, is inserted into the hollow needle. As the insulin needle is withdrawn from the eye, the prolene suture follows.

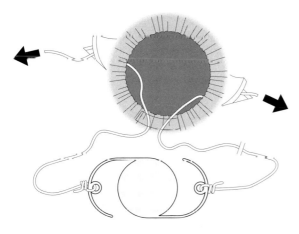

Figure 8.17 An example of a sutured intraocular lens (IOL) technique: two partial thickness scleral flaps are first constructed posterior to the limbus directly opposite each other, followed by an incision for the IOL. Prolene sutures tied to the IOL haptics are then passed through the sclera via the flaps. The IOL is positioned in the sulcus and the sutures tied.

eyes with glaucoma, abnormal angle structures, or insufficient iris support, a posterior chamber lens is preferable.

Sutured intraocular lens

Since the late 1980s, a number of different techniques have been described to fixate an IOL with 10/0 prolene (polyester) sutures placed through the ciliary sulcus.[19–21] Long and straight or curved needles are available for this purpose, and some have a loop of prolene attached, which simplifies tying the suture to the lens. A modified IOL with tying points (eyelets) ensures that the sutures do not slip on the haptic (Figure 8.16). Once tied, the knot may be buried beneath the conjunctiva and Tenon's fascia, but this may erode and is associated with endophthalmitis.[22] To minimise this risk the suture should be buried either beneath a scleral flap or within a groove cut in the sclera. Alternatively, rotating the knot has been described.[21] In most cases the lens is fixed at two points using two triangular partial thickness scleral flaps placed 180° apart, typically at 4 and 10 o'clock (Figure 8.17). It is easiest to construct these flaps before opening the incision for the IOL and reducing the intraocular pressure.

The main variable in technique focuses on whether the suture needle is passed from the ciliary sulcus (ab interno) or from the sclera (ab externo). The latter technique has been advocated as more reproducible and reliable.[20] When the sutures are first tied to the lens an ab interno technique is usually adopted, but an insulin syringe can be placed through the sclera into the sulcus (ab externo) to retrieve the

113

needle from the anterior chamber (Figure 8.18). If a 50% scleral thickness flap is used the needle should be placed through the sclera 1·2 mm behind the surgical limbus, but without a scleral flap the distance is increased to 1·5 mm. The angle of the needle should be neither perpendicular to the sclera nor parallel to the iris plane, but in an oblique direction.[23] This minimises the risk of damage to adjacent sutures reducing, for example, the risk of vitreous haemorrhage. Other complications not already mentioned include iris dialysis, damage to the angle structures with subsequent glaucoma, retinal detachment, and IOL tilt or decentration.[24–26] Despite these risks, good visual results have been reported with sutured lenses in appropriately selected cases.[27]

References

1 Kerr C. Clinical aspects of the correction of aphakia with spectacles. *Trans Ophthalmol Soc UK* 1981; **101**:440–5.

2 Apple DJ, Brems RN, Park RB, Norman DK, *et al.* Anterior chamber lenses. Part I: complications and pathology and a review of designs. *J Cataract Refract Surg* 1987;**13**:157–74.

3 Ah-Fat FG, Sharma MK, Majid MA, Yang YC. Vitreous loss during conversion from conventional extracapsular cataract extraction to phacoemeulsification. *J Cataract Refract Surg* 1998;**24**:801–5.

4 Gillies M, Brian G, La Nauze J, Le Mesurier R, *et al.* Modern surgery for global cataract blindness. *Arch Ophthalmol* 1998;**116**:90–2.

5 Harris DJ Jr, Specht CS. Intracapsular lens delivery during attempted extracapsular cataract extraction. Association with capsulorhexis. Ophthalmology 1991; **98**:623–7.

6 Pande M. Continuous curvilinear (circular) capsulorhexis and planned extracapsular cataract extraction – are they compatible? *Br J Ophthalmol* 1993; 77:152–7.

7 Blumenthal M. Manual ECCE, the present state of the art. *Klin Monatsbl Augenheilkd* 1994;**205**:266–70.

8 Ellwein LB. Kupfer C. Strategic issues in preventing cataract blindness in developing countries. *Bull World Health Organ* 1995;**73**:681–90.

9 Naeser K, Nielsen NE. Retinal detachment following intracapsular and extracapsular cataract extraction. *J Cataract Refract Surgery* 1995;**21**:127–31.

10 Lee SB, Au Eong KG, Yong VS. Management of subluxated crystalline lenses with planned intracapsular cataract extraction and anterior chamber intraocular lens implantation. *Singapore Med J* 1999;**40**:352–5.

11 Lim ES, Apple DJ, Tsai JC, Morgan RC, Wasserman D, Assia EI. An analysis of flexible anterior chamber lenses with special reference to the normalised rate of lens explanation. *Ophthalmology* 1991;**98**:243–6.

12 Hennig A, Johnson GJ, Evans JR, *et al.* Long term clinical outcome of a randomised controlled trial of anterior chamber lenses after high volume intracapsular cataract surgery. *Br J Ophthalmol* 2001;**85**:11–7.

13 Bayramlar HS, Hepsen IF, Cekic O, Gunduz A. Comparison of the results of primary and secondary implantation of flexible open-loop anterior chamber intraocular lens. *Eye* 1998;**12**:826–8.

14 Kanski JJ. Lensectomy for complicated cataract in juvenile chronic iridocyclitis. *Br J Ophthalmol* 1992;**76**: 72–75.

15 Flynn HW Jr, Davis JL, Culbertson WW. Pars plana lensectomy and vitrectomy for complicated cataracts in juvenile rheumatoid arthritis. *Ophthalmology* 1988;**95**: 1114–9.

16 Koenig SB, Mieler WF, Han DP, Abrams GW. Combined phacoemulsification, pars plana vitrectomy, and posterior chamber intraocular lens insertion. *Arch Ophthalmol* 1992;**110**:1101–4.

17 Hubbard AD, Charteris DG, Cooling RJ. Vitreolensectomy in Marfan's sydrome. *Eye* 1998;**3A**: 412–6.

18 Malinowski SM, Mieler WF, Koenig SB, Han DP, Pulido JS. Combined pars plana vitrectomy-lensectomy and open-loop anterior chamber lens implantations. *Ophthalmollogy* 1995;**102**:211–5.

19 Stark WJ, Goodman G, Goodman D, Gottsch J. Posterior chamber intraocular lens implantation in the absence of posterior capsular support. *Ophthalmic Surg* 1988;**19**:240–3.

20 Lewis JS. Ab externo sulcus fixation. *Ophthalmic Surg* 1991;**22**:692–5.

21 Lewis JS. Sulcus fixation without flaps. *Ophthalmology* 1993;**100**:1346–50.

22 Heilskov T, Joondeph BC, Olsen KR, Blankenship GW. Late endophthalmitis after transcleral fixation of a posterior chamber intraocular lens. *Arch Ophthalmol* 1989;**107**:1427.

23 Yasukawa T, Suga K. Akita J, Okamoto N. Sulcus fixation techniques. *J Cataract Refract Surg* 1998;**24**: 840–5.

24 McCluskey P, Harrisberg B. Long-term results using scleral-fixated posterior chamber intraocular lenses. *J Cataract Refract Surg* 1994;**20**:34–9.

25 Solomon K, Gussler JR, Gussler C, Van Meter WS. Incidence and management of complications of transsclerally sutured posterior chamber lenses. *J Cataract Refract Surg* 1993;**19**:488–93.

26 Lee JG. Lee JH, Chung H. Factors contributing to retinal detachment after transscleral fixation of posterior chamber intraocular lenses. *J Cataract Refract Surg* 1998;**24**:697–702.

27 Uthoff D, Teichmann KD. Secondary implanation of scleral-fixated intraocular lenses. *J Cataract Refract Surg* 1998;**24**:945–50.

9 Anaesthesia for cataract surgery

The aim of anaesthesia for cataract surgery should be to make the procedure as safe and as pleasant as possible for all concerned. Advances in anaesthesia and surgery now permit cataract extraction to be performed with minimal physiological upset to the patient. In addition to safety, analgesia, amnesia, anaesthesia, akinesia and amaurosis are all factors to be considered. This chapter outlines the options available (Box 9.1) and the risks and benefits associated with each. It emphasises the advantages of topical local anaesthesia for small incision cataract day surgery, which avoids the complications described for injectional techniques. It also recommends general anaesthesia, with carefully titrated total intravenous anaesthesia with propofol and a laryngeal mask airway, for those cases in which local anaesthesia without sedation is not possible.

Safety

The drive for maximum hospital efficiency has led to over 70% of cataract surgical procedures in the UK being performed under local anaesthesia as day surgery.[1] The very small but real morbidity and mortality associated with both local and general anaesthesia still needs to be recognised.

An obese 66 year old man with ischaemic heart disease died six days after cataract surgery in the coronary care unit. A local anaesthetic had been advised by the anaesthetist, but it appears that the anaesthetist had been persuaded by the surgeon to give a general anaesthetic.

A 68 year old man with known aortic stenosis had a cataract extraction under local anaesthesia and died thirty six hours later.

These two vignettes are the only deaths directly related to cataract surgery out of 19 816 postoperative deaths from all causes studied by the National Confidential Enquiry into Perioperative Death in 1992 and 1993.[2] The cases are mentioned to emphasise that, irrespective of the choice of anaesthesia, care is needed in making that decision. The mortality rate following cataract extraction is unknown, but the rarity of the event suggests that it is a very safe surgical procedure.

Both general and local anaesthesia are not without hazards (Tables 9.1 and 9.2).[3] Given that the average patient undergoing cataract surgery is elderly, it is not surprising that significant

---

Box 9.1 Anaesthesia options for cataract surgery

Local anaesthesia
  Topical
  Sub-Tenon's
  Peribulbar
  Retrobulbar
Local anaesthesia with sedation
General anaesthesia
  Spontaneous/assisted ventilation
  Intubated/laryngeal mask airway
General anaesthesia with local anaesthesia

Table 9.1   Hazards of local anaesthesia

Type of hazard	Examples
Drug related	Overdose
	Intravascular injection
	Allergy
	Vasovagal reaction
	Central nervous system side effects (brainstem anaesthesia/fits)
Technique related	Ecchymosis
	Chemosis
	Toxic keratopathy
	Retrobulbar haemorrhage
	Globe penetration/perforation
	Amaurosis
	Penetration of optic nerve sheath
	Optic nerve damage/atrophy
	Oculocardiac reflex
	Myotoxicity/muscle palsy

Table 9.2   Hazards of general anaesthesia

Type of hazard	Examples (where applicable)
Overdose	
Allergy	
Central nervous system	Depression, amnesia, cerebrovascular accident, awareness, agitation, confusion, disorientation
Cardiovascular	Myocardial ischaemia, myocardial infarction, arrhythmia, oculocardiac and vasovagal reflexes, hypotension, hypertension
Respiratory	Hypoxia, hypercapnia, pulmonary aspiration, barotrauma, oesophageal intubation
Gastrointestinal	Acid reflux, postoperative nausea/vomiting
Urinary	Postoperative urinary retention
Skeletomuscular	Malignant hyperpyrexia, postoperative aches and pains, fatigue
Skin	Damage to lips, teeth, gums, upper airway, extravascular injection
Endocrine	Greater physiological upset
Temperature	Impaired control, postoperative shivering, hypothermia

Table 9.3   Comorbidity in patients undergoing cataract surgery (mean age 75 years)

Percentage	Comorbidity
84%	One or more serious systemic disease
46%	Hypertension
38%	Ischaemic heart disease
18%	Hypothyroidism history
16%	Diabetes mellitus
3%	New malignancy

aortic stenosis. General anaesthesia itself poses particular risks to the patient with morbid obesity (body mass index in excess of 35 kg/m^2) or severe chronic respiratory disease.

Local anaesthesia causes less physiological disturbance to the patient and allows more rapid return to their daily routine. It also generally allows more cases to be scheduled for a given list because the turnaround time between cases is shorter. The increasing move to day surgery also favours local anaesthesia. Most physicians would therefore try to encourage suitable patients to have a local anaesthetic as a day case. Even so, serious complications have been estimated to occur once in 360 cases of local anaesthesia, and life-threatening events once in 750 cases.[3] Thus, the challenge must be to select the right anaesthesia for the patient, the surgeon, and the anaesthetist. This then allows adequate preoperative preparation (Box 9.2).[5]

Provided that patients living alone (even without a telephone) or at a distance from the site of surgery have adequate local support, they need not be excluded from day case surgery under local anaesthesia without sedation.[6] However, all patients should have a friend or relative to accompany them to and from surgery.[5]

Preoperative investigations should only be performed if they are likely to influence the assessment of risks of anaesthesia or surgery; they are not a substitute for an adequate history and examination. Many patients are assessed some time before their surgery, and it is recommended that no more than three months elapse between this assessment and surgery. On

comorbidity may be present (Table 9.3).[4] This includes, for example, occult hypertension, diabetes mellitus, ischaemic heart disease, and

---

Box 9.2 Patient preparation for cataract surgery

- History and examination of cardiac and respiratory systems (particularly orthopnoea)
- Past medical history, in particular previous surgery
- Blood pressure, urinalysis, height / weight ratio
- Allergic history and current medications: continue on the day of surgery (oral anticoagulants or insulin; see text)
- Investigations: none required unless specifically indicated
    - Electrocardiography: if significant cardiac history or examination
    - Chest radiography: if new symptoms or signs since last radiography
    - Haemoglobin: if anaemia suspected
    - Urea and electrolytes: if on diuretics, antihypertensive, or antiarrhythmic treatment, or if diabetic
    - Random blood sugar: if glycosuria present/diabetes suspected (known diabetes – check glycosylated haemoglobin)
- Determine which anaesthetic technique is likely to provide optimal results, subject to confirmation by anaesthetist (see Boxes 9.3 and 9.4)
- Preoperative information for patient and their carer on anaesthesia, surgery, and sequence of events on day of surgery (transport, timing, clothing, etc.)

---

the day of surgery any changes in medical condition or medication must be identified. Starvation is not usually necessary before local anaesthesia for cataract surgery. Patients with diabetes who are to undergo general anaesthesia should generally be placed first on an operating list so as to minimise the starvation period (six hours for food, two hours for liquids). With careful timing, little alteration to their usual treatment is required. Patients on anticoagulants should be reviewed with the aim of having an INR (international normalised ratio for prothrombin) within the therapeutic range on the day of surgery.[5]

Contraindications to local anaesthesia?

It is not possible to undertake microsurgery safely under local anaesthesia unless the patient is adequately prepared and cooperative (Box 9.3). Lack of cooperation may be predictable in infants or be less obvious because of profound deafness, lack of a common language, intellectual impairment, or psychiatric disease. Young adults, especially males, generally tolerate local anaesthesia poorly, and so in the absence of specific risks such patients are probably best dealt with under general anaesthesia.

Box 9.3 Patients who are unsuitable for local anaesthesia techniques

- Patient refusal despite adequate explanation
- Communication barrier or confusion*
- Infants and young adults
- Intractable coughing
- Tremor or abnormal body movements
- Orthopnoea or inability to lie flat
- Claustrophobia
- Uncontrolled anticoagulation
- Previous complication with local anaesthesia
- Previous reaction to local anaesthesia

* Local anaesthesia may still be the procedure of choice.

Cooperation may be unpredictable with claustrophobia, orthopnoea, intractable coughing, and musculoskeletal disorders (for example, rheumatoid arthritis and kyphoscoliosis). None of these may be evident until surgical drapes are applied, the patient has been recumbent for some time, and surgery has commenced. Patients requiring sedation should also be included in this category: these may "surface" unexpectedly and in confusion, and may therefore be less likely to follow instructions, with potentially disastrous results.[7,8]

Anticoagulation is not generally considered to be a contraindication to local techniques, provided that the INR is within the therapeutic range; the risks associated with discontinuing therapy need to be recognised.[9] Those with unstable angina may find that mental stress may exacerbate their symptoms; they may be better served by a careful general anaesthetic combined with topical anaesthesia.

If patients require cataract surgery and are suitable for peribulbar anaesthesia, then they are almost certainly also suitable for topical anaesthesia, provided that appropriate surgical skills are available. Although it makes sense to select "best case" patients when establishing experience with topical anaesthesia, continuing success will rapidly allow the selection criteria to be broadened. Indeed, if a patient is able to tolerate Goldmann applanation tonometry without the surgeon holding the eyelids open, then they are very likely to tolerate small incision cataract surgery under topical anaesthesia.[10]

Contraindications to general anaesthesia

Given the excellence of the local anaesthetic techniques, which are now available to facilitate cataract surgery (Table 9.1), general anaesthesia has increasingly become an expensive second choice, not only in terms of greater morbidity but also in terms of reduced number of cases per operating session and longer waiting lists. General anaesthesia, despite its good safety record, necessarily causes greater physiological trespass. It is associated with more risk of minor and major morbidity, especially if intubation and assisted ventilation are required (Table 9.3). Under these circumstances relative contraindications to general anaesthesia are extensive (Box 9.4). Unfortunately, general anaesthesia is all too often chosen without a full explanation of the risks and benefits of local versus general anaesthesia. The informed anaesthetist, being familiar with the advantages and disadvantages of each technique, will be the

---

Box 9.4 Relative contraindications to general anaesthesia

- Head injury, epilepsy
- Cardiac compromise
- Respiratory compromise
- Hiatus hernia, oesophageal reflux
- Severe musculoskeletal disorders
- Airway compromise
- Morbid obesity
- Diabetes mellitus

---

best guide as to which anaesthetic to use for the individual patient. However, there may be technical aspects of the surgery, such as the anticipated difficulty of the operation, which the ophthalmologist must consider.

Combined sedation with local anaesthesia

Sedation is defined as the use of drug(s) that produce a state of depression of the central nervous system enabling treatment to be performed, but throughout which constant verbal contact with the patient is maintained. As such, sedation necessarily depresses normal physiological reflexes (including upper airway protection) and differs fundamentally from anxiolysis. It may also be linked with amnesia, which may interfere with attempts to provide postoperative instructions, especially following day surgery.

Traditionally, the most popular sedatives have been benzodiazepines, for example, midazolam. These not only produce sedation but also dose dependent respiratory depression, the duration and extent of which is often unpredictable in the elderly. Additionally, impaired hepatic hydroxylation prolongs metabolism in some 5% of the population. Flumazenil is a specific benzodiazepine antagonist, but because its half-life is shorter than most benzodiazepines, late resedation is a real possibility and it cannot be recommended for routine use.

Neurolept anaesthesia is a technique that involves the administration of a sedative such as droperidol or haloperidol with an opioid, for example phenoperidine or fentanyl. A "neurovegetative block" ensues. The unpredictable extent and duration of side effects, as well as the arrival of newer improved techniques, has meant that this method is now seldom practised.

Propofol is a popular potent agent for total intravenous anaesthesia because it produces clear headed awakening following general anaesthesia. It must be used with extra caution in the elderly, in whom marked reductions in blood pressure are common if the dose is not given by infusion and carefully titrated to response. At lower dosage it has become popular among anaesthetists as a supplement to regional or local anaesthetic techniques. Unfortunately, biological variation means that a sedative dose of propofol in one patient may cause loss of consciousness in another.

In summary, the available techniques of sedation lead to an unpredictable depression of consciousness in the individual patient. This may lead to either a sudden awakening of the patient at a critical stage in the proceedings or the inadvertent production of general anaesthesia with an unprotected airway. In either case, the consequences may be disastrous. If a patient cannot tolerate ocular surgery without sedation, then a general anaesthetic is probably safer and more desirable.

General anaesthesia

Advantages of general anaesthesia for cataract surgery include amnesia and analgesia for the patient, while worries about the patient are temporarily removed for the surgeon, with benefits of an immobile eye, unhurried surgery, and freedom of speech. Significant improvements in both anaesthetic drugs and equipment are mentioned below.

- Topical amethocaine or lignocaine/prilocaine for painless intravenous cannulation represents a significant contribution to patient comfort, and is a boon for the 10% of patients who are needle phobic.

- Sevoflurane, a vapour anaesthetic agent, has become the agent of choice for gas induction because of its very rapid onset and offset. It has similar cardiovascular stability to isoflurane, making it ideal for day surgery.

- Propofol anaesthesia helps to minimise postoperative nausea and vomiting, and to maximise early clear headed awakening as compared with traditional thiopentone and inhaled vapour anaesthetics. The addition of small doses of a potent short acting opioid (alfentanil) decreases further the dose of propofol required to maintain general anaesthesia. Target plasma levels of propofol can be selected and achieved by computer controlled infusion devices, which allows rapid adjustments to the depth of anaesthesia.

- Short-acting opioid analgesics, including alfentanil, help to minimise cough reflexes in the spontaneously breathing patient or, in higher dose, obtund the hypertensive response to intubation.

- Short-acting muscle relaxants such as atracurium, vecuronium, and mivacurium have supplanted the older long-acting agents, so minimising postoperative muscle weakness due to residual partial muscle paralysis.

- Parenteral non-steroidal analgesics such as ketorolac help to minimise postoperative discomfort, without causing respiratory depression. They should, however, be used with caution in the elderly, who have reduced renal reserve and may be more prone to their gastrointestinal side effects.

- The reinforced laryngeal mask airway (Figure 9.1) has avoided the need to intubate most patients, so helping to reduce both major and minor morbidity. Insertion and removal of the airway cause less cardiovascular upset than does intubation. Intermittent positive pressure ventilation is possible if a tight seal is present and high inflation pressures are avoided.

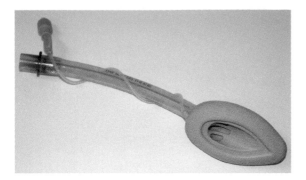

Figure 9.1   Reinforced laryngeal mask airway.

- The universal use of standard monitoring, and the more widespread use of end-tidal carbon dioxide, anaesthetic agent, pressure–volume, and muscle relaxation monitoring have all contributed to the increased safety of general anaesthesia.

When cataract surgery requires general anaesthesia and repeated general anaesthesia represents a risk to the patient, then a solution is simultaneous bilateral cataract extraction.[11] This is a controversial issue,[12,13] principally because of the potential risk of blinding bilateral postoperative endophthalmitis. To minimise risks, it is important that the operation on each eye is completely separate and that the intraocular lenses, intraocular fluids, and viscoelastics are from different batches or manufacturers. The non-disposable instruments should also be from separately sterilised sets.

Which local anaesthetic technique

The debate has traditionally centred on retrobulbar versus peribulbar anaesthesia with or without adjuncts[14] such as hyaluronidase or balloon compression devices. There is no adequate prospective trial to justify the belief that major complications, such as ocular perforation, direct optic nerve damage, and subarachnoid injection of anaesthetic (resulting in respiratory arrest), or "minor" complications

such as bruising and retrobulbar haemorrhage (which can be severe enough to result in optic atrophy) are less common after peribulbar than retrobulbar injections.[15,16] What is clear is that such eye blocks should be performed with short (25 mm) needles, or the needles should not be inserted more than 25 mm. Both techniques run the risk of direct myotoxicity to the extraocular muscles with resultant complex oculomotor disorders, which can be very difficult to manage. The routine use of facial nerve blocks is unnecessary and has largely been abandoned. Ocular compression devices should only be used for short periods at the lowest effective pressure to minimise the risks of high pressures being applied to the globe. Conventional local anaesthetic techniques have the undoubted advantages that they are widely familiar, their complications and limitations are well known (Table 9.2), and because they are often performed by anaesthetists they may reduce the time demands on the surgeon.

More recently, three innovative techniques have been described: subconjunctival anaesthesia,[17,18] sub-Tenon's anaesthesia,[19] and topical anaesthesia.[20–22] The first appears attractive, but subconjunctival haemorrhage and ocular perforation is possible. Although good analgesia ensues,[23,24] the advantages of both the sub-Tenon's (akinesia and amaurosis) and topical technique (ease and absence of needles) are lost.

Sub-Tenon's anaesthesia (Figure 9.2) starts with topical drops of local anaesthesia and a drop of epinephrine (adrenaline) to constrict conjunctival vessels.[19] An incision is then made in the inferonasal conjunctiva and a blunt needle is passed into the posterior Tenon's space, where local anaesthetic agent is delivered intraconally. This innovative technique produces deep anaesthesia, good akinesia, and good amaurosis. The technique is well tolerated as compared with peribulbar injections (Figure 9.3), and should reduce the risk of damage caused by sharp needle techniques. The specially blunted cannula may be difficult to pass behind the globe

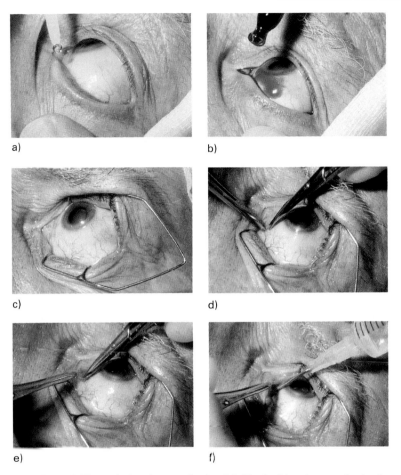

a)

b)

c)

d)

e)

f)

Figure 9.2 Technique for sub-Tenon's local anaesthetic. (a) Topical local anaesthetic drops (g.amethocaine) are administered. (b) 5% povidine drops are administered. (c) The periocular skin and lids are cleaned with povidine and a lid speculum inserted. (d) The conjunctiva and Tenon's fascia is incised approximately 3 mm posterior to the inferonasal limbus. (e) The sub-Tenon's pocket is enlarged. (f) The blunt cannula is inserted into the sub-Tenon's space, advanced, and local anaesthetic injected.

because of Tenon's adhesions, whereas the conjunctival incision may bleed or become infected. Occasionally, the amaurosis may not last as long as the akinesia and a period of marked diplopia may occur as the agent wears off. As yet, neither retrobulbar haemorrhage nor rupture of staphylomatous sclera has been reported. The technique does require somewhat greater skill and patient cooperation than does traditional local anaesthetic eye blocks, and the true place of this technique in small incision cataract surgery is not yet agreed.

Topical anaesthesia for cataract extraction was originally described using cocaine by Koller in 1884.[25] Preservative-free amethocaine or prilocaine 1% topical anaesthesia avoids all of the complications associated with injectional local anaesthetics. Successful topical anaesthesia nevertheless requires considerably more patient education than most surgeons are used to providing. As with any local anaesthetic technique in which the patient is fully awake, it is also sensible to avoid referring to cutting instruments by names that the patient will understand;

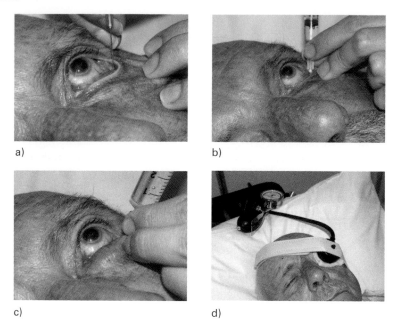

a)   b)

c)   d)

Figure 9.3 Technique for single injection transconjunctival peribulbar local anaesthetic. (a) After local anaesthetic and povidine iodine drops have been administered, the lower lid is retracted and needle (bevel toward the globe) is inserted through the inferotemporal conjunctival below the globe. (b) The needle is inserted directly posteriorly until the hub of the needle is parallel to the cornea (assuming a 25 mm needle is used and the eye has an average axial length). (c) Once the needle tip is posterior to the globe equator, it is then directed posterior to globe where the local anaesthetic injected. (d) A compression device is used to apply pressure to the eye for 5–10 minutes.

euphemisms or technical nomenclature easily overcome this problem. Advantages and limitations of topical anaesthesia are as follows:

- Need for rapport
- Analgesia without total anaesthesia
- No akinesia
- No amaurosis
- No orbicularis anaesthesia.

Pressure, touch and temperature, but not pain, appear to be relatively preserved by surface topical anaesthetics. The analogy with good quality local anaesthesia for dental surgery is useful (i.e. analgesia but not total anaesthesia). Fortunately, it is possible to demonstrate the analgesia to the patient, because the first drop to the superior fornix usually stings and the second

drop two minutes later does not. The first drop can be inserted in the anaesthetic room while an intravenous cannula and monitoring are established. Two drops are usually sufficient; additional drops may reduce corneal clarity.[26] Most patients find it amazing that two drops provide sufficient analgesia for surgery, as indeed do their doctors.

There are three avoidable causes of potential pain during topical anaesthesia:

- Pulling on the iris root
- Sudden increase in intraocular pressure (avoidable by, for example, lowering the bottle height when introducing the phaco tip into the eye)
- Subconjunctival injections (avoided by the use of prophylactic antibiotics in the irrigation fluid or oral antibiotics).

Studies have confirmed that the level of analgesia produced by topical anaesthesia is comparable with that by injectional techniques.[20,27,28] The addition of 0·5 ml intracameral unpreserved lignocaine 1% injected into the anterior chamber at the start of surgery can further minimise intraoperative discomfort.[29] The lack of akinesia makes the technique unsuitable for conventional large incision cataract surgery, but any technique with a 5 mm or smaller incision is suitable. The patient must not forcibly close the contralateral eye, because any Bell's phenomenon will disadvantage the surgeon. However, the ability to ask a patient to deviate the globe in any desired direction is an advantage,[28] removing the need for a superior rectus bridle suture, and may reduce the incidence of postoperative ptosis.

The lack of amaurosis is also both an advantage and disadvantage. Patients need to be reassured that they will not see details of their surgery. The level of microscope illumination can be increased, as the patient becomes accustomed to the bright light. This produces a significant after-image, lasting for up to two hours after surgery, and emphasises the potential danger of excessively bright coaxial illumination. In contrast, the lack of amaurosis assists early visual rehabilitation.[30]

Perioperative monitoring

Routine monitoring for all patients undergoing surgery has led to the recognition that critical incidents (events that did or, if left untreated, could have lead to harm to the patient) are common during both local and general anaesthesia (Table 9.4). In addition to a contemporaneous record of events, all patients undergoing cataract surgery with general anaesthesia should, as a minimum, have continuous electrocardiography, pulse oximetry, regular non-invasive blood pressure measurements, capnography, and vapour analysis.[31] If a sharp needle local anaesthetic technique or sedation in conjunction with local

Table 9.4 Critical incidents (n = 831) reported by the National Confidential Enquiry into Perioperative Deaths 1992–3 (of which 365 were multiple occurrences)[2]

Number	Incident
493	Hypotension (>50% fall from baseline values)
218	Cardiac arrest
150	Arrhythmia
137	Bradycardia (>50% of baseline value)
106	Hypoxia
55	Cyanosis
36	Pulmonary oedema
25	Hypertension (>150% of baseline resting systolic values)
24	Bronchospasm
18	Respiratory arrest
14	Pulmonary aspiration
14	Airway obstruction
12	Pneumothorax
10	Misplaced tube
5	Convulsions
4	Anaphylaxis
3	Wrong drug
2	Air embolism
1	Disconnected breathing tube
1	Hyperpyrexia (due to sepsis)

anaesthesia is used, then similar monitoring is required and intravenous access is essential.[5] Monitoring should always commence before induction of anaesthesia (unless it is not possible to attach a device, for example in an uncooperative child). There is an emerging consensus that where topical anaesthesia alone is applied, pulse oximetry is sufficient, provided that there is trained assistance immediately available. Indeed, monitoring is of little benefit unless those monitoring the patient have the skill and expertise to recognise and treat abnormalities before they become disasters. This person should at least be trained in basic life support.

If the "only" anaesthetic required for phacoemulsification is two drops, then is the presence of an anaesthetist essential? The role of the anaesthetist is to monitor and attend to the wellbeing of the patient; the surgeon's is to concentrate on the surgery. As the patient's "friend in court", the anaesthetist can do much to allay the patient's anxiety before the operation and to assist perioperative cooperation. The anaesthetist can also facilitate optimal surgery by constant monitoring of the patient using clinical signs supported by electrocardiography, blood pressure, oxygen saturation, and nasal end-tidal carbon dioxide measurement. In many cases, supplemental oxygen is useful to minimise claustrophobia and the effects of cardiorespiratory illness. This likewise needs to be monitored. The presence of an anaesthetist within the immediate theatre complex is mandatory, even for topical anaesthesia.

References

1 Desai P, Reidy A, Minassian DC. Profile of patients presenting for cataract surgery in the UK: national data collection. *Br J Ophthalmol* 1999;**83**:893–6.

2 Campling EA, Devlin HB, Hoile RW, Lunn JN. *The report of the National Confidential Enquiry into Perioperative Deaths 1992/1993*. London: NCEPOD, 1995.

3 Rubin AP. Complications of local anaesthesia for ophthalmic surgery. *Br J Anaesth* 1995;**75**:93–6.

4 Fischer SJ, Cunningham RD. The medical profile of cataract patients. *Geriatric Clin N Am* 1985;**1**:339–44.

5 *Local anaesthesia for intraocular surgery*. London: Royal College of Anaesthetists and Royal College of Ophthalmologists, 2001.

6 Lowe KJ, Gregory DA, Jeffery RI, Easty DL. Suitability for day case cataract surgery. *Eye* 1992;**6**:506–9.

7 Huyghe P, Vueghs P. Cataract operation with topical anaesthesia and IV sedation. *Bull Soc Belge Ophthalmol* 1994;**254**:45–7.

8 Edmeades RA. Topical anaesthesia for cataract surgery. *Anaesth Intensive Care* 1995;**23**:123.

9 Hamilton RC. The prevention of complications of regional anaesthesia for ophthalmology. In: Zahl K, Melzer MM, eds. *Ophthalmology clinics of North America. Regional anaesthesia for intraocular surgery*. Philadelphia: WB Saunders, 1990.

10 Fraser SG, Siriwadena D, Jamieson H, Girault J, Bryan SJ. Indicators of patient suitability for topical anesthesia. *J Cataract Refract Surg* 1997;**23**:781–3.

11 *Cataract surgery guidelines*. London: Royal College of Ophthalmologists, 2001.

12 Masket S, ed. Consultation section. *J Cataract Refract Surg* 1997;**23**:1437–41.

13 Responses to consultation section [letters]. *J Cataract Refract Surg* 1998;**24**:430–1.

14 Bjornstrom L, Hansen A, Otland N, Thim K, Corydon L. Peribulbar anaesthesia. A clinical evaluation of two different anaesthetic mixtures. *Acta Ophthalmol* 1994;**72**:712–4.

15 Hamilton RC, Grizzard WS. Complications. In: Gills JP, Hustead RF, Sanders DR, eds. *Ophthalmic anaesthesia*. Thorofare, NJ: Slack Inc, 1993.

16 Davis DB, Mandel MR. Efficacy and complication rate of 16,224 consecutive peribulbar blocks. A prospective mulitcentre study. *J Cataract Refract Surg* 1994;**20**: 327–37.

17 Petersen W, Yanoff M. Why retrobulbar anaesthesia? *Trans Am Ophthalmological Soc* 1990;**88**:136–47.

18 Petersen WC, Yanoff M. Subconjunctival anaesthesia: an alternative to retrobulbar and peribulbar techniques. *Ophthalmic Surg* 1991;**22**:199–201.

19 Stevens JD. A new local anaesthesia technique for cataract surgery by one quadrant sub-Tenon's infiltration. *Br J Ophthalmol* 1992;**76**:670–4.

20 Kershner RM. Topical anaesthesia for small incision self sealing cataract surgery. *J Cataract Refract Surg* 1993;**19**:290–292.

21 Burley JA, Ferguson LS. Patient responses to topical anaesthesia for cataract surgery. *Insight* 1993;**18**:24–8.

22 Shuler JD. Topical anaesthesia in a patient with a history of retrobulbar haemorrhage. *Arch Ophthalmol* 1993;**111**:733.

23 Anderson CJ. Combined topical and subconjunctival anaesthesia in cataract surgery. *Ophthalmic Surg* 1995;**26**:205–8.

24 Anderson CJ. Subconjunctival anaesthesia in cataract surgery. *J Cataract Refract Surg* 1995;**21**:103–5.

25 Koller K. Ueber die verwendung des cocain zur anasthesierung am auge. Wien Med Wochenschr 1884;**43**:1309–11.

26 Seifert HA, Nejam AM, Barron M. Regional anaesthesia of the eye and orbit. *Dermatol clin* 1992;**10**:701–8.

27 Duguid IG, Claoue CM, Thamby-Rajah Y, Allan BD, Dart JK, Steele AD. Topical anaesthesia for phakoemulsification surgery. *Eye* 1995;**9**:456–9.

28 Zehetmayer MD, Radax U, Skorpik C, *et al*. Topical versus peribulbar anaesthesia in clear corneal cataract surgery. *J Cataract Refract Surg* 1996;**22**:480–4.

29 Tseng S-H, Chen FK. A randomized clinical trial of combined topical-intracameral anesthesia in cataract surgery. 1998;**105**:2007–11.

30 Nielsen PJ. Immediate visual capability after cataract surgery: topical versus retrobulbar anaesthesia. *J Cataract Refract Surg* 1995;**21**:302–4.

31 *Recommendations for standards of monitoring during anaesthesia and recovery*. London: Association of Anaesthetists of Great Britain and Ireland, Revised 2000.

10 Cataract surgery in complex eyes

Diabetes

Diabetes is the commonest risk factor for cataract in Western countries. There is a three- to fourfold excess prevalence of cataract in patients with diabetes under 65, and up to twofold in older patients.[1] Cataract is also an important cause of visual loss in patients with diabetes, in some populations being the principal cause of blindness in older onset diabetic persons and the second commonest cause in younger onset diabetic persons.[2] The incidence of cataract surgery reflects this; estimates of the 10-year cumulative incidence of cataract surgery exceed 27% in younger onset diabetic persons aged 45 years or older, and 44% in older onset diabetic persons aged 75 years or older.[3]

The visual outcome of such surgery, however, depends on the severity of retinopathy and may be poor (Figure 10.1).[4] Cataract may prevent recognition or treatment of sight threatening retinopathy before surgery, and after surgery visual acuity may be impaired by severe fibrinous uveitis,[5] capsular opacification,[6] anterior segment neovascularisation,[7] macular oedema,[8] and deterioration of retinopathy.[9] Appropriate management of cataract in patients with diabetes therefore represents a process incorporating meticulous pre- and postoperative monitoring and treatment of retinopathy,

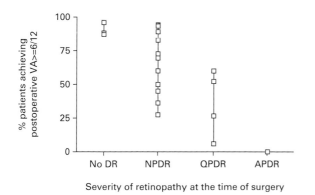

a)

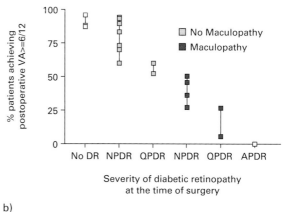

b)

Figure 10.1   Meta-analysis of visual acuity following extracapsular cataract extraction in patients with diabetes. (a) Relationship between preoperative severity of retinopathy and proportion of patients achieving a postoperative visual acuity of 6/12 or better. (b) Effect of maculopathy on relationship between preoperative severity of retinopathy and proportion of patients achieving a postoperative visual acuity of 6/12 or better. APDR, active proliferative diabetic retinopathy; No DR, no diabetic retinopathy; NPDR, non-proliferative diabetic retinopathy; QPDR, quiescent proliferative diabetic retinopathy. Modified from Dowler et al.[4]

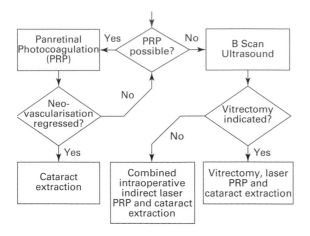

Figure 10.2 Algorithm for the management of proliferative diabetic retinopathy in the presence of cataract.

carefully timed and executed surgery, and measures to preserve postoperative fundus view. Close cooperation between retinal specialist, diabetologist, and cataract surgeon is essential.

Preoperative management

Cataract surgery in eyes with clinically significant macular oedema (CSME)[10] or high risk proliferative retinopathy[11] is associated with poor postoperative visual acuity. The outcome may be better if laser therapy can be applied before surgery.[12] However, even minor cataract may impede clinical recognition of retinal thickening or neovascularisation, and degrade angiographical images. Furthermore, even if sight threatening retinopathy can be diagnosed, lens opacity may obstruct laser therapy. In these cases it may be necessary to use a longer wavelength, for example dye yellow (577 nm) or diode infrared (810 nm), that is better suited to penetrating nuclear cataract than is argon green (514 nm). Panretinal photocoagulation may also be easier to apply with the indirect ophthalmoscope or trans-scleral diode probe. In eyes with proliferative retinopathy and cataract that is sufficiently dense to prevent any preoperative laser, if ultrasound reveals vitreous

haemorrhage or traction macular detachment then a combination of cataract extraction, vitrectomy, and endolaser may be required. By contrast, if ultrasound reveals no indication for vitrectomy then it may be necessary to apply indirect laser panretinal photocoagulation during cataract surgery, because this may reduce the incidence and severity of surgical complications (Figure 10.2).

Indications and timing of surgery

Symptomatic visual loss or disturbance is the major indication for cataract surgery in patients without diabetes. In those with diabetes, however, the need to maintain surveillance of retinopathy, and where necessary to carry out laser treatment, represents an additional indication. The high morbidity and poor postoperative visual acuity described by some authors in association with cataract surgery in patients with diabetes have led to recommendations that surgery in eyes with retinopathy should either be deferred until visual acuity has deteriorated greatly[8] or not be undertaken at all.[13] With this approach, however, cataract may become so dense as to preclude recognition or treatment of sight threatening retinopathy before surgery, and the outcome of surgery may therefore be poor. By contrast, if surgery is undertaken before the cataract reaches the point where diagnosis and treatment of retinopathy are significantly impeded, then it may be possible to maintain uninterrupted control of retinopathy, and the outcome of surgery may thereby be improved. Overall, cataract surgery should be performed early in patients with diabetes.

Surgical technique and intraocular lens implantation

Posterior segment complications are frequently major determinants of visual acuity after cataract extraction in diabetics. Surgical technique and the choice of intraocular lens (IOL) are thus governed by the need to maintain postoperative fundus visualisation. Rigid, large optic diameter polymethylmethacrylate (PMMA) lenses permit peripheral retinal visualisation, which may be valuable if panretinal photocoagulation or vitreoretinal surgery is required. They also allow wide posterior capsulotomy early in the postoperative course; this is important in eyes with more severe retinopathy, in which the risk of retinopathy progression[11] and capsular opacification is greatest.[6] They tend, however, to accumulate surface deposits,[14] and require a large incision, which may delay refractive stabilisation and exacerbate postoperative inflammation. Foldable silicone lenses can be implanted through a small incision, but plate haptic designs may not be sufficiently stable to permit early capsulotomy, and the incidence of anterior capsular aperture contracture (capsulophimosis) appears high.[15] All silicone lenses have the disadvantage that if vitrectomy surgery is required then fundus visualisation may be compromised by droplet adherence, temporarily during fluid–gas exchange[16] or more permanently by silicone oil.[17] Square edged acrylic lenses, which may also be implanted through a small incision, appear stable, show less adherence of silicone oil,[18] and in patients without diabetes they have a reduced tendency to contraction of the anterior capsular aperture[15] and opacification of the posterior capsule.[19]

Extracapsular cataract surgery using "can opener" capsulotomy eliminates the risk of anterior capsular aperture contraction, but the tissue damage associated with a large incision and nucleus expression may further exacerbate the tendency in diabetic eyes to severe postoperative inflammation. A randomised paired eye comparison of phacoemulsification with foldable silicone lens versus extracapsular surgery with 7 mm PMMA lens was conducted in patients with diabetes.[20] It identified a higher incidence of capsular opacification and early postoperative inflammation in eyes undergoing extracapsular surgery, and slightly worse postoperative visual acuity. No significant difference was identified between techniques in respect of

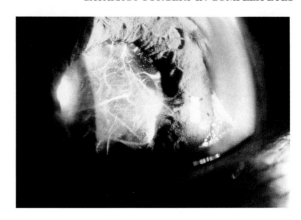

Figure 10.3 Fibrinous uveitis complicating cataract surgery in a patient with active proliferative diabetic retinopathy.

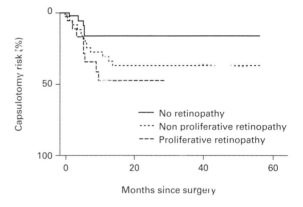

Figure 10.4 Relationship between capsulotomy risk over time and retinopathy severity in patients with diabetes undergoing extracapsular cataract surgery.

incidence of CSME, requirement for macular laser therapy, severity or progression of retinopathy, or requirement for panretinal photocoagulation.

Postoperative management

Anterior segment complications

Eyes of patients with diabetes appear especially susceptible to severe fibrinous uveitis after cataract surgery (Figure 10.3).[5] Iris vascular permeability is increased in proportion to retinopathy severity, and cataract surgery may permit larger proteins such as fibrinogen to enter

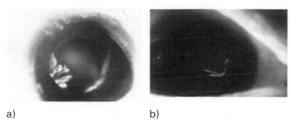

a)   b)

Figure 10.5 Anterior segment fluorescein angiogram of anterior hyaloidal fibrovascular proliferation after cataract surgery. (a) Before and (b) after panretinal photocoagulation.

the anterior chamber. Fibrin membranes may form on the IOL, anterior hyaloid face, posterior capsule, or across the pupil, giving rise to pseudophakic pupil block glaucoma. Capsular opacification may be commoner in diabetic persons, its incidence appearing to correlate with severity of retinopathy (Figure 10.4).[6] Neovascularisation derived from the anterior segment may encroach over the iris (rubeosis iridis), the anterior surface of the posterior lens capsule (rubeosis capsulare[21]) or, more rarely, new vessels derived from the posterior segment may arborise over the posterior surface of the posterior lens capsule (anterior hyaloidal fibrovascular proliferation;[7] Figure 10.5). These complications may result from the action of soluble retina derived factors, such as vasoactive endothelial growth factor. These leave the eye through the trabecular meshwork, but en route they may stimulate neovascularisation, cellular proliferation of the posterior capsule, and increased iris vascular permeability.

Postoperative uveitis may require intensive therapy with topical or periocular steroid, non-steroidal anti-inflammatory agents, atropine, and tissue plasminogen activator (TPA) if fibrin is prominent. Capsular opacification requires examination with retroillumination to exclude anterior hyaloidal fibrovascular proliferation, and as early and as wide a capsulotomy as is consistent with IOL stability, because marginal cellular proliferation may subsequently

compromise fundus visualisation. Neovascular complications mandate urgent panretinal photocoagulation because both anterior and posterior segment neovascularisation may progress extremely rapidly, and secondary neovascular glaucoma is commonly refractory to treatment. If anterior hyaloidal fibrovascular proliferation is present, then associated capsular opacification may preclude panretinal photocoagulation, and capsulotomy in this context may precipitate haemorrhage. Direct closure of anterior hyaloidal vessels with argon laser may permit safe capsulotomy and panretinal photocoagulation.

Posterior segment complications

Macular oedema is a common cause of poor visual acuity after cataract surgery in diabetics.[8] It may represent diabetic macular oedema that was present at the time of surgery (but unrecognised or untreated because of the presence of cataract or diabetic) or macular oedema that was precipitated or exacerbated by cataract surgery. Alternatively, it may be the typically self-limiting Irvine–Gass type macular oedema, which occurs in a proportion of both diabetic and non-diabetic persons after cataract surgery. This presents a therapeutic conundrum, because laser therapy that is appropriate to diabetic macular oedema present at the time of surgery or developing afterward is inappropriate to Irvine–Gass macular oedema, in which spontaneous resolution may be anticipated. In recent studies,[10] no patient with CSME during the immediate postoperative period showed spontaneous resolution of oedema over the subsequent year, and thus it would seem reasonable to consider treatment in such patients. By contrast CSME developing within six months of surgery resolved within six months of surgery in half of the eyes affected, and by one year in three quarters. Spontaneous resolution was commoner in eyes with less severe retinopathy at the time of surgery and in eyes showing angiographical improvement by six months. In such eyes a conservative approach seems justified. It is important to recognise that the presence of optic disc hyperfluorescence in eyes with postoperative macular oedema does not necessarily imply that spontaneous resolution will occur.[10] In addition, postoperative fluorescein leakage arising from diabetic microvascular abnormalities may resolve spontaneously.[10]

Progression of retinopathy after cataract surgery is best documented by paired eye comparisons; one such study showed progression of non-proliferative retinopathy in 74% of operated eyes and 37% of unoperated fellow eyes.[9] Deterioration appears particularly common in eyes with severe non-proliferative or proliferative retinopathy at the time of surgery, and preoperative or intraoperative panretinal photocoagulation may be considered. If high risk proliferative retinopathy develops after surgery, then panretinal photocoagulation should be applied as soon as possible because progression of retinopathy may be rapid. However, this may prove difficult because of photophobia, therapeutic contact lens intolerance, poor mydriasis, IOL deposits and edge effects, capsulophimosis, or capsular opacification. If high risk proliferative retinopathy and CSME develop after surgery it seems appropriate to apply both macular and panretinal laser because the latter carries the risk of exacerbating macular oedema. Close postoperative surveillance of the retina is essential in all patients with diabetic retinopathy undergoing cataract surgery, and close cooperation between retinal specialist and cataract surgeon should be encouraged in order to optimise management of macular oedema and visual outcome.

Visual outcome

A meta-analysis carried out in 1995 demonstrated a direct relationship between the severity of diabetic retinopathy at the time of extracapsular cataract surgery and postoperative visual acuity, and an association between poor visual outcome and the presence of maculopathy (Figure 10.1).[4] In that study, between 0 and 80% of eyes with diabetic retinopathy achieved a postoperative visual acuity of 6/12 or more. More than 80% of patients in recent studies,[20,22,23] however, have achieved postoperative visual acuity of 6/12 or better. A number of possible factors may account for this improvement, including earlier intervention since the advent of phacoemulsification, recognition of the importance of glycaemic control, and careful preoperative and postoperative management of retinopathy.

Future developments

Much information about cataract surgery in diabetics has yet to be gathered. The optimal timing of surgery, the ideal surgical technique, the most appropriate IOL, the role of glycaemic and blood pressure control in postoperative deterioration of retinopathy, and the optimal management of postoperative macular oedema remain uncertain. Significant research effort is currently devoted to the elucidation of these issues. These efforts must, however, be accompanied by more widespread recognition of the need to offer patients with diabetes undergoing cataract surgery the pre- and postoperative care that is appropriate to their condition, rather than that afforded to the bulk of patients with age-related cataract, whose need is much less. Only through an appreciation of the unique problems of cataract surgery in can diabetics good results be obtained.

Uveitis related cataract

The development of cataract in eyes with uveitis is common and may occur as a result of both the inflammatory process and its treatment with topical, periocular, or systemic corticosteroids. Uveitis primarily affects young adults with high visual requirements who in the past may have been advised against surgical intervention until the cataract was considerably advanced because of the significant risk of complications. Although these risks have not been abolished, advances in surgical technique, better control of inflammation, careful patient selection, and meticulous perioperative management have significantly improved the outcome of surgery for uveitis related cataracts during the past 20 years.

Preoperative management

The rationale of prophylactic systemic steroid therapy is to minimise the risks of rebound inflammation in the posterior segment during the immediate postoperative period, and to optimise the outcome of surgery with minimum visual and systemic morbidity.

Eyes with acute recurrent episodes of inflammation confined to the anterior segment and with no history of macular oedema do not, as a rule, require prophylactic systemic steroids. However, patients of Asian ethnic origin with chronic anterior uveitis are at risk of postoperative macular oedema even when this has not previously been detected.[24,25] Steroid prophylaxis is not required for cataract surgery in patients with Fuchs' heterochromic cyclitis[26] unless macular oedema has previously been recognised, and preferably confirmed by fluorescein angiography. When there has been a panuveitis or documented posterior segment involvement, steroid prophylaxis is indicated for cataract and posterior segment surgery (Table 10.1). Patients already receiving systemic steroids and/or immunosuppressive therapy such as cyclosporin will usually need to increase their steroid dose before surgery because maintenance systemic treatment is normally kept to the minimum required to control inflammation.[27]

Prophylactic steroid therapy is commenced between one to two weeks before surgery at a dose of 0·5 mg/kg per day prednisolone (or equivalent for other steroid preparations, for example prednisone or methylprednisolone).[27] This dose is maintained for approximately

Table 10.1   Systemic steroid prophylaxis for uveitis related cataract surgery

Pattern of uveitis	Previous macular oedema or posterior segment disease	Steroid prophylaxis
Acute anterior uveitis, recurrent	No	None
Chronic anterior uveitis	No	Yes
Fuchs' heterochromic cyclitis	No	None
Intermediate uveitis	Yes	Yes
Posterior uveitis or panuveitis	Yes	Yes

one week after surgery and then tapered according to clinical progress. A reduction of 5 mg prednisolone per week is usually possible. Intravenous steroid administration at the time of surgery has been used as an alternative to oral steroids, employing a dose of 500–1000 mg methylprednisolone. This is delivered by slow intravenous infusion, and can be repeated if necessary during the immediate postoperative period. The major risk from intravenous steroid infusion is acute cardiovascular collapse, and caution should be exercised in older patients or if there is a history of cardiac disease. Periocular depot steroid (triamcinolone or methylprednisolone) injection may be given at the time of surgery, but is best avoided if there is a history of raised intraocular pressure or documented pressure response to steroids. The introduction of slow release intravitreal steroid devices[28] may in future offer the prospect of intraocular surgery in uveitic eyes without systemic steroid prophylaxis or postoperative therapy.

Indications and timing of surgery

The most common indication for surgery is visual rehabilitation. In eyes with sufficient lens opacity to preclude an adequate view of the posterior segment, cataract surgery may prove necessary to allow monitoring or treatment of underlying inflammation. Phacolytic glaucoma and lens induced uveitis are less common indications for lens extraction in eyes with established uveitis.

It is a generally accepted maxim that elective cataract surgery in eyes with uveitis should only be performed when the inflammation is in complete remission.[27,29,30] In the ideal situation there should be no signs of inflammatory activity, and this is particularly appropriate for those patterns of uveitis that are characterised by well defined acute episodes, for example HLA-B27 associated acute anterior uveitis. When the intraocular inflammation is of a more chronic and persistent pattern, for example in juvenile idiopathic arthritis (previously know as juvenile chronic arthritis) associated uveitis, complete abolition of intraocular inflammation may only be achievable through profound immunosuppression.[31] This poses significant risks for the patient, and may not be absolutely necessary for a successful surgical outcome.[32,33] The use of prophylactic corticosteroid therapy to suppress intraocular inflammation is widely endorsed, although the optimum regimen regarding dose, duration, and route of administration has not been universally defined. The absolute period of disease remission or suppression before elective surgery is a matter of debate among surgeons, but a minimum of three months of quiescence has broad acceptance. The timing of surgical intervention will also depend on individual patient factors, including the level of vision in the other eye, coexisting systemic inflammatory or other disorders, and social factors, for example the educational needs of a child or young adult.

Surgical technique and intraocular lens selection

Phacoemulsification

Although there is a paucity of reliable data confirming that phacoemulsification has a lesser propensity to exacerbate inflammation in uveitic eyes, this is generally perceived to be the case

and is supported by studies in non-inflamed eyes.[34] Phacoemulsification has the advantage of a smaller wound with minimal or no conjunctival trauma, the latter being particularly important if glaucoma filtration surgery must subsequently be undertaken. A clear corneal tunnel has been shown to cause less intraocular inflammation than a sclerocorneal tunnel in eyes without uveitis.[35] In addition, a wide variety of foldable IOL implants manufactured from different materials are now available that may have specific advantages in eyes with uveitis (see below). Except in the most severely bound down pupil, it is usually possible to enlarge the pupil sufficiently to perform an adequate capsulorhexis, which is the most critical element during this type of surgery in uveitic eyes. Fibrosis of the anterior capsule with subsequent constriction (capsulophimosis or capsular contraction syndrome[36,37]) occurs more commonly in eyes with uveitis, and the risk of this developing can be avoided by performing a generous capsulorhexis either at the time of the primary capsulorhexis or by enlarging the capsulorhexis after lens implantation.

Extracapsular cataract extraction

Extracapsular cataract extraction (ECCE) remains an important surgical method, particularly where phacoemulsification facilities are less readily available and uveitis is common, for example in the developing world. Although the extracapsular approach offers good access to the pupil, refinements in the surgical techniques for managing small pupils during phacoemulsification have reduced the need to use extracapsular surgery solely for this reason. The larger wound is more likely to cause problems, particularly during combined procedures, for example aqueous leak when combined with pars plana vitrectomy. This is also associated with more induced astigmatism, and the slower rate of visual recovery[27] as compared with that after phacoemulsification is frustrating for patients.

Lensectomy

Lensectomy is most frequently performed when cataract surgery is combined with pars plana vitrectomy.[29] It remains the method of choice for removal of cataracts in juvenile idiopathic arthritis related uveitis, in which an anterior or complete vitrectomy is also performed to prevent the development of a cyclitic membrane and subsequent hypotony.[32,33] However, phacoemulsification and IOL implantation is an alternative in these patients if the pupil is mobile.

Lensectomy has almost been superseded by phacoemulsification when vitrectomy and cataract surgery are combined in other patterns of uveitis. Following phacoemulsification, a deep anterior chamber can easily be maintained during vitrectomy, and retention of the capsular bag allows insertion of a posterior chamber lens implant at the end of the procedure if indicated.[38] Lensectomy does retain the anterior capsule, which can support a sulcus placed lens implant, either as a primary or secondary procedure.

Management of small pupils

Careful management of the small pupil is the key to success in uveitis cataract and vitreoretinal surgery. Management of pupils that do not dilate or dilate poorly is dealt with below.

Lens materials

Although there have been exciting developments in IOL technology, the ideal material for lens implants in eyes with uveitis has not yet been identified. Small cellular deposits and giant cells can be observed on the IOL implant surface in normal eyes after cataract surgery,[39] and these changes are more marked in uveitic eyes.[40] Heparin surface modification of PMMA lenses reduces the number and extent of these deposits but does not completely prevent their formation.[26,39] Acrylic and hydrogel lens implants are associated with fewer surface deposits than are unmodified PMMA lenses,

and these materials are flexible, which allows the lens to be foldable. The tendency of foldable silicone lenses to develop surface deposits depends on whether they are first or second generation silicone. The surface of all types of lens implants can be damaged during folding or by rough handling during insertion.[41] Rauz et al.[42] noted scratch marks on 40% of lens implants (predominantly hydrophobic and hydrophilic acrylic lenses) in a study of uveitis related cataract, but did not comment on whether these implants were more likely to develop cell deposits. Overall, they found no significant difference in lens performance between acrylic and silicone lens implants.

Patients undergoing surgery for uveitis related cataract are commonly pre-presbyopic, and may have normal vision in the other normally accommodating eye. These patients may therefore be considered for a multifocal lens implant (see Chapter 7). Lens cellular deposits are more likely to occur in eyes in which there is continuing inflammatory activity, for example in chronic anterior uveitis or Fuchs' heterochromic cyclitis (Figure 10.6). The deposits can be "polished" off the lens surface by low energy yttrium aluminium garnet (YAG) laser, although care must be exercised to avoid pitting the surface, which may promote further cellular deposition.

Posterior capsule opacification (PCO) is more common in uveitic eyes primarily because of the younger age of patients,[43,44] and this tendency may be exacerbated by some lens materials and designs. Acrylic lenses appear to have the lowest propensity to cause PCO, in comparison with PMMA and hydrogel lenses. PCO is, however, related not only to the material from the lens is manufactured but also to the design of the lens and the degree of contact between the optic and the posterior capsule.

There is no conclusive evidence that the type of material used for the IOL implant has any influence on the development of macular oedema. A recent comparative study[45] of acrylic

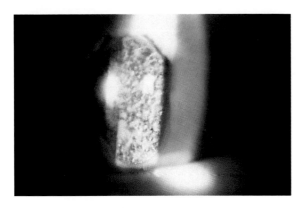

Figure 10.6 Extensive cellular deposits on a polymethylmethacrylate intraocular lens implant.

and silicone lens implants in combined cataract and glaucoma surgery in non-uveitic eyes demonstrated higher intraocular pressure, particularly in the immediate postoperative period, in the acrylic lens group. It is important, therefore, that the surgeon remains vigilant for potential problems when using newer lens materials in "at risk" eyes.

Postoperative management

Uveitis patients should be reviewed on the first postoperative day and again within one week of surgery to identify early any excessive inflammation that may not be apparent on the first day.

Anterior uveitis should be treated with topical steroid (for example betamethasone, dexamethasone, prednisolone acetate, rimexolone, loteprednol) given with sufficient frequency to control anterior chamber activity. The spectrum of activity will vary considerably between patients, typically being minimal in Fuchs' heterochromic cyclitis and greatest in eyes that have required the most iris manipulation. In uncomplicated procedures, four to six times daily administration during the first week will usually suffice, but following complex anterior segment surgery topical steroid drops should be administered every one to two hours, and adjusted according to clinical progress. Topical

non-steroidal anti-inflammatory agents (for example, indomethacin, ketorolac, flurbiprofen) can also be administered postoperatively. Severe postoperative anterior uveitis is associated with an increased risk of macular oedema and should be managed intensively.[24]

The necessity for and frequency of mydriatic agents depends on preoperative pupillary mobility and intraoperative iris manipulation. In Fuchs' heterochromic cyclitis eyes mydriatics are rarely required but should be used when synechiolysis, iris stretching, or iris surgery has been undertaken. It is important to ensure that the pupillary margin and anterior capsule margin are not closely apposed because synechiae may rapidly develop and cause acute iris bombé. For this reason, it is advisable to avoid pupillary stasis by using short acting mydriatics such as cyclopentolate 1% once or twice daily, or to use an additional agent such as phenylephrine 2·5% once daily.

Fibrin deposition in the anterior chamber, especially within the visual axis (Figure 10.7), is an indication for more intensive topical steroid therapy, mydriatics, and lysis with recombinant TPA, for example alteplase. This can be injected via a paracentesis and should be performed at an early stage, well before cellular invasion of the membrane occurs. Periocular depot steroid (triamcinolone or methylprednisolone) can also be administered unless the intraocular pressure is or has been elevated.

The presence of a hypopyon in the immediate postoperative period may be due to severe inflammation or endophthalmitis. It is prudent to manage these eyes as suspected endophthalmitis, and to give intravitreal antibiotics (vancomycin 1–2 mg and ceftazidime 1 mg or amikacin 400 µg) after obtaining aqueous and vitreous samples for microscopy, culture, and polymerase chain reaction.

Macular oedema may develop despite or in the absence of steroid prophylaxis, and should be confirmed by fluorescein angiography. If prophylaxis has not been used, then combined

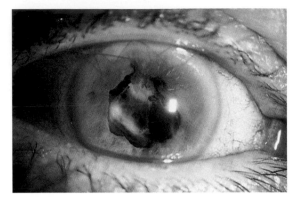

Figure 10.7 Postoperative fibrin deposits on intraocular lens implant surface following extracapsular cataract and pupil surgery.

Table 10.2 Ocular comorbidity influencing visual outcome

Ocular region	Pathology	Clinical disease example
Macula	Macular oedema	Pars planitis, intermediate uveitis
	Macula ischaemia	Behçet's disease
	Subfoveal choroidal neovascularisation	PIC, POHS, birdshot choroidoretinopathy
	Macular scar	Toxoplasmosis
	Full thickness macula hole	Older patients
	Epiretinal membrane	Toxoplasmosis
Optic nerve	Optic nerve ischaemia	Behçet's disease
	Papillitis	Sarcoidosis
	Optic neuritis	Multiple sclerosis
	Glaucoma	Sympathetic ophthalmia
Cornea	Band keratopathy	JIA associated uveitis

JIA, juvenile idiopathic arthropathy; PIC, punctate inner choroidopathy; POHS, presumed ocular histoplasmosis syndrome.

treatment with a topical steroid (dexamethasone, prednisolone acetate, or betamethasone), a non-steroidal anti-inflammatory drug (ketorolac, flurbiprofen, or indomethacin), and periocular (sub-Tenon's or orbital floor injection) depot steroid (methylprednisolone or triamcinolone) should be initiated. If there is no clinical or angiographical response in three to four weeks, then systemic steroids should be added in a dose of 0·5 mg/kg per day. If the patient is already receiving systemic steroids, then the dose should be increased to 1 mg/kg per day and titrated according to clinical response. In rare occasions, additional therapy with cyclosporin or other immunosuppressive agents may be required.

Postoperative visual acuity

The majority of patients undergoing surgery for uveitis related cataract obtain significant visual improvement. Macular and optic nerve comorbidity are the major vision limiting factors (Table 10.2) but most series of mixed patterns of uveitis report that 80–90% of eyes achieve a visual acuity of 6/12 or better.[24,30,42,46] It is important to advise uveitis patients considering cataract surgery of the increased risk of postoperative inflammation and to indicate a realistic expectation of outcome, particularly in those with known posterior segment involvement.

Small pupils

The pupil may fail to dilate after long-term miotic treatment for glaucoma, in conditions such as pseudoexfoliation, or following trauma. Posterior synechiae may prevent mydriasis in patients with uveitis and may also be present in patients who have previously undergone trabeculectomy. The management of a small pupil can present a surgical challenge, particularly because they often coexist with other ocular features that increase the difficulty of cataract surgery.

Preoperative management

Patients whose pupils do not dilate well should, if possible, be identified as part of their first consultation when dilated fundus examination takes place. This allows adequate surgical planning and ensures that the surgeon has adequate experience. Short acting mydriatic agents, given before surgery, are usually effective in dilating the pupils in the majority of patients. In the elderly, there is potential for cardiovascular side effects with topical phenylepherine, in most circumstances 2·5% phenylepherine is as effective as 10%,[47] although with dark or poorly dilating irides 10% may be useful.[48]

Topical non-steroidal anti-inflammatory drugs, given before cataract surgery, have no mydriatic properties but reduce intraoperative miosis. Diclofenac sodium and flurbiprofen are thought to be equally effective in maintaining intraoperative mydriasis,[49] but ketorolac appears better than fluribiprofen.[50] Avoiding intraoperative iris trauma my prevent pupil constriction during cataract surgery and intraocular irrigation with epinephrine (adrenaline) 1 : 1 000 000 (1 ml of 1 : 1000 epinephrine in 1000 ml of irrigation solution) is a safe and effective means of maintaining mydriasis.[51,52]

Surgical technique

Releasing posterior synechiae and injecting viscoelastic into the anterior chamber may be all that is required to enlarge the pupil. An excessively large pupillary aperture is not always required, and successful cataract surgery can be undertaken through a 4–5 mm pupil by an experienced surgeon.[53] Stripping of fibrous bands around the pupil margin with fine forceps (for example, capsulorhexis forceps) may also allow sufficient enlargement of the pupil to give access to the lens. If this is insufficient and stretching of the iris sphincter does not result in an adequate pupillary aperture, then iris retractors or a pupil expanding device should be used.

Pupil stretch

When stretching the pupil[54] (stretch pupilloplasty) two instruments (for example, Kruglen hooks) are typically used to engage the iris margin at separate points 180° apart (Figure 10.8). Using a simultaneous bimanual movement the pupil is stretched toward the limbus. This may be repeated in different directions,[55] although a single stretch may be sufficient. Devices are available that perform the same function but simultaneously stretch the iris in more than one direction, for example the Beehler pupil dilator. The pupil stretch

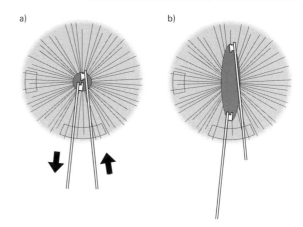

Figure 10.8 Pupil stretch technique. (a) The pupil margin is engaged with a pair of Kruglen hooks. (b) The pupil is stretched towards the limbus.

technique is quick and simple to perform but may not always be successful and does not prevent subsequent intraoperative pupil constriction. It may also result in an atonic pupil, particularly if the failure to dilate was due to previous inflammation or trauma.

Iris hooks

A variety of ingenious devices are now available to enlarge and then maintain the pupil size during cataract surgery. These range from self-retaining iris hooks to devices placed within the pupil, such at the implantable grooved rings decribed by Graether.[56] First described for use during vitrectomy,[57] flexible iris hooks are typically made of polypropylene with a hook at one end and an adjustable rubber or silicone retaining sleeve (Figure 10.9), although others are made of wire. In addition to retracting the iris during cataract surgery,[58] iris hooks can be used to support and protect the capsulorhexis margin, which is at greater risk in small pupil surgery or if zonular dehiscence occurs.[59] The use of multiple iris hooks to control iridoschisis during cataract surgery has also been described.[60]

Iris hooks are inserted through paracenteses made perpendicularly at the limbus (Figure 10.10). It is important to avoid placing the iris

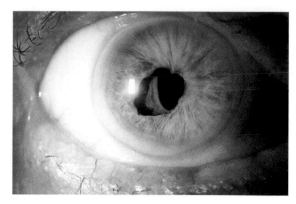

Figure 10.11 Inferotemporal iris tear following the use of self-retaining iris hooks for phacoemulsification in chronic anterior uveitis.

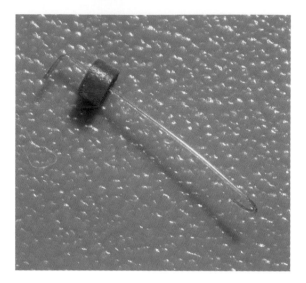

Figure 10.9 A typical nylon iris hook (Synergetic Inc.).

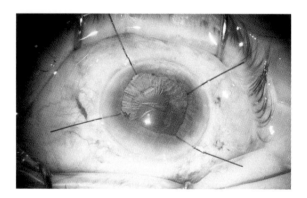

Figure 10.10 Iris hooks in use. Note the square pupil and limbal placement.

hooks anteriorly because the iris becomes "tented" forward and this may impede the insertion of instruments into the eye or lead to iris damage. Usually four iris hooks are used, placed 90° apart around the limbus, which when in position form a square pupil. It is important not to stretch the pupil excessively with the retractors because radial tears of the iris may occur (Figure 10.11), especially if fibrosis involves a sector of the pupil. This is of particular relevance to patients with rubeosis or those at risk of bleeding (for example, anticoagulation or

chronic uveitis).[61] Gradually enlarging the pupil may reduce the risk of iris trauma. Pupillary function is more likely to be impaired where the pupil has been stretched beyond 5 mm.[61,62] If the hooks are not placed accurately around the limbus, then a non-square pupil results that has an increased circumference without increasing the pupil area.[63] This may be avoided by using a 90° limbus marking instrument. Alternatively, by using a fifth hook to form a pentagon shape, the pupil circumference can be decreased while maximising the pupil area.[63]

Iris spincterotomies

If iris retractors or pupil expanders are not available, then multiple small spincterotomies (Figure 10.12) can be performed with capsule or retinal scissors, the latter having the advantage of allowing access through a side port incision during phacoemulsification. Multiple partial spincterotomies may also be combined with pupil stretching.[64] Large sphincterotomies cause an atonic or irregular shaped pupil and, if phacoemulsification is planned, the mobile tags of iris can be aspirated and traumatised by the phaco needle. Where extracapsular or intracapsular lens extraction is planned, a single large superior radial iridotomy allows excellent access to the lens. Subsequently, the iris can be sutured with Prolene to improve cosmesis and reduce the visual

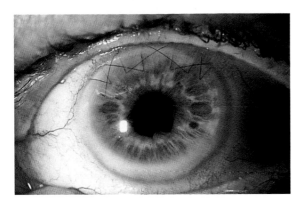

Figure 10.12 Extracapsular cataract surgery with multiple small inferior sphincterotomies.

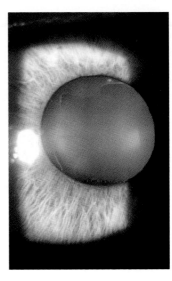

Figure 10.14 Pseudoexfoliation syndrome.

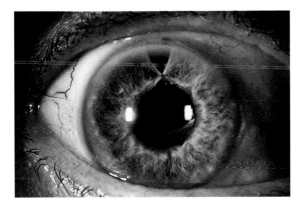

Figure 10.13 Endocapsular cataract surgery with sutured superior radial iridotomy and inferior sphincterotomies.

problems associated with a large and irregular pupil (Figure 10.13). During lensectomy, the vitreous cutter can be used to enlarge the pupil if iris retractors are not available, although care should be taken to avoid removing iris tissue.

Postoperative management

It is important to minimise iatrogenic trauma to the iris as much as possible because this disrupts the blood–aqueous barrier, and bleeding from the iris leads to the deposition of fibrin at the pupil and on the lens implant. This increases the risk of synechiae formation

to the edge of the anterior capsule and pupillary membrane development. Any patient who undergoes iris manipulation of the iris for a small pupil is likely to require increased topical steroids after surgery and should be kept under close review. Postoperative fibrin deposition in the anterior chamber is best treated by injection of recombinant TPA (5–25 µg in 100 µl), in combination with mydriatics and intensive topical steroids. Injections of recombinant TPA can be repeated if fibrin deposition recurs.

Subluxed lenses and abnormal zonules

A number of ocular conditions, such as high myopia, pseudoexfoliation (Figure 10.14), Marfan's syndrome, and Ehlers–Danlos syndrome (Figure 10.15), have weak or fragile zonules that may coexist with cataract and require surgery. Zonule disruption may also follow pars plana vitrectomy or ocular trauma. In many of these conditions glaucoma can be present and surgery may be complicated by poor pupil dilatation, zonule dehiscence, capsule rupture, and vitreous loss. Lens subluxation can

137

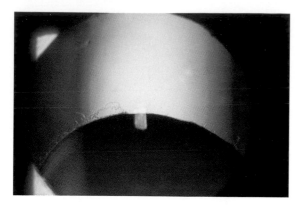

Figure 10.15 Lens subluxation in a patient with Ehlers–Danlos syndrome.

Table 10.3 Phacoemulsification and unstable zonules: troubleshooting

Objective	Actions
Avoid posterior pressure on the lens	Do not overfill the anterior chamber with viscoelastic Lower infusion rate (reduce bag/bottle height) Stabilise lens with a second instrument Use sufficient phaco power to avoid lens movement
Use tangential forces	Initiate and propagate the capsule tear avoiding radial forces Use chopping techniques rather than divide and conquer Commence aspiration of cortex in area of least zonule instability (strip cortex toward area of zonule)
Stabilise the capsular bag	Capsular tension ring ± suture in ciliary sulcus Iris hooks to support the capsular rhexis
Careful hydrodissection	Multiple sites Low hydrostatic force Decompress injected fluid with gentle posterior lens pressure

cause myopia and astigmatism that is impossible to correct optically, and clear lens extraction may be indicated. Surgery in these circumstances is challenging and selection of technique depends on the extent of lens instability. IOL choice and site of implantation is also important, particularly because decentration or subluxation may occur postoperatively.

Preoperative management

Before routine cataract surgery, a past history of ocular trauma, surgery, or conditions that predispose to zonule disruption should always be sought. In patients who have sustained trauma, problems such as glaucoma, retinal injury, and inflammation may restrict the visual prognosis irrespective of the technical success of cataract surgery. Preoperative examination of the anterior segment should include assessment for features of pseudoexfoliation and signs such as phacodonesis and iridonesis. If the lens is particularly unstable then it may move with posture and, although located in the anatomical position at a slit lamp, it may fall posteriorly when supine. Such patients should be examined sitting and lying.

Surgical technique and intraocular lens implantation

Surgical technique depends on lens stability. With limited zonule loss phacoemulsification (or

ECCE) can be performed. If the lens is very unstable, then surgery may cause additional zonule damage and risks dislocation of the lens into the vitreous. In these circumstances either intracapsular cataract extraction (ICCE) or lensectomy may be required.

Phacoemulsification

Phacoemulsifcation can often be performed safely in the presence of an unstable lens with modifications in technique that help support the lens and reduce further zonule damage (Table 10.3). During capsulorhexis, overfilling the anterior chamber with viscoelastic should be avoided because it may cause excessive posterior pressure on the lens. Similarly, infusion pressure (bottle or bag height) should be reduced. Radial forces on the capsular bag should be avoided, particularly in the region of zonular weakness. During initiation of the rhexis, and propagation of the tearing flap, only tangential forces should be applied to the anterior capsule. A small rhexis may make phacoemulsification difficult and

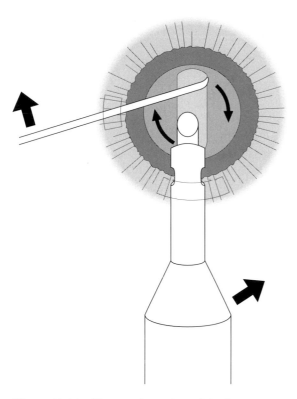

Figure 10.16   Bimanual rotation of the lens.

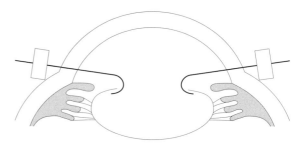

Figure 10.17   Iris hooks supporting the capsulorhexis and the capsular bag in an eye with unstable zonules.

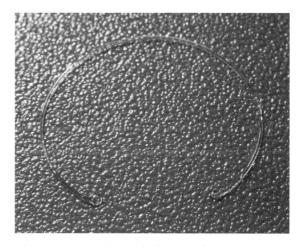

Figure 10.18   A typical capsule tension ring (Morcher).

predispose to postoperative anterior capsule contraction. However, the rhexis can be enlarged if required following IOL insertion.

During hydrodissection, only gentle hydrostatic pressure should be applied to the lens and over-inflation of the capsular bag avoided. This may be achieved by hydrodissecting at multiple sites and using gentle posterior pressure on the lens to decompress injected fluid. The same factors apply during hydrodelamination. As always, it is useful to confirm that the nucleus and lens rotate with ease before commencing phaco. Rotating the lens with a bimanual technique, for example using both the phaco probe and a second instrument, minimises stress on the zonules (Figure 10.16).

Once the rhexis is completed, the capsule and lens complex may be stabilised with iris hooks.[65] These are inserted through the limbus in the same manner as is described for small

pupils, but are placed under the rhexis edge (Figure 10.17). The site of zonule loss and extent of lens instability determine the position and number of hooks used. Four hooks placed at 90° intervals can create a tenting effect that supports the entire unstable bag. During phacoemulsification, force directed posteriorly must be reduced and sufficient ultrasound power used to prevent the needle tip moving the lens. Engaging the lens with a second instrument may help to stabilise and limit its movement while sculpting. During nucleus disassembly a technique that minimises capsular bag distortion is preferred, and chopping has been advocated as safest.[66]

Capsule tension rings are open PMMA rings that are placed into the capsular bag and transfer

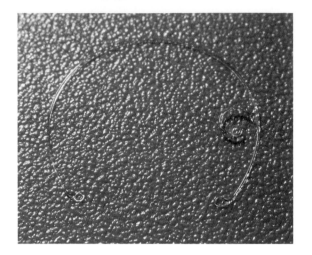

Figure 10.19 A modified capsule ring with arm and eyelet for ciliary sulcus suturing (Morcher).

support from areas of normal to abnormal zonule integrity (Figure 10.18). In eyes with zonule damage or weakness, they may be useful during phacoemulsification, cortical aspiration, and before IOL implantation. They may be inserted if a dialysis is noted during surgery or at any stage depending on the extent of lens instability.[67] In soft cataracts the ring may be inserted directly following capsulorhexis but hydrodissection makes this manoeuvre easier, particularly in harder lenses. Capsule tension ring insertion may be simplified by using an injection instrument, alternatively, inserting the ring through the second instrument paracentesis aids control. When the zonule is severely unstable or if a capsule tear is suspected, then a 10/0 nylon suture may be temporarily tied to one of its eyelets. This enables the ring to be removed if required and, by placing the suture on the leading eyelet, it may also be used to prevent it from snagging the equatorial capsule as it is inserted. In cases of severe or progressive zonule loss a capsule ring alone may be insufficient to maintain the capsular bag, leading to postoperative IOL decentration or pseudophacodonesis. Using a trans-scleral suture to secure the ring in a manner similar to that used when fixating a sutured IOL can provide additional support.[68] This requires passing a suture through the capsule, and in order to avoid the risk of tearing it may be performed as secondary procedure,[69] after capsule scarring has occurred. Rings have been designed that have a side arm or arms with anchor points that project outside the capsular bag to allow suturing without capsule perforation (Figure 10.19).[70]

Cortex aspiration risks zonule damage and needs to proceed with caution. It should commence in areas of normal zonule support and initially avoid areas of dialysis. Stripping of aspirated cortex should employ tangential rather that radial movements, and where possible it should be directed toward the areas of weakness. A capsular tension ring may trap cortical matter in the equatorial capsular bag and make it difficult to aspirate. This is reduced if thorough hydrodissection has preceded ring insertion. Inserting the IOL into the capsular bag before cortical removal may also help to reduce zonule damage but similarly may trap cortical material.

Extracapsular cataract extraction

Expression extracapsular techniques, with preservation of the capsule for either IOL insertion in the bag or sulcus fixation have been largely superceded by phacoemulsifcation. In patients with pseudoexfoliation phacoemulsification is thought to have a lower risk of posterior capsule rupture and vitreous loss.[71] To minimise zonule stress during nucleus expression, the incision should be large enough to accommodate the lens easily. Also, thorough hydrodissection and delamination loosens the lens from the capsular bag. Zonule rupture usually becomes apparent after nucleus expression and typically involves the capsular bag opposite the incision. A lens glide can be used to push the involved capsule back toward the ciliary sulcus and provide sufficient support to allow cortical aspiration and in the bag IOL implantation.[72]

Intracapsular cataract extraction

Intracapsular cryoextraction of dislocated and partially dislocated lenses has a high reported incidence of vitreous loss, haemorrhage, and retinal detachment.[73] However, in hard severely unstable lenses, in which lensectomy may be difficult, ICCE may be the treatment of choice. Even in severe zonule weakness α-chymotrypsin should be injected to ensure that the lens is removed easily. The use of a lens glide and anterior chamber maintainer may allow intracapsular lens extraction through a smaller incision.[74]

Lensectomy

Several studies have shown that subluxed lenses in children can be successfully treated by lensectomy.[75,76] Where lens instability prevents phaco or ECCE, and ICCE carries a increased risk of retinal detachment, lensectomy is procedure of choice, particularly if the cataract is soft.[77]

Lens implantation

Retention of the capsular bag helps to support a posterior chamber lens implant and may allow in the bag foldable lens implantation. Because of the risk of capsule contraction, an IOL with rigid haptic material and larger overall diameter is ideal. Plate haptic implants should be avoided. The use of a capsular ring or rings may reduce the risk of capsule contraction, which is particularly prevalent in eyes with pseudoexfoliation.[78,79] If the capsule has been retained but zonule integrity is in doubt, then the IOL can be placed in the ciliary sulcus. Lensectomy may also provide sufficient capsular support for a sulcus placed lens, but following ICCE the options for lens implantation are either anterior chamber placement or an IOL sutured into the ciliary sulcus. In the past anterior chamber lenses gained a poor reputation because of their association with complications such as late corneal decompensation. More recent open loop designs have a much lower risk

profile and, as compared with sutured lenses, are simple and easy to implant. In younger patients and those with established glaucoma, an IOL sutured into the ciliary sulcus may be preferable to an angle supported anterior chamber lens. The techniques of anterior chamber IOL implantation and sutured IOL fixation in the context of both ICCE and lensectomy are discussed in Chapter 8.

Postoperative management

Zonule weakness may be progressive and, despite an initially stable IOL, lens decentration or pseudophacodonesis may cause visual symptoms. In some cases pupil constriction with a miotic such as pilocarpine may reduce problems, particularly those that occur at night. Surgical options include lens repositioning or explantation (see Chapter 7). An alternative is to fixate the haptic of a tilted lens[80] or the capsular tension ring if one was used,[69] by attaching it to the ciliary sulcus with a trans-scleral 10/0 prolene suture. Capsule contraction may account for some IOL decentration, and this may be associated with capsulophimosis. If this affects visual acuity then a neodymium (Nd):YAG anterior capsulotomy may be required.[81]

Eyes with pseudoexfoliation syndrome have a higher risk of blood–aqueous barrier breakdown and postoperative inflammation. They are also at higher risk of corneal decompensation and raised intraocular pressure, which should be monitored in the early postoperative period.

Vitrectomised eyes

Cataract is a frequent complication of pars plana vitrectomy, occurring in up to 80% of patients with diabetes[82] and almost invariably in eyes in which silicone oil tamponade has been used.[83] Following pars plana vitrectomy, a number of problems often coexist that make cataract surgery challenging. Pupil dilatation may be poor, particularly in the presence of posterior synechiae, and zonule damage may result in capsular bag instability and an increased risk of vitreous loss. The lack of anterior hyaloid may cause increased lens–iris diaphragm mobility and altered intraocular fluid dynamics, similar to that found in high myopes.[84]

Phacoemulsification, extracapsular and intracapsular surgery, and lensectomy have all been described in the management of cataract in vitrectomised eyes.

Preoperative management

Before cataract extraction the visual prognosis of surgery needs to be assessed in the context of any existing retinal pathology and conditions such as glaucoma or uveitis. If silicone oil is present in the posterior segment then a decision needs to be reached on whether to remove it.[85] This may either be at the time of surgery or as a separate procedure before cataract extraction. The presence of oil can alter the selection of surgical technique, as well as the type and strength of the IOL implanted. If silicone oil remains in situ following cataract surgery, then it may cause severe posterior capsule opacification that is refractory to Nd:YAG capsulotomy[86] and oil may leak into the anterior chamber with resulting oil keratopathy. If it is deemed necessary that silicone oil should remain, then it may be preferable to delay cataract surgery until such a time that it can be removed.

Surgical technique and intraocular lens selection

Phacoemulsification

Phacoemulsification has the advantage, when compared with ECCE, that it avoids the potential difficulties associated with nucleus expression following removal of the anterior hyaloid (Table 10.4). As such it is considered the technique of choice following vitrectomy, but aspects of surgery may require extra care or modification.[6] Small pupils or unstable zonules often coexist but they can usually be dealt with

Table 10.4 Phacoemulsification and vitrectomised eyes: troubleshooting

Problem	Action
Conjunctival and scleral scarring	Use a clear corneal incision in preference to a scleral tunnel
Risk of small pupil	Pupil stretch, or Multiple microsphincterotomies, or Iris hooks, or Pupil expansion device
Unstable iris–lens diaphragm	Reduce infusion rate (lower bottle/bag) Reduce aspiration rate Protect posterior capsule with second instrument
Risk of zonule weakness	See Table 10.3

using the techniques described previously. Pars plana sclerostomies cause conjunctival and scleral scarring that make the construction of a scleral tunnel incision difficult, and a clear corneal incision is safer and easier to perform. In the absence of the vitreous base, fluctuation of the anterior chamber depth and movement of the lens–iris diaphragm may be a problem during phacoemulsification. This is particularly important because the flaccid posterior capsule can then become aspirated and damaged. Decreasing the rate of the infusion (lowering the bottle height) minimises this problem. Using a second instrument to protect the posterior capsule (Figure 5.11) and reducing the aspiration rate may also be helpful. In addition, care needs to be exercised during removal of the lens cortex. If silicone oil tamponade is present, then a posterior capsulotomy or capsulectomy allows oil–fluid exchange without the need for additional pars plana incisions.[88]

Non-phacoemulsification surgery

Before the widespread adoption of phacoemulsification, expression extracapsular surgery was used for the removal of cataracts in vitrectomised eyes, particularly where silicone oil had been removed or not used. Lens expression is difficult in the absence of vitreous support, but this may be partly overcome by extensive

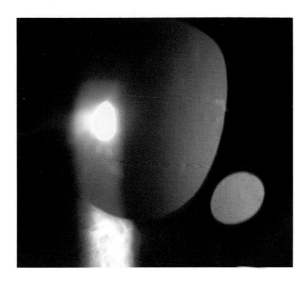

Figure 10.20   An inferior peripheral iridectomy in a pseudophakic eye with silicone oil in situ.

hydrodissection and hydrodelamination.[5] If silicone oil is removed during an ECCE, then a pars plana infusion allows oil–fluid exchange and provides posterior pressure, which aids nucleus expression. It has been suggested that a peroperative posterior capsulotomy is an effective method of maintaining a clear visual axis and preventing the dense PCO associated with silicone oil left in situ.[86] ICCE has been advocated where silicone oil is not removed from the posterior segment, and the cataract is mature. However, cryoextraction may be impeded by silicone oil in the anterior segment, and a vectis or capsule forceps may be required to remove the lens. Using an intracapsular technique, an inferior peripheral (6 o'clock) iridectomy should always be performed to prevent pupil block from the silicone oil (Figure 10.20), although this may cause optical problems such as diplopia.

When the patient is young and the cataract soft, an alternative to ICCE is lensectomy. However, lensectomy can leave little or no support for IOL implantation, and therefore this technique may be preferred where IOL insertion is not planned or if the eye has poor visual potential.[86]

Intraocular lens selection

Biometry is substantially altered by silicone oil tamponade within the posterior segment, and the choice of IOL design and material needs careful consideration, particularly if the oil is not removed (see Chapters 6 and 7). Lenses with an optic constructed of silicone should be avoided if contact with silicone oil may occur.[89]

An unstable capsular bag or damaged zonules may dictate IOL selection, but in the majority of patients, who have previously had a vitrectomy, the ability to visualize the fundus fully takes priority. In this respect IOL choice is governed by factors similar to those discussed above in the context of diabetes. A large optic IOL with a low rate of PCO and anterior capsule opacification is highly desirable. Although postoperative inflammation may be reduced by small incision surgery with a folding IOL, good biocompatibility is also of importance.

Postoperative management

Recurrent retinal detachment may occur following cataract extraction in eyes that have previously undergone pars plana vitrectomy, and this is probably most common in those that have had an ICCE performed. Patients with previous retinal detachment treated with vitrectomy need to be observed carefully.

Following ECCE in vitrectomised eyes the commonest complication is PCO, requiring Nd:YAG laser capsulotomy in up to 80% of cases in one series.[86] As mentioned above, if silicone oil has been used or is in situ, high levels of laser energy may be required. Cataract surgery in previously vitrectomised eyes may also be more prone to other postoperative complications such as uveitis and glaucoma, and may require more frequent monitoring.

Corneal and ocular surface disorders

Corneal opacity and ocular surface disease, particularly that associated with conjunctival

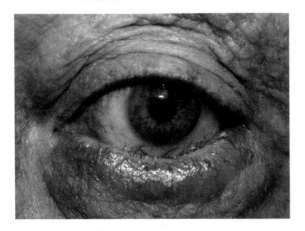

Figure 10.21   Entropion.

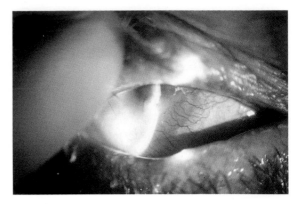

Figure 10.23   Corneal melt in a patient with rheumatoid arthritis.

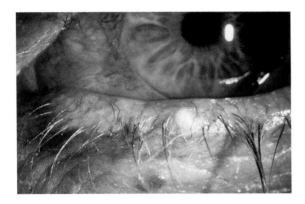

Figure 10.22   Blepharitis.

cicatrisation, makes cataract surgery a technical challenge. Eyes with a pre-existing corneal graft or reduced endothelial cell count also present difficulties. In other circumstances, cataract extraction may be combined with penetrating keratoplasty. Control of active ocular surface disorders and any associated systemic disease, which may require systemic immunosuppression, forms an important part of both pre- and postoperative management.

Preoperative management

Cataract surgery in patients with ocular surface disease is associated with a higher incidence of postoperative infective and non-infective complications. Where possible, attempts should be made to reduce coexisting risk factors. Lid malpositions such as entropion (Figure 10.21) and trichiasis, which may be a result of cicatrising conjunctival disease, should be treated before intraocular surgery. Blepharitis (Figure 10.22) can be managed with a combination of lid hygiene, oral tetracycline drugs and topical antibiotics, such as fusidic acid. If severe blepharoconjunctivitis exists then swabs should also be taken for microbiological analysis and a course of oral azithromycin prescribed (500 mg/day for three days). Dry eyes may be improved preoperatively by using punctual plugs or cautery if indicated. Other adnexal disease, such as a nasolacrimal sac mucocoele, should also be addressed. Sjögren's syndrome may be associated with several systemic disorders, for example rheumatoid arthritis (Figure 10.23), and ideally these should be controlled fully before surgery. Similarly ocular ciciatricial pemphigoid should be rendered inactive using immunosuppression where necessary. However, in this context, increased systemic immunosuppression as prophylaxis before cataract extraction is not usually required.

If significant corneal opacity coexists with cataract, then keratoplasty at the same time as cataract surgery and lens implantation should be considered (i.e. a "triple procedure"). This may also be relevant if corneal endothelial function is poor in the presence of cataract. Evidence of guttata or corneal oedema on slit lamp examination and a history of painless blurring on waking that improves during the day should alert the clinician to the possibity of Fuchs' endothelial dystrophy or endothelial dysfunction. Corneal pachmetry (> 600 μm after waking) and specular microscopy also aid diagnosis and help in the decision to perform a triple procedure. It should be noted that, in an eye with early cataract, penetrating keratoplasty and postoperative treatment with topical steroids is likely to cause progression of lens opacity.

Surgical technique and lens implantation

Corneal opacity, endothelial dysfunction, and penetrating keratoplasty

Where corneal grafting is considered certain to fail, removal of cataract alone may result in a significant improvement in acuity despite corneal opacity. In such cases corneal scarring can substantially impede visualisation of the anterior segment and may make cataract surgery difficult. Visually insignificant corneal opacity, thought at slit lamp examination to be relatively mild, may unexpectedly and disproportionately reduce the operating microscope view of the anterior segment. In spite of a limited anterior segment view, phacoemulsification may be possible by an experienced surgeon if capsulorhexis can be performed. The use of a capsule dye, such as trypan blue, makes this manoeuvre substantially easier. Hypromellose placed on the anterior corneal surface may smooth irregularities and also improve the view. If capsulorhexis is not possible then it is unlikely that phacoemulsification can succeed and an expression extracapsular technique should be adopted. Over-sizing the incision allows direct visualisation of the cataract and capsular bag at key stages in surgery, for example during irrigation and aspiration of lens cortex or IOL implantation.

Any intraocular procedure has a detrimental effect on the endothelium, and in eyes with reduced endothelial function it is important to minimise iatrogenic injury. This is particularly relevant to cataract surgery following penetrating keratoplasty, where a risk of graft rejection also exists. Viscoelastic must be used to protect the intraocular structures and the use of two agents, one cohesive and the other dispersive, may minimise endothelial injury (see Chapter 7). Phacoemulsification and ECCE have been shown to have similar consequences for the endothelium.[90] However, if phacoemulsification is performed utilising chopping techniques, using less ultrasound energy, then endothelial damage is thought to be reduced when compared with nucleus sculpting.[91] Scleral tunnels rather than corneal incisions may also be advantageous in terms of endothelial cell loss,[92] and phacoemulsification should be performed in the posterior rather than the anterior chamber.

When cataract is present with corneal disease, such as decompensated Fuchs' endothelial dystrophy, a triple procedure may be indicated. The removal of the cataract is best managed by an open sky approach following removal of the corneal button, although phacoemulsification through the partly trephined cornea has been described.[93] A stable capsular bag with a continuous anterior capsulorhexis facilitates "in the bag" posterior chamber lens implantation, which is an important consideration in graft surgery. If the view of the anterior segment allows, capsulorhexis is ideally performed before the host cornea is trephined.[94] A small limbal paracentesis allows injection of viscoelastic into the anterior chamber and capsulorhexis can then be performed using a needle without compromising the subsequent surgery. Removal of the corneal epithelium or use of a capsule stain may improve the view of the capsule. If corneal opacity makes capsulorhexis impossible, then an open sky method can be adopted. To reduce posterior pressure and the risk of a radial anterior capsule tear, counter-pressure can be

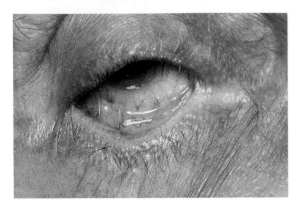

Figure 10.24 Conjunctival scarring and forniceal shortening in a case of ocular cicatricial conjunctivitis.

applied to the centre of the lens with a large spatula while the rhexis is performed.

Once capsulorhexis has been performed and the corneal button removed, open sky cataract extraction can proceed. Phacoemulsification may be used to reduce the size of the lens[95] but, assuming the capsulorhexis is not too small, the lens can usually be removed from the capsular bag by visco- or hydroexpression. This should be performed with care because intracapulsar cataract extraction may occur. Extensive hydrodissection and hydrodelamination minimises this risk, as does prechopping the lens with, for example, a pair of Nagahara chopping instruments.

Cicatrising conjunctivitis and dry eye

Dry eyes are associated with blepharoconjunctivitis, punctate epitheliopathy, and filamentary keratitis. These patients are subsequently at higher risk of persistent epithelial defects, infective corneal ulceration, and stromal melting after cataract surgery.[96] The precise aetiology of these complications is unclear, although the use of topical steroids following surgery and localised corneal denervation caused by the incision have been implicated. Small incision phacoemulsification therefore offers an advantage over extracapsular surgery.

Cicatrising conjunctival diseases may suffer the same spectrum of complications as a severe dry eye,[97] and a small incision is probably also advantageous. Unfortunately, corneal opacity and vascularisation may make this impossible. In addition, access to the globe may be severely limited by conjunctival scarring and forniceal shortening (Figure 10.24), which makes insertion of a speculum virtually impossible. To reduce the risk of reactivating the disease process in ocular cicatricial pemphigoid, conjunctival surgery to reform the fornices is usually not encouraged. Lateral cantholysis and stay sutures placed into the tarsal plate via the skin minimise trauma to the conjunctiva and usually provide an adequate view of the eye. This also reduces the force that a speculum places on the posterior segment, which can increase vitreous pressure. Hypromellose, placed on the corneal surface during surgery, protects the delicate epithelium, prevents drying, and, as mentioned above, may improve the anterior segment view.

Lens implantation

A key factor when considering lens implantation is its effect on the corneal endothelium. As stated above, open loop anterior chamber IOLs have a better record than do closed loop lenses;[98] but a higher rate of endothelial cell loss is associated with any lens placed in the anterior chamber as compared with those in the posterior chamber. When endothelial function is known to be poor the lens should ideally be inserted into the capsular bag or alternatively the ciliary sulcus.[99] Some lens materials have been reported to cause less damage when in contact with the endothelium.[100] Because all implants should be carefully inserted, using a viscoelastic agent to protect the endothelium, this should be a theoretical rather than a real advantage. Coating the anterior surface of a PMMA lens optic with viscoelastic may aid lens implantation and further protect the endothelium.

If no capsule support exists, then the choice of IOL is either an open loop anterior chamber IOL or a posterior chamber sutured lens. Despite the technical complexity of suturing an

IOL into the sulcus, endothelial loss is initially similar to that with posterior chamber lens implantation[101] and should subsequently be lower than that with an anterior chamber IOL. However, the risks associated with a sutured IOL (see Chapter 8) usually only make this the preferred option in young patients, in whom long term preservation of the endothelial cell count takes priority.

Implant power in triple procedures

The inaccuracy associated with lens implant power calculation during a triple procedure reflects the unpredictability of keratometry following corneal grafting. The options to minimise this source of error are discussed in Chapter 6. The variation in refractive outcome has led to the suggestion that non-simultaneous penetrating keratoplasty, cataract extraction, and lens implantation (or two-stage surgery) should be adopted.[102,103] As mentioned above, cataract surgery as a second procedure inevitably causes some endothelial damage and may cause graft rejection. A two-stage operation also has the disadvantage that keratometry does not stabilise until graft sutures are removed (up to two years after surgery), which delays visual rehabilitation. In addition, many graft patients have to wear a contact lens to correct residual astigmatism irrespective of spherical error. As a result, two-stage surgery may only be advisable when early cataract is present and its visual significance is uncertain.[104]

Postoperative management

In patients with dry eyes or cicatrising conjunctival disease, intensive preservative free topical lubricants should be used in conjunction with the usual topical antibiotics and steroids (also preservative free if available). Close and regular follow up is essential in these patients, who have a high rate of serious complications. Persistent epithelial defects should be treated with a soft bandage contact lens or tarsorrhaphy. In cases refractory to this treatment, amniotic membrane transplantation may be required and cyanoacrylate glue is useful if perforation occurs. Dry eyes associated with a systemic connective tissue disorder have more frequent complications, such as corneal melting, infective keratitis, and endophthalmitis, following cataract extraction. In ocular cicatricial pemphigoid the disease may reactivate after surgery. Close review allows systemic immunosuppression to be commenced early if necessary.

Herpes simplex keratitis, a common indication for penetrating keratoplasty, may be reactivated following intraocular surgery. This is of particular concern because of the need for topical steroids after cataract extraction. In such cases postoperative prophylactic oral antiviral treatment is advisable (aciclovir 400 mg twice a day).

Glaucoma

Glaucoma and cataract may coexist in a wide variety of situations. This includes patients who have controlled open angle glaucoma but may require drainage surgery in the future, or those who have uncontrolled open angle glaucoma and require drainage. Other glaucoma patients with cataract may have had a trabeculectomy to lower intraocular pressure or peripheral iridotomies to prevent or treat acute angle closure glaucoma. Glaucoma also occurs in association with extremes of axial length and conditions such as pseudoexfoliation. Cataract surgery in these patients, like in those who have had previous procedures, presents a surgical challenge. In addition, phacomorphic and phacolytic glaucoma are caused by hypermature cataract and treatment is by lens extraction.

Preoperative management

Miotics such as pilocarpine are in decline as a topical treatment for glaucoma, but historically many patients have been treated with these agents. A small pupil may accentuate the effect of early cataract, and simply changing to a different

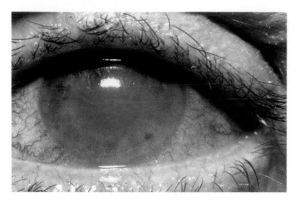

Figure 10.25 Angle closure glaucoma with a phacomorphic component.

medication may be sufficient to delay the need for cataract surgery. Stopping miotic treatment may also improve pupil dilatation if cataract surgery is planned. When a patient with narrow angles and cataract is examined at the preoperative stage, the intraocular pressure should be measured following dilated fundoscopy. If a significant increase in pressure occurs, then medical treatment or peripheral iridotomy to lower it may be required in the perioperative period.

The presence of cataract may affect the accuracy of both field testing and optic disc examination, which complicates the assessment of glaucoma progression. This may have implications for the timing of cataract and drainage surgery. Trabeculectomy may accelerate the development of cataract because of intraoperative lens trauma, inflammation, and the use of topical steroids following surgery. This should be borne in mind if early cataract exists and drainage surgery alone is planned. The patient should be informed of the possible need for cataract extraction in the future, or that a combined procedure may be indicated.

Lens induced glaucoma

Lens induced glaucoma is usually caused by an advanced hypermature cataract. Phacolytic glaucoma may also follow traumatic capsule rupture, and is caused by leakage of high molecular weight lens proteins from the capsular bag that obstruct the trabecular meshwork. Phacomorphic glaucoma results from a tumescent lens that causes pupil block and acute angle closure (Figure 10.25). In both phacolytic and phacomorphic glaucoma the intraocular pressure may be very high in conjunction with a marked inflammatory response and corneal oedema. Phacomorphic glaucoma appears to be more common in patients with pseudoexfoliation syndrome, reflecting zonular laxity and anterior movement of the lens–iris diaphragm.

Treatment in the first instance is medical, using topical and systemic agents to lower intraocular pressure as well as to treat inflammation. Where angle closure exists temporary success has been reported using Nd:YAG laser peripheral iridotomy.[105] Topical miotics may reduce intraocular pressure but they may also exacerbate pupil block, and dilatation is required before cataract extraction.

Surgical technique and lens implantation

Controlled open angle glaucoma

Clear corneal phacoemulsification with posterior chamber IOL implantation is associated with a significant sustained drop in intraocular pressure in the order of 1–3 mmHg in normal patients as well as glaucoma suspect and glaucoma patients.[106] This may prove to be beneficial, allowing a reduction in topical glaucoma medication. Surgery that involves the conjunctiva is known to compromise the success of future drainage surgery,[107] and phacoemulsification through a clear corneal incision minimises disturbance to the ocular surface. If patients have been treated with miotics then the pupil may fail to dilate or dilate only poorly, and techniques to enlarge the pupil may be required.

Uncontrolled glaucoma (combined drainage and cataract surgery)

Patients with progressive glaucoma, uncontrolled with topical medications, may

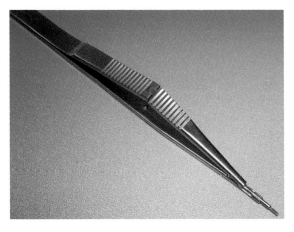

Figure 10.27 Kelly sclerostomy punch (Altomed).

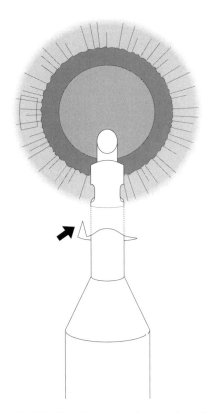

Figure 10.26 Single site phacotrabeculectomy: lateral relieving incision in a scleral tunnel (arrow) to aid phaco probe movement and reduce the risk of phacoburn.

require drainage surgery. When cataract is also present the surgical options are sequential trabeculectomy and cataract extraction or combined surgery. Combined trabeculectomy and cataract extraction offers the advantage of a single operation. However, trabeculectomy combined with ECCE is not as effective as trabeculectomy alone.[108] Phacoemulsification combined with trabeculectomy may be performed at a single site using a modified scleral tunnel incision, and this has been shown to provide better long term postoperative control of intraocular pressure than does ECCE combined with trabeculectomy.[109] Although phacotrabeculectomy may be performed under general or local anaesthesia, topical anaesthesia requires the addition of subconjunctival anaesthetic.[110] Numerous phacotrabeculectomy techniques have

been described, but a fornix based conjunctival flap combined with a scleral tunnel incision is easiest to perform and does not compromise outcome.[111] To provide an adequate superficial scleral flap, the tunnelled incision should be commenced more posteriorly than usual. This may reduce movement of the phaco probe and cause compression of the irrigation sleeve, with heating of the wound and phaco burn. A lateral scleral relieving incision, partly opening the superficial scleral flap, reduces these problems (Figure 10.26). Following phacoemulsification and folding lens implantation, the scleral flap is produced by incising anteriorly from the lateral edges of the incision. A sclerostomy is most easily produced using a scleral punch (Figure 10.27), and a peripheral iridectomy is then performed with scissors. The scleral flap may then be sutured with adjustable or releasable 10/0 nylon sutures. The conjunctiva is closed in a manner similar to any trabeculectomy with either absorbable or non-absorbable sutures.

Studies of single site phacotrabeculectomy have suggested that its success may be lower than that with trabeculectomy performed in isolation.[112] This may be due to trauma, inflammation, and subsequent scarring caused by phacoemulsification at the trabeculectomy site. A single intraoperative application of an antimetabolite, such as 5-fluorouracil (5FU), modifies the healing response and improves the outcome of trabeculectomy alone.[113] Antimetabolites have therefore been used as an adjunct to improve the performance of phacotrabeculectomy. Comparison of phacotrabeculectomy and 5FU with trabeculectomy and 5FU followed later by phacoemulsification has shown similar long term results in terms of intraocular pressure.[114] Mitomycin C has also been shown to be effective in conjunction with phacotrabeculectomy,[115] but this antimetabolite has more potential for early and late complications. To minimise tissue manipulation that occurs with a single site phacotrabeculectomy, two site surgery may offer advantages. Typically, a temporal clear corneal incision is used for phacoemulsification and a separate trabeculectomy is performed superiorly.[116] Although good results have been reported using this approach, it does require the surgeon to move position during surgery.

Previous glaucoma surgery

Patients who have undergone trabeculectomy may develop cataract, or pre-existing cataract may progress following filtration surgery. Poorly dilating pupils or a shallow anterior chamber may then complicate cataract extraction. Cataract surgery must also avoid damage to a functioning bleb and, as far as possible, must not compromise long term control of intraocular pressure. Unless bleb revision is planned as part of surgery, a corneal incision anterior to the bleb is usually adopted during ECCE. This avoids injury to the bleb, but the anterior position of the incision makes postoperative astigmatism and endothelial cell loss more likely. In patients who have had filtration surgery and subsequently had cataract extraction, intraocular pressure is better controlled by phacoemulsification than by ECCE.[117] Clear corneal phacoemulsification using a temporal approach minimises the risk to the filtering bleb and is the operation of choice.

Lens induced glaucoma

Cataract surgery is the definitive treatment for lens induced glaucoma, which should ideally be performed soon after intraocular pressure is controlled. This is particularly relevant in phacomorphic glaucoma, in which permanent peripheral anterior synechiae may develop and prevent a return to normal pressures. If permanent peripheral anterior synechiae are present, then a combined procedure is usually required. Corneal oedema, the risk of unstable zonules, and difficulty in obtaining a capsulorhexis may be indications for an ECCE.[118] Capsulorhexis is complicated both by the lack of red reflex and the tension a tumescent lens places on the anterior capsule. Puncture of the anterior capsule with a standard rhexis needle or cystotome may then result in a rapidly propagating radial tear. This can usually be overcome by using a suitable viscoelastic to tamponade the anterior chamber and aspiration of lens material through a narrow (30 G) needle (see Chapter 3).[119] Although poor pupil dilatation and unstable zonules may also be present, phacoemulsification may then be possible and provide the advantages of small incision surgery with "in the bag" IOL implantation.

Lens implantation

In most glaucoma patients anterior chamber lens implantation should be avoided, and the ideal position for the IOL is the posterior chamber within the capsular bag. Phacoemulsification allows the use of a foldable posterior chamber lens implanted through a small incision. During phacotrabeculectomy a foldable lens can be inserted either through the trabeculectomy opening or a separate corneal incision without the need for wound enlargement. Foldable silicone lens implantation in conjunction with single site phacotrabe-culectomy does not appear to impact negatively on bleb formation or control of intraocular pressure when compared with the use of a PMMA lens.[120] Anterior chamber inflammation, as measured by the laser flare meter, is more prolonged after phacoemulsification than after trabeculectomy.[121] Postoperative inflammation may be a relevant factor in the failure of drainage procedures, and the biocompatibility of the IOL material is therefore of particular importance in combined procedures (see Chapter 7).[122] Implant biocompatibility and IOL selection is also relevant following cataract surgery in eyes that may be associated with increased postoperative inflammation, for example those with phacomorphic or phacolytic glaucoma.

Postoperative management

It is important that all viscoelastic is removed from the anterior chamber at the end of surgery because this is recognised to cause a postoperative pressure rise.[123] Despite this the intraocular pressure frequently elevates during the first 24 hours following cataract surgery and may exceed 35 mmHg.[124] In patients with existing glaucoma and optic nerve damage, medical prophylaxis to prevent this pressure spike is required, such as a single dose of oral Diamox SR 250 mg (Wyeth). Six hours after cataract surgery, intraocular pressure has been shown to be statistically higher in patients with a scleral tunnel incision as compared with a clear corneal incision.[125] Following cataract surgery, patients with glaucoma may be more likely to have additional postoperative inflammation, particularly those that have suffered an episode of acute angle closure glaucoma. Topical steroids may be required at a higher concentration or frequency. These patients should be carefully followed up in view of the risk of a steroid response and intraocular pressure elevation.

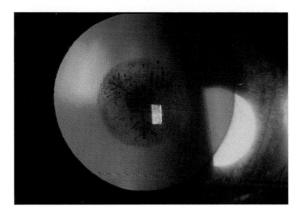

Figure 10.28 Altered red reflex in a typical congenital cataract.

Paediatric cataract

The treatment of paediatric cataract is a complex subspeciality area. It often requires a multidisciplinary team of doctors and eye professionals to work closely with the child and parents. Ocular examination may be difficult and surgery is technically challenging. At all stages of treatment it is imperative that the child's parents fully understand the relevant issues and are able to be actively involved in the decision making process. This is particularly important because intensive management of amblyopia and refractive error after surgery are the key to effective treatment. Despite this, a successful outcome is not guaranteed, particularly in unilateral cataract.

Preoperative management

Ophthalmologist, optometrist, orthoptist, and paediatric anaesthetist all play important roles in the management of paediatric cataract. A geneticist and paediatrican may also be required if a cataract is associated with a systemic disorder. Clear information should be provided to the parents of the affected child from the outset. It is often difficult to determine the visual impact of a cataract on a preverbal infant. The

151

appearance of the red reflex (Figure 10.28) and fixation pattern may be useful indicators, but fixed choice preferential looking and visual evoked potentials provide a subjective assessment of acuity. Examination under anaesthesia allows the appraisal of cataract morphology, which may also be an indicator of its visual significance. Features that favour surgery include large, axial, dense, or posterior cataracts. Pupil dilatation may benefit eyes with less significant cataract but success can be limited by loss of accommodation and glare.

Patients with bilateral visually significant cataracts should undergo surgery within three months of age to minimise the risk of developing irreversible amblyopia and nystagmus.[126] The second eye should have surgery within one week of the first (intermittently patching the operated eye in the interim). The management of unilateral visually significant cataract is more controversial.[127] The results of cataract surgery in these circumstances are variable and good outcomes are only obtainable with early surgery (as early as six weeks of age[128]) and intensive treatment of amblyopia. This has a risk of inducing amblyopia in the non-affected eye and requires substantial long term commitment from the child's parents. Surgery is unlikely to be effective if there is a coexisting ocular disorder such as retinopathy of prematurity or sclerocornea. The decision to operate on unilateral cataract should also be carefully considered if severe systemic disease is present or if the parents or child are unlikely to manage amblyopia treatment.

Cataract presenting later in infancy poses a management problem because surgery may be of little use if visually significant cataract has existed since birth but has gone undetected. Lack of strabismus or nystagmus in an older infant with a substantial lens opacity may indicate that an initially insignificant cataract has progressed, and surgery may be worthwhile in such cases.

Surgical technique

Spin-off techniques from phacoemulsification have been incorporated into paediatric cataract

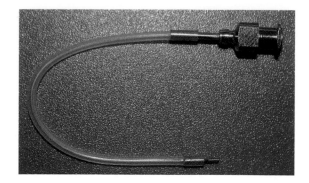

Figure 10.29 A self-retaining Lewicky anterior chamber maintainer (BD Ophthalmic Systems).

extraction, but there are several aspects of this surgery that differ from that in adults. These relate to the soft lens, anatomical differences, and the need to address the high incidence of posterior capsular and anterior hyaloid opacity found postoperatively.[129] Scleral or corneal tunnelled incisions can be used in infants but have a tendency to leak and should be sutured at the end of the procedure.

The thin flexible sclera in the paediatric eye is thought to account for the tendency of the anterior chamber to collapse during surgery, particularly when instruments are removed from the eye. This may be minimised by using an anterior chamber maintainer (Figure 10.29) throughout surgery and ensuring that anaesthesia is deep enough to prevent extraocular muscle contraction. The lens capsule is also highly elastic as compared with that in adults, and this makes anterior continuous curvilinear capsulorhexis difficult. Alternative techniques that have been suggested include radiofrequency diathermy capsulorhexis[130] and central anterior capsulotomy performed with a vitrector. The vitrector can then be used to aspirate the lens and perform a posterior capsulotomy with anterior vitrectomy. This removes the need for secondary surgical intervention to clear the visual axis. Posterior capsulorhexis has been reported as an effective alternative, which allows "in the bag" IOL implantation.[131] Although a phacoemulsification probe can be used for lens removal, irrigation and aspiration equipment, especially bimanual instruments, are probably less traumatic and safer. An aspiration port with a diameter larger than that usually found on a standard instrument (0·35 mm) may be more effective.

Pars plana lensectomy has been used to remove paediatric cataracts,[132] but the long term risk of posterior segment complications are largely unknown and usually little capsule remains to support an IOL. Intracapsular surgery is not appropriate in children because of the strong attachments between the posterior capsular and the anterior vitreous, which may cause substantial vitreous loss and risk retinal detachment.

Lens implantation and selection of power

Lens implantation as a primary procedure is increasingly common in all children.[133] The long term complications of anterior chamber lenses preclude their use, and the ideal site for an IOL is within the capsular bag in the posterior chamber. PMMA is the only implant material that has sufficient follow up to allow safe implantation in infants. Although lenses with optics constructed from highly biocompatible foldable materials may offer advantages, at present their long term outcomes are unknown. Lenses designed specifically for the paediatic eye are available but adult lenses can be used, providing their overall diameter is not greater than 12 mm.

During the first six to eight years of life the infant eye undergoes a substantial myopic shift from hypermetropia to emmetropia.[134] There is general agreement that an IOL implant should aim to anticipate this with an initial hypermetropic over-correction.[133] The extent of intentional hypermetropia depends on the age of the child at time of surgery. Residual refractive error must then be corrected with spectacles (bifocals), contact lenses, or a combination (to prevent amblyopia). Relative contraindications to IOL implantation are anatomical ocular abnormalities such as microphthalmos or persistent hyperplastic primary vitreous. Contact lenses are the main alternative to IOL implantation, although aphakic spectacles may be used. Refractive corneal techniques, for example epikeratophakia, have largely been abandoned in favour of lens implantation.

Postoperative management

The key to the treatment of paediatric cataract is the postoperative management of amblyopia and refractive error. This requires a major input from the child's parents that may put a strain on family life. The parents may need supervision and help in many aspects of postoperative care including, for example, contact lens care and handling. In young infants incremental part time patching reduces the risk of inducing amblyopia in the better or normal eye. Daily wear or extended wear contact lenses can be used to correct refractive error, usually with a lens power designed to achieve near vision (i.e. induce a low degree of myopia).

Refraction and postoperative assessment may require multiple examinations under general anaesthesia. Intraocular inflammation commonly complicates paediatric cataract surgery, and may require intensive topical steroids and, in some cases, recombinant TPA. Other frequent complications include glaucoma and, as previously mentioned, posterior capsule and anterior hyaloid opacification.[135] The latter requires either Nd:YAG capsulotomy or a surgical procedure to clear the visual axis. Because of the lifetime risk of glaucoma and retinal detachment, patients should be monitored in the long term.[136]

References

1 Ederer F, Hiller R, Taylor HR. Senile lens changes and diabetes in two population studies. *Am J Ophthalmol* 1981;**91**:381–95.
2 Klein R, Klein BE, Moss SE. Visual impairment in diabetes. *Ophthalmology* 1984;**91**:1–9.
3 Klein BE, Klein R, Moss SE. Incidence of cataract surgery in the Wisconsin Epidemiologic Study of Diabetic Retinopathy. *Am J Ophthalmol* 1995;**119**:295–300.

4   Dowler JG, Hykin PG, Lightman SL, Hamilton AM. Visual acuity following extracapsular cataract extraction in diabetes: a meta-analysis. *Eye* 1995;**9**:313–7.

5   Krupsky S, Zalish M, Oliver M, Pollack A. Anterior segment complications in diabetic patients following extracapsular cataract extraction and posterior chamber intraocular lens implantation. *Ophthalmic Surg* 1991;**22**:526–30.

6   Ionides A, Dowler JG, Hykin PG, Rosen PH, Hamilton AM. Posterior capsule opacification following diabetic extracapsular cataract extraction. *Eye* 1994;**8**:535–7.

7   Ulbig MR, Hykin PG, Foss AJ, Schwartz SD, Hamilton AM. Anterior hyaloidal fibrovascular proliferation after extracapsular cataract extraction in diabetic eyes. *Am J Ophthalmol* 1993;**115**:321–6.

8   Pollack A, Leiba H, Bukelman A, Oliver M. Cystoid macular oedema following cataract extraction in patients with diabetes. *Br J Ophthalmol* 1992;**76**:221–4.

9   Jaffe GJ, Burton TC. Progression of nonproliferative diabetic retinopathy following cataract extraction. *Arch Ophthalmol* 1988;**106**:745–9.

10 Dowler JGF, Sehmi KS, Hykin PG, Hamilton AM. The natural history of macular edema after cataract surgery in diabetes. *Ophthalmology* 1999;**106**:663–5.

11 Hykin PG, Gregson RM, Stevens JD, Hamilton PA. Extracapsular cataract extraction in proliferative diabetic retinopathy. *Ophthalmology* 1993;**100**:394–9.

12 Benson WE, Brown GC, Tasman W, McNamara JA, Vander JF. Extracapsular cataract extraction with placement of a posterior chamber lens in patients with diabetic retinopathy. *Ophthalmology* 1993;**100**:730–8.

13 Schatz H, Atienza D, McDonald HR, Johnson RN. Severe diabetic retinopathy after cataract surgery. *Am J Ophthalmol* 1994;**117**:314–21.

14 Borgioli AM, Coster DJ, Fan RFT, Henderson J. Effect of heparin surface modification of polymethylmethacrylate intraocular lenses on signs of post-operative inflammation after extracapsular cataract extraction. *Ophthalmology* 1992;**99**:1248–55.

15 Hayashi K, Hayashi H, Nakao F, Hayashi F. Reduction in the area of the anterior capsule opening after polymethylmethacrylate, silicone, and soft acrylic intraocular lens implantation. *Am J Ophthalmol* 1997;**123**:441–7.

16 Francese JE, Christ FR, Buchen SY, Gwon A, Robertson JE. Moisture droplet formation on the posterior surface of intraocular lenses during fluid/air exchange. *J Cataract Refract Surg* 1995;**21**:685–9.

17 Apple DJ, Federman JL, Krolicki TJ, *et al*. Irreversible silicone oil adhesion to silicone intraocular lenses. A clinicopathologic analysis. *Ophthalmology* 1996;**103**:1555–61.

18 Apple DJ, Isaacs RT, Kent DG, *et al*. Silicone oil adhesion to intraocular lenses: an experimental study comparing various biomaterials. *J Cataract Refract Surg* 1997;**23**:536–44.

19 Hollick EJ, Spalton DJ, Ursell PG, *et al*. The effect of polymethylmethacrylate, silicone, and polyacrylic intraocular lenses on posterior capsular opacification three years after cataract surgery. *Ophthalmology* 1999;**106**:49–54.

20 Dowler JG, Hykin PG, Hamilton AM. Phakoemulsification versus extracapsular cataract surgery in diabetes. *Ophthalmology* 2000;**107**:457-62.

21 Eifrig DE, Hermsen V, McManus P, Cunningham R. Rubeosis capsulare. *J Cataract Refract Surg* 1990;**16**:633–6.

22 Henricsson M, Heijl A, Janzon L. Diabetic retinopathy before and after cataract surgery. *Br J Ophthalmol* 1996;**80**:789–93.

23 Wagner T, Knaflic D, Rauber M, Mester U. Influence of cataract surgery on the diabetic eye: a prospective study. *Ger J Ophthalmol* 1996;**5**:79–83.

24 Okhravi N, Lightman SL, Towler HMA. Assessment of visual outcome after cataract surgery in patients with uveitis. *Ophthalmology* 1999;**106**:703–9.

25 Okhravi N, Towler HMA, Lightman SL. Cataract surgery in patients with uveitis. *Eye* 2000;**14**:689–90.

26 Jones NP. Cataract surgery using heparin surface-modified intraocular lenses in Fuchs' heterochromic uveitis. *Ophthalmic Surg* 1995;**26**:49–52.

27 Barton K, Hall AJH, Rosen PH, Cooling RJ, Lightman S. Systemic steroid prophylaxis for cataract surgery in patients with uveitis. *Ocular Immunol Inflamm* 1994;**2**:207–16.

28 Cheng CK, Berger AS, Pearson PA, Ashton P, Jaffe GJ. Intravitreal sustained-release dexamethasone device in the treatment of experimental uveitis. *Invest Ophthalmol Vis Sci* 1995;**36**:442–53.

29 Diamond JG, Kaplan HJ. Lensectomy and vitrectomy for complicated cataract secondary to uveitis. *Arch Ophthalmol* 1978;**96**:1798–804.

30 Foster CS, Fong LP, Singh G. Cataract surgery and intraocular lens implantation in patients with uveitis. *Ophthalmology* 1989;**96**:281–8.

31 Ceisler EJ, Foster CS. Juvenile rheumatoid arthritis and uveitis: minimizing the blinding complications. *Int Ophthalmol Clin* 1996;**36**:91–107.

32 Kanski JJ. Lensectomy for complicated cataract in juvenile chronic iridocyclitis. *Br J Ophthalmol* 1992;**76**:72–5.

33 Flynn HW Jr, Davis JL, Culbertson WW. Pars plana lensectomy and vitrectomy for complicated cataracts in juvenile rheumatoid arthritis. *Ophthalmology* 1988;**95**:1114–9.

34 Oshika T, Yoshimura K, Miyata N. Postsurgical inflammation after phacoemulsification and extracapsular extraction with soft or conventional intraocular lens implantation. *J Cataract Refrac Surg* 1992;**18**:356–61.

35 Dick HB, Schwenn O, Krummenauer F, Krist R, Pfeiffer N. Inflammation after sclerocorneal versus clear corneal tunnel phacoemulsification. *Ophthalmology* 2000;**107**:241–7.

36 Davison JA. Capsule contraction syndrome. *J Cataract Refract Surg* 1993;**19**:582–9.

37 Luke C, Dietlein TS, Jacobi PC, Konen W, Krieglstein GK. Massive anterior capsule shrinkage after plate-haptic silicone lens implantation in uveitis. *J Cataract Refract Surg* 2001;**27**:333–6.

38 Koenig SB, Mieler WF, Han DP, Abrams GW. Combined phacoemulsification, pars plana vitrectomy, and posterior chamber intraocular lens insertion. *Arch Ophthalmol* 1992;**110**:1101–4.

39 Shah SM, Spalton DJ. Comparison of the post-operative inflammatory response in the normal eye with heparin-surface-modified and polymethyl methacrylate intraocular lenses. *J Cataract Refract Surg* 1995;**21**:579–85.

40 Percival SPB, Pai V. Heparin-modified lenses for eyes at risk for breakdown of the blood- aqueous barrier during cataract surgery. *J Cataract Refract Surg* 1993;**19**:760–5.

41 Dick B, Kohnen T, Jacobi KW. Alterationen der heparinbeschichtung auf intraokularlinsen durch implantationsinstrumente. *Klin Monatsbl Augenheilkd* 1995;**206**:460–6.

42 Rauz S, Stavrou P, Murray PI. Evaluation of foldable intraocular lenses in patients with uveitis. *Ophthalmology* 2000;**107**:909–19.

43 Apple DJ, Solomon KD, Tetz MR, *et al*. Posterior capsule opacification. *Surv Ophthalmol* 1992;**37**: 73–116.

44 Dana MR, Chatzistefanou K, Schaumberg DA, Foster CS. Posterior capsule opacification after cataract surgery in patients with uveitis. *Ophthalmology* 1997; **104**:1387–94.

45 Lemon LC, Shin DH, Song MS, *et al*. Comparative study of silicone versus acrylic foldable lens implantation in primary glaucoma triple procedure. *Ophthalmology* 1997;**104**:1708–13.

46 Estafanous MF, Lowder CY, Meisler DM, Chauhan R. Phacoemulsification cataract extraction and posterior chamber lens implantation in patients with uveitis. *Am J Ophthalmol* 2001;**131**:620–5.

47 Tanner V, Casswell AG. A comparative study of the efficacy of 2·5% phenylephrine and 10% phenylephrine in pre-operative mydriasis for routine cataract surgery. *Eye* 1996;**10**:95–8.

48 Duffin MR, Pettit TH, Straatsma BR. 2·5% v 10% phenylephrine in maintaining mydriasis during cataract surgery. *Arch Ophthalmol* 1983;**101**:1903–9.

49 Roberts CW. Comparison of diclofenac sodium and flurbiprofen for inhibition of surgically induced miosis. *J Cataract Refract Surg* 1996;**22**(suppl 1):780–7.

50 Solomon KD, Turkalj JW, Whiteside SB, Stewart JA, Apple DJ. Topical 0·5% ketorolac vs 0·03% flurbiprofen for inhibition of miosis during cataract surgery. *Arch Ophthalmol* 1997;**115**:1119–22.

51 Corbett MC, Richards AB. Intraocular adrenaline maintains mydriasis during cataract surgery. *Br J Ophthalmol* 1994;**78**:95–8.

52 Fell D, Watson AP, Hindocha N. Plasma concentrations of catecholamines following intraocular irrigation with adrenaline. *Br J Anaesth* 1989;**62**:573–5.

53 Joseph J, Wang HS. Phacoemulsification with poorly dilated pupils. *J Cataract Refract Surg* 1993;**19**:551–6.

54 Shepherd DM. The pupil stretch technique for miotic pupils in cataract surgery. *Ophthalmic Surg* 1993;**24**. 851–2.

55 Dinsmore SC. Modified stretch technique for small pupil phacoemulsification with topical anesthesia. *J Cataract Refract Surg* 1996;**22**:27–30.

56 Graether JM. Graether pupil expander for managing the small pupil during surgery. *J Cataract Refract Surgery* 1996;**22**:530-5.

57 De Juan E Jr, Hickingbotham D. Flexible iris retractor [letter]. *Am J Ophthalmol* 1991;**111**:776–7.

58 Nichamin LD. Enlarging the pupil for cataract extraction using flexible nylon iris retractors. *J Cataract Refract Surg* 1993;793–6.

59 Novak J. Flexible iris hooks for phacoemulsification. *J Cataract Refract Surg* 1997;**23**:828–31.

60 Smith GT, Liu CS. Flexible iris hooks for phacoemulsification in patients with iridoschisis. *J Cataract Refract Surg* 2000;**26**:1277–80.

61 Masket S. Avoiding complications associated with iris retractor use in small pupil cataract extraction. *J Cataract Refract Surg* 1996;**22**:168–71.

62 Yuguchi T, Oshika T, Sawaguchi S, Kaiya T. Pupillary function after cataract surgery using flexible iris retractor in patients with small pupil. *Jpn J Ophthalmol* 1999;**43**:20–4.

63 Birchall W, Spencer AF. Misalignment of flexible iris hook retractors for small pupil cataract surgery: effects on pupil circumference. *J Cataract Refract Surg* 2001;**27**:20–4.

64 Fine IH. Pupilloplasty for small pupil phacoemulsification. *J Cataract Refract Surg* 1994;**20**:192–6.

65 Merriam JC, Zheng L. Iris hooks for phacoemulsification of the subluxed lens. *J Cataract Refract Surg* 1997;**23**:1295–7.

66 Fine IH, Hoffman RS. Phacoemulsification in the presence of pseudo-exfoliation: Challenges and options. *J Cataract Refract Surg* 1997;**23**:160–5.

67 Menapace R, Findl O, Georgopoulos M, *et al*. The capsular tension ring: designs, applications and techniques. *J Cataract Refract Surg* 2000;**26**:898–912.

68 Lam DS, Young AL, Leung AT, *et al*. Scleral fixation of a capsular tension ring for severe ectopia lentis. *J Cataract Refract Surg* 2000;**26**:609–612.

69 Fischel JD, Wishart MS. Spontaneous complete dislocation of the lens in pseudo-exfoliation syndrome. *Eur J Implant Refract Surg* 1995;**7**:31–3.

70 Cionnin RJ, Osher RH. Management of profound zonular dialysis or weakness with a new endocapsular ring designed for scleral fixation. *J Cararact Refract Surg* 1998;**24**:1299–306.

71 Shastri L, Vasavada A. Phacoemulsification in Indian eyes with pseudo-exfoliation syndrome. *J Cataract Refract Surg* 2001;**27**:1629–37.

72 Isakov I, Bartov E. Managing inferior zonule tears during manual extracapsular extraction. *J Cataract Refract Surg* 1998;**24**:300–2.

73 Demler U, Sautter H. Surgery in sub-luxated lenses in adults. *Dev Ophthalmol* 1985;**11**:162–5.

74 Blumenthal M, Kurtz, Assia EI. Hydroexpression of subluxed lenses using a glide. *Ophthalmic Surg* 1994; **25**:34–7.

75 Hakin KN, Jacobs M, Rosen P, *et al*. Management of the subluxed crystalline lens. *Ophthalmology* 1992;**99**:542–5.

76 Plager DA, Parks MM, Helveston EM, Ellis FD. Surgical treatment of subluxed lenses in children. *Ophthalmology* 1992;**99**:1018–21.

77 Hubbard AD, Charteris DG, Cooling RJ. Vitreolensectomy in Marfan's syndrome. *Eye* 1998;**3Λ**: 412–6.

78 Gimbel HV. Role of capsular tension rings in preventing capsule contraction. *J Cataract Refract Surg* 2000;**26**: 791–2.

79 Liu C, Eleftheriadis H. Multiple capsular tension rings for the prevention of capsule contraction syndrome. *J Cataract Refract Surg* 2001;**27**:342–3.

80 Berger RR, Kenyeres A, Van Coller BM, Pretorius CF. Repositioning a tilted ciliary-sulcus-fixated intraocular lens. *J Cataract Refract Surg* 1995;**21**:497–8.

81 Davison JA. Capsule contraction syndrome. *J Cataract Refract Surg* 1993;**19**:582–9.

82 Blankenship GW. Stability of pars plana vitrectomy results for diabetic retinopathy complications; a comparison of five-year and six-month post-vitrectomy findings. *Arch Ophthalmol* 1981;**99**:1009–12.

83 McCuen B, de Juan E, Landers MB, Machemer R. Silicone oil in vitreoretinal sugery II. Results and complications. *Retina* 1985;**5**:198–205.

84 Wilbrandt HR, Wilbrant TH. Pathogenesis and management of the lens-diaphragm retropulsion syndrome during phacoemulsification. *J Cataract Refract Surg* 1994;**20**:48–53.

85 Franks WA, Leaver PK. Removal of silicone oil: rewards and penalties. *Eye* 1991;**5**:333–7.

86 Baer RM, Aylward WG, Leaver PK. Cataract extraction following vitrectomy and silicone oil tamponade. *Eye* 1995;**9**:309–12.

87 Lacelle VD, Garate FJO, Alday NM, *et al.* Phacoemulsification cataract surgery in vitrectomised eyes. *J Cataract Refract Surg* 1998;**24**:806–9.

88 Grey R, Horsborough B. Cataract extraction following vitrectomy and silicone oil tamponade. *Eye* 1996;**10**:151–2.

89 Apple DJ, Federman JL, Krolicki TJ, *et al.* Irreversible silicone oil adhesion to silicone intraocular lenses. A clinicopathologic analysis. *Ophthalmology* 1996;**103**: 1555–61.

90 Ravalico G, Tognetto D, Palomba MA, Lovisato A, Baccara F. Corneal endothelial function after extracapsular cataract extraction and phacoemulsification. *J Cataract Refract Surg* 1997;**23**:1000–5.

91 Hayashi K, Nakao F, Hayashi F. Corneal endothelial cell loss after phacoemulsification using nuclear cracking procedures. *J Cataract Refract Surg* 1994; **20**:44–7.

92 Oshima Y, Tsujikawa K, Oh A, Harino S. Comparative study of intraocular lens implantation through 3·0mm temporal clear corneal and superior scleral tunnel self-sealing incisions. *J Cataract Refract Surg* 1997;**23**:347–53.

93 Malbran ES, Malbran E, Buonsanti J, Adrogue E. Closed-system phacoemulsification and posterior chamber implant combined with penetrating keratoplasty. *Ophthalmic Surg* 1993;**24**:403–6.

94 Caporossi A, Traversi C, Simi C, Tosi GM. Closed-system and open-sky capsulorhexis for combined cataract extraction and corneal transplantation. *J Cataract Refract Surg* 2001;**27**:990–3.

95 Lindquist TD. Open-sky phacoemulsification during corneal transplantation. *Ophthalmic Surg* 1994;**25**: 734–6.

96 Ram J, Sharma A, Pandav SS, Gupta A, Bambery P. Cataract surgery in patients with dry eyes. *J Cataract Refract Surg* 1998;**24**:1119–24.

97 MacLeod JD, Dart JK, Gray TB. Corneal and cataract surgery in chronic progressive conjunctival cicatrisation. *Dev Ophthalmol* 1997;**28**:228–39.

98 Lim ES, Apple DJ, Tsai JC, *et al.* An analysis of flexible anterior chamber lenses with special reference to the normalised rate of lens explanation *Ophthalmology* 1991;**98**:243–6.

99 Ohguro N, Matsuda M, Kinoshita S. Effects of posterior chamber lens implantation on the endothelium of transplanted corneas. *Br J Ophthalmol* 1997;**81**:1056–9.

100 Barrett G, Constable IJ. Corneal endothelial loss with new intraocular lenses. *Am J Ophthalmol* 1984;**98**: 157–65.

101 Lee JH, Oh SY. Corneal endothelial cell loss from suture fixation of a posterior chamber intraocular lens. *J Cataract Refract Surg* 1997;**23**:1020–2.

102 Rosen ES. Combined or sequential keratoplasty and cataract surgery? *J Cataract Refract Surg* 1998;**24**: 1283–4.

103 Hsiao CH, Chen JJ, Chen PY, Chen HS. Intraocular lens implantation after penetrating keratoplasty. *Cornea* 2001;**20**:580–5.

104 Epstein RJ. Combining keratoplasty and cataract surgery. *J Cataract Refract Surg* 1999;**25**:603.

105 Tomey KF, Al-Rajhi AA. Neodymium YAG laser iridotomy in the initial management of phacomorphic glaucoma. *Ophthalmology* 1992;**99**:660–5.

106 Shingleton BJ, Gamell LS, O'Donoghue MW, *et al.* Long-term changes in intraocular pressure after clear corneal phacoemulsification: Normal patients versus glaucoma suspect and glaucoma patients. *J Cataract Refract Surg* 1999;**25**:885–90.

107 Broadway DC, Grierson I, Hitchings RA. Local effects of previous conjunctival incisional surgery and the subsequent outcome of filtration surgery. *Am J Ophthalmol* 1998;**125**:805–18.

108 Murchinson JF Jr, Shields MB. An evaluation of three surgical approaches for coexisting cataract and glaucoma. *Ophthalmic Surg* 1989;**20**:393–8.

109 Kosmin AS, Wishart PK, Ridges PJG. Long-term intraocular pressure control after cataract extraction: phacoemulsification versus extracapsular technique. *J Cataract Refract Surg* 1998;249–55.

110 Vicary D, McLennan S, Sun XY. Topical plus subconjunctival anesthesia for phacotrabeculectomy: one year follow-up. *J Cataract Refract Surg* 1998;**24**: 1247–51.

111 Shingleton BJ, Chaudhry IM, O'Donoghue MW, *et al.* Phacotrabeculectomy: limbus-based versus fornix-based conjunctival flaps in fellow eyes. *Ophthalmology* 1999;**106**:1152–5.

112 Naveh N, Kottass R, Glovinsky J, *et al.* The long-term effect on intraocular pressure of a procedure combining trabeculectomy and cataract surgery, as compared with trabeculectomy alone. *Ophthalmic Surg* 1990;**21**:339–45.

113 Smith MF, Sherwood MB, Doyle JW, Khaw PT. Results of intra-operative 5-fluorouracil supplementation on trabeculectomy for open-angle glaucoma. *Am J Ophthalmol* 1992;**114**:737–41.

114 Donoso R, Rodriguez A. Combined versus sequential phacotrabeculectomy with intra-operative 5-fluorouracil. *J Cataract Refract Surg* 2000;**26**:71–4.

115 Cohen JS, Greff LJ, Novack GD, Wind BE. A placebo-controlled, double-masked evaluation of mitomycin C in combined glaucoma and cataract procedures. *Ophthalmology* 1996;**103**:1934–42.

116 El Sayyad F, Helal M, El Maghraby A, Khalil M, El Hamzawey H. One-site versus 2-site phacotrabeculectomy: a randomized study. *J Cataract Refract Surg* 1999;**25**:77–82.

117 Manoj B, Chako D, Khan MY. Effect of extracapsular cataract extraction and phacoemulsification performed after trabeculectomy on intraocular pressure. *J Cataract Refract Surg* 2000;**26**:75–8.

118 McKibbin M, Gupta A, Atkins AD. Cataract extraction and intraocular lens implantation in eyes with phacomorphic or phacolytic glaucoma. *J Cataract Refract Surg* 1996;**22**:633–6.

119 Rao SK, Padmanabhan R. Capsulorhexis in eyes with phacomorphic glaucoma. *J Cataract Refract Surg* 1998; **24**:882–4.

120 Braga-Mele R, Cohen S, Rootman DS. Foldable silicone versus polymethyl methacrylate intraocular lenses in combined phacoemulsification and trabeculectomy. *J Cataract Refract Surgery* 2000;**26**:1517–22.

121 Siriwardena D, Kotecha A, Minassian D, Dart JK, Khaw PT. Anterior chamber flare after trabeculectomy and after phacoemulsification. *Br J Ophthalmol* 2000;**84**:1056–7.

122 Samuelson TW, Chu YR, Kreiger RA. Evaluation of giant-cell deposits on foldable intraocular lenses after combined cataract and glaucoma surgery. *J Cataract Refract Surg* 2000;**26**:817–23.

123 Tanaka T, Inoue H, Kudo S, Ogawa T. Relationship between post-operative intraocular pressure elevation and residual sodium hyaluronate following phacoemulsification and aspiration. *J Cataract Refract Surg* 1997;**23**:284–8.

124 Barak A, Desatnik H, Ma-Naim T, *et al.* Early post-operative intraocular pressure pattern in glaucomatous and nonglaucomatous patients. *J Cataract Refract Surg* 1996;**22**:607–11.

125 Schwenn O, Dick HB, Krummenauer F, *et al.* Intraocular pressure after small incision cataract surgery: temporal sclerocorneal versus clear corneal incision. *J Cataract Refract Surg* 2001;**27**:421–5.

126 Lesueur LC, Arne JL, Chapotot EC, Thouvenin D, Malecaze F. Visual outcome after paediatric cataract surgery: is age a major factor? *Br J Ophthalmol* 1998;**82**:1022–5.

127 Taylor D, Wright KW, Amaya L, Cassidy L, Nischal K, Russell-Eggitt I. Should we aggressively treat unilateral congenital cataracts? *Br J Ophthalmol* 2001;**85**:1120–6.

128 Birch EE, Stager DR, Leffler J, Weakley D. Early treatment of congenital unilateral cataract minimises unequal competition. *Invest Ophthalmol Vis Sci* 1998;**39**:1560–6.

129 Koch DD, Kohnen T. Retrospective comparison of techniques to prevent secondary cataract formation after posterior chamber intraocular lens implantation in infants and children. *J Cataract Refract Surg* 1997;**23**:657–63.

130 Comer RM, Abdulla N, O'Keefe M. Radiofrequency diathermy capsulorhexis of the anterior and posterior capsules in paediatric cataract surgery: preliminary results. *J Cataract Refract Surg* 1997;**23**:641–4.

131 Gimbel HV. Posterior continuous curvilinear capsulorhexis and optic capture of the intraocular lens to prevent secondary opacification in paediatric cataract surgery. *J Cataract Refract Surg* 1997;**23**:652–6.

132 Ahmadieh H, Javadi MA, Ahmady M, *et al.* Primary capsulectomy, anterior vitrectomy, lensectomy and posterior chamber lens implantation in children: limbal versus pars plana. *J Cataract Surg* 1999;**25**:768–75.

133 Dahan E. Intraocular lens implantation in children. *Curr Opin Ophthalmol* 2000;**11**:51–5.

134 Flitcroft DI, Knight-Nanan D, Bowell R, *et al.* Intraocular lenses in children: changes in axial length, corneal curvature and refraction. *Br J Ophthalmol* 1999;**83**:265–9.

135 Keech RV, Tongue AC, Scott WE. Complications after surgery for congenital and infantile cataracts. *Am J Ophthalmol* 1989;**108**:136–41.

136 Brady KM, Atkinson CS, Kilty LA, Hiles DA. Glaucoma after cataract extraction and posterior chamber lens implantation in children. *J Cataract Refract Surg* 1997;**23**:669–74.

11 Vitreous loss

Vitreous loss is the most common serious intraoperative complication of phacoemulsification and extracapsular cataract surgery, occurring in approximately 2–4% of contemporary procedures.[1,2] Incidences of up to and around 10% have been reported, particularly from surgeons in training[3–6] and in the older literature. Vitreous loss usually results from iatrogenic intraoperative rupture of the posterior capsule, although it can also arise from intraoperative zonule dehiscence or pre-existing injuries or anomalies of the capsule and zonule.

The importance of vitreous loss is its association with increased surgical morbidity and a poorer postoperative visual outcome[7–9] as compared with uncomplicated cataract surgery (Box 11.1). If vitreous loss cannot be prevented, then appropriate and careful management at the time of initial surgery can ameliorate problems. It is essential to have a systematic approach to the variety of causes and consequences of vitreous loss, and familiarity with the additional instrumentation that may be required.

Box 11.1 Consequences of vitreous loss

- Uveitis
- Glaucoma
- Macular oedema
- Corneal oedema
- Rhegmatogenous retinal detachment
- Endophthalmitis
- Pupil irregularity and distortion
- Vitreous wick syndrome

Box 11.2 Risk factors for vitreous loss

- Small pupil (diabetes, uveitis, age, previous intraocular surgery, chronic pilocarpine)
- Intraoperative miosis (secondary to iris trauma)
- Lens subluxation (iridodonesis and phacodonesis)
- Irregularity of capsulorhexis
- Radial tears of anterior capsule
- Very dense cataracts
- Pseudoexfoliation syndrome
- Previous blunt trauma
- Poor wound construction
- Extraocular pressure on globe (lid speculum, large volume peribulbar local anaesthetic)
- Retrobulbar haemorrhage
- Vitreous loss in previous eye
- Surgical inexperience: the "learning curve"
- Uncooperative patient

Prevention

Identification of eyes that are especially at risk of capsular rupture or zonular dehiscence is important (Box 11.2). This may allow the surgery to be undertaken by a more experienced surgeon in eyes with, for example, pseudoexfoliation syndrome (Figure 11.1)[10] or very dense/white cataracts (Figure 11.2). Alternatively, it may be more appropriate to employ a different surgical method, such as pars plana vitreolensectomy for subluxed cataractous lenses following ocular injury or in patients with Marfan's syndrome (Figure 11.3). Small pupils (Figure 11.4) are associated with a significantly

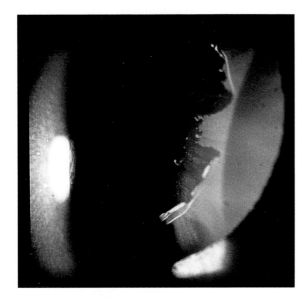

Figure 11.1   Pseudoexfoliation.

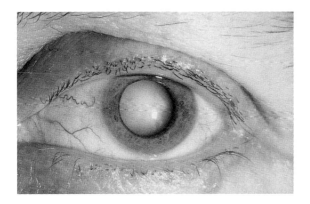

Figure 11.2   Mature white cataract.

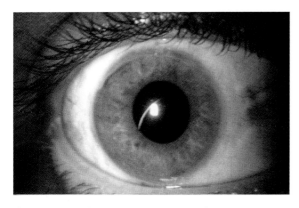

Figure 11.3   Lens subluxed inferiorly.

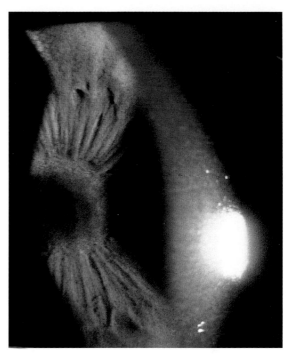

Figure 11.4   Posterior synechiae and a small pupil in an eye with recurrent anterior uveitis.

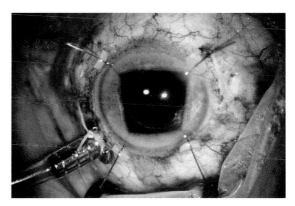

Figure 11.5   Iris hooks being used during pars plana vitrectomy and cataract extraction.

increased risk of capsule rupture and vitreous loss,[11] and this underlines the value of intraoperative enlargement of the pupil using surgical iridotomies, iris hooks (Figure 11.5), or stretching.

Radial tears of the anterior capsule incurred during capsulorhexis may extend peripherally through the zonule into the posterior capsule if subjected to undue pressure. In the absence of an intact capsulorhexis, phacoemulsification of a hard nucleus requires a technique that does not transmit forces to the capsule in a manner that is likely to extend the radial tear posteriorly. A high index of suspicion in "at risk" eyes can help to identify capsular rupture at an earlier stage, before vitreous loss or dislocation of lens fragments has occurred, and allow appropriate remedial action to be taken. The surgeon needs to be alert for subtle signs that may indicate the development of capsular rupture, such as unexpected deepening of the anterior chamber. If the surgeon is faced with a zonular dehiscence, or a situation in which zonular support is suspect, such as in pseudoexfoliation, then the insertion of an endocapsular tension ring will redistribute forces throughout the lens equator and stabilise the situation.[12]

General principles of management

During phacoemulsification the combination of gravity and the posteriorly directed force of the infusion fluid conspire to encourage lens material to fall backward into the vitreous cavity (the "dropped nucleus"). In extracapsular surgery, however, capsular catastrophes are usually associated with forward movement of the vitreous through the pupil into the anterior chamber, the surgical wound, and beyond.

Once vitreous loss has been recognised, the immediate priority is to prevent the posterior loss of the nucleus or its fragments into the vitreous. The next priority is to clear the wound, anterior chamber, and pupil of vitreous and lens material, while preserving the anterior and posterior lens capsule to allow, if appropriate, the insertion of an intraocular lens implant. When topical anaesthesia has been used, supplementary anaesthesia by intracameral, subconjunctival, or sub-Tenon's routes may be required.

Removal of remaining nuclear fragments from the anterior chamber or capsular bag

will usually require conversion from phacoemulsification to an extracapsular extraction, although it may be possible for the experienced surgeon to remove these by phacoemulsification if the vitreous can be adequately controlled. Vitreous should be removed using a suction cutter either with an integral irrigation sleeve or a separate anterior chamber infusion, and using a high cut rate and low (<150 mmHg) suction. An experienced vitreoretinal surgeon should deal with posteriorly dislocated lens material, and the timing of this intervention will vary according to the individual circumstances and available facilities.

Expulsive choroidal haemorrhage is a very serious intraoperative complication, but is fortunately much rarer than vitreous loss. It is important to remember that vitreous loss may be the first sign of expulsive choroidal haemorrhage, and the surgeon must always be alert to this possibility, especially when no other cause of vitreous loss can be identified. Shallowing of the anterior chamber and disappearance of the red reflex usually precede expulsive haemorrhage. Rapid wound closure is required and this may be successful in preserving some vision if the retina can be preserved. Expulsive haemorrhage during phacoemulsification is much more readily controlled because of the ability to achieve prompt wound closure.

Vitreous loss during phacoemulsification surgery

Vitreous loss during phacoemulsification most commonly arises as a result of the radial extension of an anterior capsular tear through the zonule into the posterior capsule, or through direct injury of the posterior capsule by the tip of the phaco needle.[13] This latter scenario typically occurs during the "learning curve", while the surgeon in training is learning the volume and shape of the endocapsular space. It is important to remember that the posterior lens surface is curved and that the tip of the phaco needle must therefore be lifted anteriorly as the equator is approached when sculpting a groove. Extension of capsular tears may occur early during hydrodissection or at the commencement of phacoemulsification, allowing the entire lens to dislocate into the vitreous. Smaller tears of the capsule may only be apparent after the nucleus has been cracked, when a lens fragment can drop through the capsular rent into the vitreous. If this is not accompanied by forward displacement of vitreous, loss of small lens fragments may not be noticed by the surgeon and not come to light unless complications ensue. It is therefore imperative that all eyes complicated by posterior capsule rupture be examined carefully for retained lens fragments. Unrecognised loss of lens fragments can result in patients presenting with severe uveitis, possibly with hypopyon, which may be mistaken for endophthalmitis.[14]

Capsule rupture in the presence of a complete nucleus or nuclear fragments is discussed below. If a capsule tear with vitreous loss occurs during cortex aspiration or becomes apparent at the end of phacoemulsification, then all soft lens matter should be removed while avoiding traction on the vitreous. In practice this is not achievable with either an automated or manual irrigation and aspiration instrument. An alternative is a dry aspiration technique using a syringe and a cannula (typically a lacrimal cannula). The soft lens matter is fully engaged with the cannula tip and aspirated; if the anterior chamber begins to collapse then it is reformed using a viscoelastic. This can be a protracted procedure, and because vitreous traction may still occur cortical lens matter may be better removed as part of a vitrectomy.

An anterior vitrectomy using a separate cutter and infusion (or bimanual) technique (Figure 11.6a) is preferable to a suction cutter with an integral (coaxial) infusion (Figure 11.6b).[15] The anterior chamber may not act as a closed system when using a coaxial infusion and cutter, particularly if the main incision has been

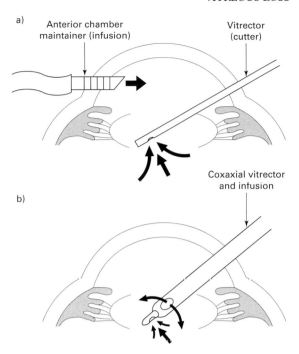

Figure 11.6 Comparison of anterior vitrectomy techniques. (a) Separate cutter and infusion (or bimanual). (b) Suction cutter with an integral (coaxial) infusion.

enlarged. The delivery of the infusion to the tip of the cutter and loss of fluid around the instrument can then force vitreous anteriorly and out of the eye. A bimanual technique affords better access, less corneal distortion, and less forward displacement of vitreous. Using this technique, the vitreous cutter should be inserted through a limbal paracentesis, avoiding the main incision, to produce a closed anterior chamber. A second paracentesis, opposite that initially made for the second instrument, enables the vitreous cutter to access 360° of the capsular bag. The vitreous cutter can then be used in aspirate mode to gently remove residual soft lens material attached to the lens capsule. If vitreous is aspirated, cutting mode can then be used but not in proximity to the capsule. The infusion can either be held in the other paracentesis or a self-retaining anterior chamber maintainer can be inserted through a third paracentesis. The anterior segment and wound should be cleared of vitreous, avoiding damage to the iris and minimising traction on the vitreous in order to reduce the risk of retinal tears. The lens capsule should be carefully preserved, unless it is obvious that neither the anterior or posterior capsule are capable of supporting a posterior chamber lens implant, in which case the capsule remnants can be excised.

To ensure that no vitreous strands persist to the internal aspect of the wound, an intracameral injection of acetylcholine or carbachol should be given to constrict the pupil; if this is peaked then vitreous is likely to be the cause and can be dealt with. If a sulcus intraocular lens (IOL) is to be inserted then this should precede the use of any miotic agent. Gently sweeping a second instrument or an iris repositor across the pupil can then help to identify vitreous. Similarly, the external aspect of the wound needs to be meticulously checked with a cellulose sponge to exclude vitreous herniating through the wound (even with a round pupil). Again, this should be undertaken as gently as possible. Any iris movement implies the presence of vitreous from the posterior segment through the wound, and risk of a vitreous wick syndrome or chronic macular oedema. If there is any doubt that the incision may not self-seal, it should be sutured. This prevents a postoperative wound leak, which may become incarcerated with vitreous.

Small pieces of retained soft lens material may frequently be reabsorbed spontaneously and do not always require surgical removal if the eye remains quiet and the intraocular pressure normal during follow up. In these cases outpatient review needs to be frequent and assiduous. Larger retained pieces of soft lens matter are more frequently associated with a moderate to severe uveitis with raised intraocular pressure that necessitates their removal.

Management of impending dislocation of nuclear fragment

In the presence of a sudden unexpected deepening of the anterior chamber or suspicion that vitreous loss has occurred, the natural human response is denial. This is of course the worst possible response because continuing surgery is likely to further compromise the outcome. If vitreous loss is suspected then stop everything and assess the situation. The aims of the surgeon should now be modified to avoid losing the entire nucleus or large nuclear fragments into the vitreous cavity.

The precise action to take will depend on the stage of surgery and the experience of the operator. Junior surgeons must never hesitate to seek advice. Whatever strategy is undertaken, the bottle height should immediately be lowered to avoid flushing the nucleus into the posterior segment. Should the nucleus or nuclear fragment(s) appear to be dropping posteriorly, they can first be supported using the second instrument. Then a high density viscoelastic can be injected beneath them, pushing back any vitreous and supporting the lens. If nuclear sculpting has only just been started, then it may be appropriate to convert to extracapsular approach, enlarge the wound (see Chapter 2), and remove the nucleus with an irrigating vectis after making relieving incisions in the rhexis. An experienced surgeon might consider pars plana transfixation of the lens or passing a Sheets glide beneath the lens,[16] followed by phacoemulsification in the anterior chamber.

Continuing with a basic unmodified "Divide and conquer" technique will inevitably result in loss of large fragments of nucleus into the posterior segment. If the nucleus has already been divided into segments then the danger is greater because smaller fragments are more likely to migrate through the capsule defect. In this situation it may be possible to use a narrow width irrigating vectis (Figure 11.7) to remove the fragments through the unenlarged (or minimally enlarged) incision. Alternatively, after low infusion pressure vitrectomy, the fragments may be secured with high vacuum phaco and removed from the eye (although the anterior chamber must be completely clear of vitreous). If the nucleus or a fragment of it falls posteriorly,

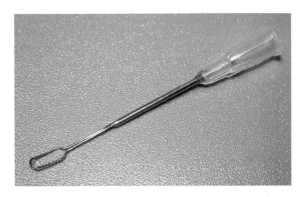

Figure 11.7 Pearce small incision irrigating vectis (BD Ophthalmic Systems).

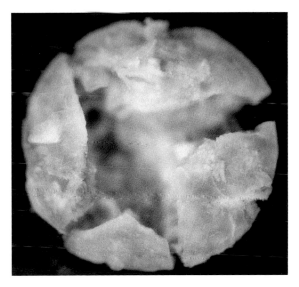

Figure 11.8 Entire lens nucleus retrieved from the posterior segment in a patient with Stickler's syndrome. Note the nuclear sculpting grooves.

they should not be pursued into the vitreous cavity by a surgeon without vitreoretinal experience because this will increase the risk of retinal detachment, particularly giant retinal tears.[17] Once all nuclear fragments are removed from the anterior segment, cortical lens matter and vitreous can then be dealt with using one of the methods already described.

Retained lens fragments in the vitreous may result in raised intraocular pressure, uveitis, corneal and macular oedema, vitreous opacification, and retinal detachment.[18,19] Small fragments (less than 25%) may be reabsorbed without causing complications, allowing a policy of observation to be followed. Larger fragments or the entire nucleus (Figure 11.8) in the vitreous cavity require removal, the timing of which will be dictated by a variety of factors (see below). Retinal detachment is the most significant complication affecting visual outcome following retained lens fragments, occurring in approximately one in six eyes (16%), either before or after vitrectomy.[19–22]

Vitreous loss during extracapsular cataract surgery

Vitreous loss during planned extracapsular surgery is infrequently associated with posterior displacement of the lens nucleus or fragments, and typically occurs during cortex aspiration.[13] Subsequent vitreoretinal surgical intervention is uncommon in the absence of the development of rhegmatogenous retinal detachment or chronic macular oedema. However, the larger wound results in more extensive vitreous loss, over a greater area, which requires meticulous removal to minimise visual morbidity.

Removal of obvious vitreous from the wound with scissors and cellulose sponges should be avoided because this puts traction on the vitreous base, which increases the risk of retinal tears and subsequent retinal detachment. A suction cutter with an integral infusion sleeve or separate anterior chamber infusion should be used, the former being more suitable during extracapsular surgery. When the wound has been cleared of vitreous, one or two temporary sutures can be inserted to close the section, which helps reduce further vitreous loss and corneal endothelial damage. Vitreous should then be cleared from the anterior chamber and pupil, working steadily toward the posterior capsule, while trying to avoid enlarging any capsular tears or unnecessarily removing residual lens capsule. If a large tear in the posterior capsule is present, then the vitrector should be cautiously advanced through the tear to assist removal of all prolapsing vitreous. Care should be taken to avoid inserting an irrigating cutter too far into the vitreous cavity because the infusion fluid may promote forward vitreous displacement and increase the risk of retinal damage. Sterile filtered air can be used instead of an irrigating fluid during anterior vitrectomy,[23] which has the advantage of promoting posterior displacement of the vitreous due to the surface tension of the gas, and facilitates identification of vitreous strands caught in the wound or distorting the pupil margin. Alternatively, the techniques discussed above as part of vitrectomy in the context of phacoemulsification can be used.

Intraocular lens implantation in the presence of vitreous loss

Before IOL insertion all vitreous must be cleared from the anterior segment. The style and position of lens implant will be determined by the amount of residual lens capsule that is available for support. When posterior capsule rupture results in vitreous loss during extracapsular surgery, there is usually less residual capsule to support a lens implant than with phacoemulsification, particularly if a "can opener" or endocapsular (intercapsular) capsulotomy has been performed. In most situations in which phacoemulsification results in vitreous loss, it should be possible to place a posterior chamber IOL in the ciliary sulcus.[13] An intact capsulorhexis provides an excellent platform to support a posterior chamber lens in the sulcus. Providing the lens haptic diameter is suitable ($\geq 12\cdot5$ mm), there is no reason not to insert a foldable IOL. This allows the patient to benefit from the advantages of small incision surgery despite vitreous loss. Whichever IOL is used, it is important to ensure that the haptics are located in the sulcus and not posterior to the capsule. This is aided by first injecting viscoelastic between the iris and the residual capsule. When implanting a sulcus placed lens, reducing the optimal IOL power by $0\cdot5$ dioptres should compensate for the relative anterior

position of the IOL. If a different type of IOL is to be implanted, then the lens power should be appropriately modified in accordance with the difference in A constants.

When part or all of the nucleus has been dropped into the vitreous, the decision of whether to implant an IOL depends on the technique used to remove them, and liaison with the local vitreoretinal service before problems are encountered is recommended. In general, if the entire lens nucleus or large fragments (25% or more) have fallen into the vitreous cavity, then insertion of a lens implant may be best deferred until these have been removed. Pseudophakia in these circumstances can cause difficulties in visualising the posterior segment, preclude transpupillary removal of the nucleus, and may compromise subsequent vitreoretinal surgery.

In the absence of sufficient capsule to support a sulcus placed IOL, either an open loop anterior chamber lens or a sutured posterior chamber lens can be used (see Chapter 8). In the context of vitreous loss a sutured lens is best performed as a secondary elective procedure, leaving the patient aphakic in the interim. An anterior chamber lens can be usually be inserted without the need for a second procedure.[24] This may first require the incision to be enlarged to match the optic diameter. The technique for anterior chamber lens insertion is described in Chapter 8 and, as mentioned, a peripheral iridectomy must be performed to prevent pupil block glaucoma. Diplopia may occur unless this is placed in the superior peripheral iris. Although a forceps and scissors can be used, performing a peripheral iridectomy through a temporal phacoemulsification wound is easiest using the vitrector. Iris is aspirated in the selected site for the peripheral iridectomy and the iris is excised using a low cut rate.

Surgical management of the dropped nucleus

The most significant factor in determining the timing of surgery to remove retained lens

Table 11.1 Factors influencing the timing of vitrectomy for retained lens fragments

Timing of vitrectomy	Factor
Immediate/early	Single procedure for patient (immediate only) Possible reduced risk of glaucoma (<3 weeks) Uveitis less severe Macular oedema less severe
Late	Better fundus visualisation Posterior vitreous detachment more likely Lens material softer Possible lower risk of retinal complications

fragments is the clarity of the fundus view through the cornea (Table 11.1). This is optimal at the time of the primary cataract surgery, and whenever possible vitrectomy should be undertaken then. However, delay in surgical intervention to allow control of raised intraocular pressure and clearing of corneal oedema does not appear to affect the final visual outcome adversely.[19–22] Unfortunately, there have to date been no prospective, randomised studies comparing early versus delayed intervention, and the conclusions of published retrospective series with regard to visual outcome and complications have often been contradictory.

When dealing with a dropped nucleus, the vitreoretinal surgeon is frequently confronted with the problem of a small pupil. This is most easily overcome by the use of self-retaining iris hook retractors inserted through the peripheral cornea. In addition to improving the view of the fundus, residual lens material is more readily identified and removed without compromising the remaining lens capsule.

A thorough three-port pars plana vitrectomy should be performed, ensuring that all vitreous is removed from around the lens fragments, which can be debulked of any adherent soft lens material. Residual vitreous gel in the anterior chamber or around the lens capsule should be removed, while avoiding any further capsular damage. If it is planned to deliver the nucleus through the pupil with the aid of perfluorocarbon heavy liquid,[25] then residual anterior vitreous gel may ensnare the nucleus and increase the risk of damage to peripheral retina. Hence, the vitreous base should be cleared as extensively as possible, which also allows an opportunity to inspect closely the peripheral retina for any breaks. An attached posterior hyaloid face can be left to act as a cushion over the retina at this stage, but should be removed later when all lens fragments have been dealt with. If the retina is detached then heavy liquid can be used to flatten the retina, which reduces the risk of iatrogenic damage.

Small lens fragments may be crushed between the cutter and the endoilluminator, but this is a very laborious means of dealing with larger fragments, and is inappropriate for very dense nuclei. These can be either be fragmented with ultrasound or removed intact via a corneolimbal incision. Floating the lens fragments on a layer of heavy liquid allows the use of ultrasound fragmentation in the mid-vitreous cavity. This may prove difficult because of the mobility of the fragments and, in addition, hard nuclear fragments can tear the retina during ultrasound fragmentation or careless manipulation. A snare can be fashioned from a flute needle and a 6/0 prolene suture to catch and stabilise lens fragments, which can then be safely fragmented in the mid-vitreous without risk to the retina. It is critical to ensure that all vitreous has been removed before using ultrasound fragmentation because this instrument does not cut vitreous and can result in serious retinal injury.

If ultrasound fragmentation is not available or the nucleus is too hard or too large to fragment safely in the vitreous cavity, then the lens can be delivered to the anterior chamber through the pupil by floating it up with heavy liquid.[25] Here, the fragment can be removed by phacoemulsification, allowing the operator to use a bimanual technique with direct illumination, but at risk of trauma to the endothelium and iris. Alternatively, the entire nuclear fragment can be removed through a limbal or corneal incision. If an anterior or posterior chamber lens implant has previously been inserted, this must first be removed. It is important to make the incision large enough to allow the nuclear fragment to be removed easily because excessive manipulation in the anterior chamber will further compromise the corneal endothelium. Viscoelastic should be injected into the anterior chamber, after which the nucleus can be floated into the plane of the pupil and removed with, for example, an irrigating vectis.

The peripheral retina should then be carefully examined and any identifiable breaks treated by cryopexy or laser photocoagulation. If retinal detachment has already occurred, then gas tamponade with or without scleral buckling may be required. Approximately half of retinal detachments associated with retained fragments have been observed to develop after vitrectomy.[20–22]

If no retinal complications have been identified, then a lens implant can be inserted at this stage. Should there be insufficient capsule to support a sulcus fixated posterior chamber lens, then either an anterior chamber lens or a scleral sutured posterior chamber lens can be placed. In the presence of retinal problems, lens implantation is best avoided at this stage. Aphakia can be corrected by a contact lens or a secondary lens implant performed as a separate procedure when retinal integrity has been established.

Postoperative management

Following successful removal of dislocated lens fragments, raised intraocular pressure and inflammation usually respond well to topical medication, which can subsequently be withdrawn. Patients with pre-existing glaucoma may be at risk of more sustained elevation of intraocular pressure and require filtration surgery.[22] There is a significant risk of retinal detachment during the postoperative period, of which the patient must be warned and the ophthalmologist should be alert.

166

References

1   Courtney P. The National Cataract Surgery Survey: 1. Method and descriptive features. *Eye* 1992;**6**:487–92.

2   Desai P, Minassian DC, Reidy A. National cataract surgery survey 1997–8: a report of the results of the clinical outcomes. *Br J Ophthalmol* 1999;**83**:1336–40.

3   Browning DJ, Cobo LM. Early experience in extracapsular cataract surgery by residents. *Ophthalmology* 1985;**92**:1647–53.

4   Cruz OA, Wallace GW, Gay CA, Matoba AY, Koch DD. Visual results and complications of phacoemulsification with intraocular lens implantation performed by ophthalmology residents. *Ophthalmology* 1992;**99**:448–52.

5   Heaven CJ, Davison CRN, Boase DL. Learning phacoemulsification; the incidence of complications and the outcome in these cases. *Eur J Implant Refract Surg* 1994;**6**:324–7.

6   Tabandeh H, Smeets B, Teimory M, Seward H. Learning phacoemulsification: the surgeon-in-training. *Eye* 1994;**8**:475–7.

7   Claoue C, Steele A. Visual prognosis following accidental vitreous loss during cataract surgery. *Eye* 1993;**7**:735–9.

8   Frost NA, Sparrow JM, Strong NP, Rosenthal AR. Vitreous loss in planned extracapsular cataract extraction does lead to a poorer visual outcome. *Eye* 1995;**9**:446–51.

9   Ionides A, Minassian D, Tuft S. Visual outcome following posterior capsule rupture during cataract surgery. *Br J Ophthalmol* 2001;**85**:222–4.

10 Lumme P, Laatikainen L. Exfoliation syndrome and cataract extraction. *Am J Ophthalmol* 1993;**116**:51–5.

11 O'Donuel FE, Santos BA. Prospective study of posterior capsule-zonular disruption during extracapsular cataract extraction: eliminating iatrogenic disruption. *J Cataract Refract Surg* 1990;**16**:329–32.

12 Cionni RJ, Osher RH. Endocapsular ring approach to the subluxed cataractous lens. *J Cataract Refract Surg* 1995;**21**:245–9.

13 Ah-Fat FG, Sharma MK, Majid MA, Yang YC. Vitreous loss during conversion from conventional extracapsular cataract extraction to phacoemulsification. *J Cataract Refract Surg* 1998;**24**:801–5.

14 Irvine WD, Flynn HW, Murray TG, Rubsamen PE. Retained lens fragments after phacoemulsification manifesting as marked intraocular inflammation with hypopyon. *Am J Ophthalmol* 1992;**114**:610–4.

15 Kusaka S, Tsujioka M, Mano T, Tsuboi S, Ohashi Y. Two-port vitrectomy for vitreous loss during sutureless cataract surgery. *Am J Ophthalmol* 1994;**117**:533–4.

16 Michelson MA. Use of a Sheets glide as a pseudoposterior capsule in phacoemulsification complicated by posterior capsule rupture. *Eur J Implant Refract Surg* 1993;**5**:70–2.

17 Aaberg TM Jr, Rubsamen PE, Flynn HW Jr, Chang S, Mieler WF, Smiddy WE. Giant retinal tear as a complication of attempted removal of intravitreal lens fragments during cataract surgery. *Am J Ophthalmol* 1997;**124**:222–6.

18 Gilliland GD, Hutton WL, Fuller DG, Topping TM. Retained intravitreal lens fragments after cataract surgery. *Ophthalmology* 1992;**99**:1263–9.

19 Kim JE, Flynn HW Jr, Smiddy WE, *et al.* Retained lens fragments after phacoemulsification. *Ophthalmology* 1994;**101**:1827–32.

20 Borne MJ, Tasman W, Regillo C, Malecha M, Sarin L. Outcomes of vitrectomy for retained lens fragments. *Ophthalmology* 1996;**103**:971–6.

21 Wang D, Briggs MC, Hickey-Dwyer MU, McGalliard JN. Removal of lens fragments from the vitreous cavity. *Eye* 1997;**11**:37–42.

22 Vilar NF, Flynn HW, Smiddy WE, Murray TG, Davis JL, Rubsamen PE. Removal of retained lens fragments after phacoemulsification reverses secondary glaucoma and restores visual acuity. *Ophthalmology* 1997;**104**:787–92.

23 Ansons AM, Atkinson PL, Wang D. A closed microsurgical technique for anterior vitrectomy using a continuous air infusion. *Eye* 1980;**3**:704–5.

24 Bayramlar HS, Hepsen IF, Cekic O, Gunduz A. Comparison of the results of primary and secondary implantation of flexible open-loop anterior chamber intraocular lens. *Eye* 1998;**12**:826–8.

25 Lewis H, Blumenkranz MS, Chang S. Treatment of dislocated crystalline lens and retinal detachment with perfluorocarbon liquids. *Retina* 1992;**12**:299–304.

12 Postoperative complications

The wide variety of postoperative complications following cataract surgery are summarised in Table 12.1.

Table 12.1 Postoperative complications

Complication	Examples
Infection	Endophthalmitis
Haemorrhage	Hyphaema
	Uveitis–glaucoma–hyphaema syndrome
	Suprachoroidal haemorrhage
Raised intraocular pressure/glaucoma	Open angle
	Viscoelastic induced
	Steroid related
	α-Chymotrypsin induced
	Retained lens matter
	Closed angle
	Pupil block
	Malignant glaucoma (aqueous misdirection)
	Rubeosis
	Chronic uveitis
	Epithelial ingrowth
Wound related	Wound leak/dehiscence
	Suture related/surgically induced astigmatism
	Sclerokeratitis/corneal melt
Corneal	Oedema
	Endothelial trauma
	Intraocular lens or vitreous touch
	Brown–McClean
	Toxicity
	Descemet's membrane detachment
Intraocular lens related	Capsule opacification
	Decentration and subluxation
	Refractive error
Retinal	Macula oedema
	Retinal detachment
	Retinal light toxicity
Miscellaneous	Atonic pupil
	Ptosis

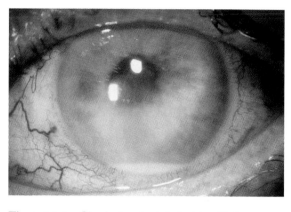

Figure 12.1   Classical endophthalmitis with hypopyon.

Endophthalmitis

Intraocular infection (endophthalmitis) is a devastating complication of cataract surgery (Figure 12.1) that shows no signs of eradication. Although the incidence is low, occurring in between 0·1 and 0·3% of cases,[1,2] it remains one of the most feared complications because of its unpredictability and variable response to treatment. Consideration of endophthalmitis as a possible differential diagnosis in eyes with postoperative inflammation is crucial to early diagnosis and the implementation of appropriate treatment in order to minimise the risk of a poor visual outcome. Endophthalmitis occurring within the first 6 weeks is termed "acute", and endophthalmitis presenting more than 6 weeks after surgery is termed "chronic" or "delayed".

Table 12.2   Risk factors for endophthalmitis

Risk factors	Examples
Preoperative	Ocular surface disease
	Keratoconjunctivitis sicca
	Blepharitis
	Rosacea
	Atopic blepharoconjunctivitis
	Lid malposition
	Entropion
	Poor eyelid closure
	Previous ocular surgery
	Corneal graft
	Trabeculectomy
	Nasolacrimal disease
	Partial obstruction
	Subclinical dacryocystitis
	Systemic
	Diabetes mellitus
	Immunosuppressive therapy
	Advanced age
	Male sex
Intra-operative	Inadequate ocular surface disinfection
	Inadequate isolation of the surgical field
	Vitreous loss
	Inappropriate handling of instruments and materials
	Inadequate cleansing of non-disposable equipment
	Contamination of intraocular fluids, viscoelastics, or lens implants
	Poor wound construction
Postoperative	Wound leak
	Iris prolapse
	Vitreous wick
	Removal or breakage of corneal sutures
	Systemic infection
	Poor personal hygiene

Pathogenesis and risk factors

Risk factors for endophthalmitis are listed in Table 12.2.

Bacteria can be isolated from the surgical field during cataract surgery and from intraocular fluids even in the presence of adequate surface disinfection and draping of the eyelids.[3] Most endophthalmitis is due to commensals from the ocular surface,[4] but on occasion bacteria or fungi may be introduced from contaminated fluids,[5] intraocular lenses (IOLs),[6,7] and cataract equipment,[8] or from distal sites of infection.[2]

Pre-existing ocular surface disease, blepharitis and eyelid malposition, and nasolacrimal infection are well recognised risk factors for endophthalmitis. These should be corrected where possible before consideration of cataract surgery. Occult nasolacrimal obstruction without evidence of infection is common in patients undergoing cataract surgery and does not require any additional measures. Systemic immunosuppressive treatment, diabetes mellitus, advanced age, and male sex have also been found to be statistically significant risk factors for endophthalmitis.

Intraoperative risk factors for endophthalmitis include capsule rupture with vitreous loss necessitating anterior vitrectomy, secondary versus primary IOL implantation,[2] poor wound construction and wound leak, and ocular surface contact of the IOL implant during insertion.[7] Intracapsular cataract extraction is associated with an increased risk of endophthalmitis,[9] but there is no evidence for any significant difference in risk between small incision phacoemulsification and extracapsular cataract surgery.

Incidence

The reported incidence of endophthalmitis in cataract surgery is variable but most commonly within the range 0·1–0·5%.[1,2,9] It is likely that the true incidence of endophthalmitis is underestimated because of the combination of failure to isolate the infecting organism, variable follow up of patients, and on some occasions self-limiting disease.

Prevention

The most common source of the infecting organisms in eyes without other identifiable risk factors is the ocular surface,[4] and hence most prophylactic measures have been directed toward this.

Preoperative administration of topical antibiotics has been shown to reduce the numbers of organisms in the conjunctival sac,[10] but this effect is short lived. In addition, the administration of topical antibiotics may selectively increase the numbers of resistant organisms on the ocular surface. Preoperative eye cultures have no significant predictive value because many healthy eyes have been demonstrated to harbour *Staphylococcus aureus* and other potential intraocular pathogens.[11] As a consequence, the routine administration of preoperative antibiotic eye drops has fallen out of favour, other than in eyes with manifest risk factors such as blepharitis or chronic nasolacrimal infection, in which their benefit is unproven. Routine use of preoperative norfloxacin was not shown to reduce the incidence of

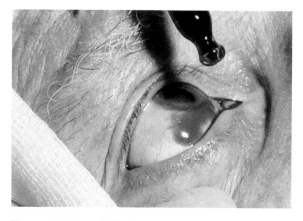

Figure 12.2 5% Povidine iodine placed into the conjunctival sac before surgery.

aqueous contamination in one study.[12] Ocular surface disinfection at the time of surgery with 5% povidone iodine (Figure 12.2) significantly reduces bacterial counts[13,14] and the risk of endophthalmitis,[15] and this is considered the most reliable method of surface decontamination for intraocular surgery. Isolation of the eyelids and eyelashes from the surgical field by careful draping is advisable (Figure 12.3), and unnecessary contact of instruments or lens implants with the ocular surface should be avoided.

Addition of antibiotics to infusion fluids has been shown to reduce the incidence of positive cultures from aqueous fluids at the end of surgery,[16,17] but there is little evidence to show a real reduction in the risk of endophthalmitis with this strategy. A persuasive argument against the unnecessary use of vancomycin in a hospital setting is the increasing spread of resistance to vancomycin among bacteria, and the problem of methicillin resistant *S. aureus* (MRSA).

Addition of heparin[18,19] to the infusion or use of heparin surface modified lens implants[20] is reported to be associated with less intraocular inflammation. However, these theoretical benefits have not been shown to have a significant effect on the incidence of endophthalmitis.

Postoperative administration of antibiotics via the topical or subconjunctival route has little

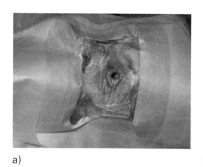
a)

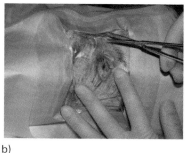
b)

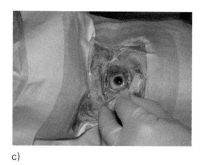
c)

Figure 12.3   Draping the eye. (a) The drape (BD Ophthalmic Systems) is applied to remove the lashes from the operative field. (b) An aperture is cut through the drape in the palpebral aperture. (c) A speculum is carefully inserted to ensure the edges of the cut drape fold around the lid margins.

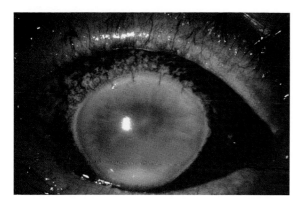

Figure 12.4 Endophthalmitis with hypopyon after extracapsular cataract surgery.

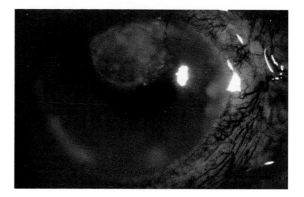

Figure 12.5 Bacterial endophthalmitis with keratitis.

proof of benefit other than in exceptional circumstances. Many surgeons have stopped using subconjunctival antibiotic injections after uncomplicated cataract surgery without detriment, and the same is likely to apply to antibiotic drops. Unfortunately, the fear of endophthalmitis and possible litigation perpetuates old habits, and it likely that postoperative antibiotic drop use will persist for some time.

In conclusion, it should be borne in mind that there is no absolutely certain and reliable method of preventing endophthalmitis, and that every ophthalmic surgeon can expect to deal with this condition at some time in their career. It is therefore incumbent on all ophthalmologists to have a well defined strategy of management of eyes suspected to have developed intraocular infection following intraocular surgery.[21]

Diagnosis

Clinical presentation (Figure 12.4)

It is crucial to maintain a high index of suspicion during after care for the cataract surgery patient. Early diagnosis of endophthalmitis is dependent on the awareness and detection of the often subtle and non-specific symptoms and signs of inflammation in the postoperative period. This is especially important in infections caused by organisms of lower virulence, in which the severity and speed of

onset may be much less. In the Endophthalmitis Vitrectomy Study,[22] blurred vision, conjunctival injection, pain, and lid swelling were the predominant presenting symptoms in order of prevalence. However, the absence of ocular pain or hypopyon did not exclude a diagnosis of endophthalmitis, these being present in only 75% of patients in that study.[23]

The presence of significant intraocular inflammation in an eye after cataract surgery or secondary lens implantation always requires an explanation. It should always be remembered that major intraoperative complications such as capsule rupture with vitreous loss are associated with an increased risk of endophthalmitis, and so it is unwise to attribute postoperative inflammation to additional surgical trauma alone.

Eyes that require manipulation of the iris, for example posterior synechie in uveitis eyes, are also likely to have greater postoperative inflammation, but they may also occasionally develop endophthalmitis and so it is essential to be vigilant. The earlier and the greater the severity of the signs of inflammation after surgery, the more virulent an infecting organism is likely to be.[24] Streptococci, S. aureus, and Gram negative organisms are common pathogens in endophthalmitis, which presents within the first two days after surgery and is often associated with corneal infiltrates (Figure 12.5),

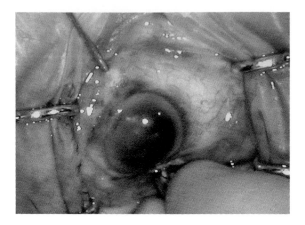

Figure 12.6 Vitreous biopsy with vitrector during vitrectomy.

wound abnormalities, a relative afferent pupil defect, loss of red reflex or view of the fundus, and profound visual loss.[24]

As soon as the diagnosis of endophthalmitis has been considered, it is necessary to investigate and treat the patient accordingly. Because endophthalmitis cannot be unequivocally excluded by negative investigations,[25] a mild to moderately inflamed eye after cataract surgery may be treated with intensive anti-inflammatory therapy (topical steroids with or without non-steroidal anti-inflammatory agents) under close clinical supervision for 24–48 hours. However, if there is any suggestion of deterioration then an endophthalmitis protocol should be initiated. The endophthalmitis management protocol should include the following:

- Tissue samples: aqueous and vitreous biopsy (Figure 12.6)
- Corneal, conjunctival, and wound scrapes if clinically infected
- Gram and periodic acid–schiff stain of the above
- Microbiology cultures, both aerobic and anaerobic, and fungal plates
- Where available, polymerase chain reaction analysis of aqueous and vitreous fluids

- Intravitreal broad spectrum antibiotics
- Fibrinolytic agents if there is extensive fibrin deposition in the anterior chamber.

Differential diagnosis

The differential diagnosis of endophthalmitis includes the following.

- Non-infectious inflammation. The distinction may only be evident in hindsight because there is no absolutely reliable method of excluding infection from sterile, endogenous inflammation.
- Lens induced uveitis. This encompasses the terms "phacoanaphylactic uveitis" and "phacotoxic uveitis", which represent an immune mediated reaction to lens protein of varying severity. It differs from phacolytic glaucoma, in which where macrophages are characteristically full of lens protein that has been phagocytosed. Lens material may be sequestered in the capsular bag or drainage angle, or fragments of lens nucleus may fall into the vitreous cavity if capsule rupture occurs. This diagnosis may only be evident if gonioscopy is performed or vitrectomy is undertaken.
- Toxic lens syndrome. This rather non-specific term has been applied to the inflammatory reaction associated with poorly manufactured or sterilised IOL implants. This is extremely rare now but should always be considered if more than one case of endophthalmitis develops in a unit within a few days or weeks. For this reason, it is essential to have good clinical records that allow IOL use to be quickly traced to individual patients.

Tissue sampling and analysis

Aqueous biopsy An aqueous tap can be easily performed with the patient sitting at the slit lamp under topical anaesthesia with amethocaine or a similar anaesthetic agent.

Following instillation of 5% povidone iodine drops into the conjunctival fornices, 100–200 μl of aqueous should be aspirated using an insulin syringe, which combines a sharp 27-guage needle with minimum dead space. Although vitreous samples are more likely to yield a positive culture, aqueous may occasionally be the only positive source.[21]

Vitreous biopsy (Figure 12.6) Vitreous biopsy with a needle or mechanized cutter (vitrector) is equally effective.[26] The Endophthalmitis Vitrectomy Study[22] showed that pars plana vitrectomy was only beneficial when the visual acuity was poorer than hand movements, and thus the majority of endophthalmitis cases can be managed without primary vitrectomy. A needle tap may be performed under topical, subconjunctival, or other local anaesthetic using a 2–5 ml syringe and 23- to 27-guage needle, providing a sample of 250–500 μl. In the pseudophakic eye, the needle should be inserted 4 mm behind the limbus.

Pars plan vitrectomy facilitates the collection of a larger vitreous sample and, in addition, the vitreous infusion fluid can be collected and filtered to assist with the detection of organisms. Vitrectomy in these severely infected eyes is technically demanding, and does not improve the visual outcome except in eyes with vision poorer than hand movements.[22]

Intravitreal antibiotics should be administered after all ocular samples have been obtained.

Wound and corneal cultures Scrapes of infected wounds or cornea should be obtained by conventional methods and may provide valuable results.

Conjunctival cultures Cultures from the conjunctiva may yield organisms but these may not be relevant to the intraocular pathogen. Okhravi *et al.*[20] noted that only in three out of ten culture positive cases did the conjunctival organism correspond with the vitreous cultures, and all were coagulase negative staphylococci.

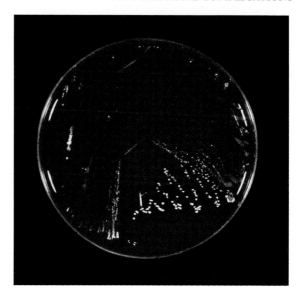

Figure 12.7 *Propionibacterium acnes* growth after anaerobic culture

Microbiology It is advisable to liaise with microbiology colleagues as closely as possible because they have the greatest experience in the preparation of cultures and handling the specimens that may be of very limited volume.

It is important to perform aerobic and anaerobic cultures of specimens, particularly in cases of delayed endophthalmitis, in which there is a high incidence of *Propionibacterium acnes* infection. Culture media may include blood and chocolate blood agar (Figure 12.7), Robertson's cooked meat broth, brain heart infusion broth, and thioglycolate broth.[21] If microbiology assistance and culture plates are unavailable, then ocular specimens can be injected into blood culture bottles with successful results.[27]

Polymerase chain reaction The identification of DNA and RNA from infecting organisms by the application of polymerase chain reaction is likely to be increasingly helpful in the next few years.[28–32] These techniques have been shown to detect bacterial and fungal DNA reliably in cases of culture proven endophthalmitis, and to distinguish between species of bacteria. Furthermore, polymerase chain reaction may assist in the early identification of microbial resistance to antibiotics.

Treatment

Antibiotic therapy

Intravitreal antibiotic injection Intravitreal antibiotic injections are mandatory for effective management of acute postoperative endophthalmitis. All other routes of administration (topical, subconjunctival, intravenous, or oral) should be considered adjuncts only. The antibiotics should be bactericidal and effective against the range of likely infecting organisms, which include staphylococci (S. aureus and S. epidermidis), Streptococci, Haemophilus, Spp., Neisseria, Spp., Proteus Spp., Pseudomonas Spp., Enterococcus Spp., Bacillus Spp., and Propionibacterium Spp. Because no single antibiotic provides adequate cover against this spectrum of organisms, combined treatment with two agents is necessary until positive cultures (at least two plates or other media) have been obtained to guide the optimum choice of therapy. The most useful choices of antibiotics[21,22,33,34] are vancomycin 1–2 mg in 100 µl plus ceftazidime 2·25 mg in 100 µl, or vancomycin 1–2 mg in 100 µl plus amikacin 400 µg in 100 µl.

The antibiotics must not be mixed together in the same syringe for intravitreal injection. During intravitreal injection of antibiotic, it is recommended to aim the needle away from the macula to minimise the risk of macular damage. It is advisable for the antibiotics to be prepared by an experienced pharmacologist to avoid the risk of error in diluting antibiotic solutions.

Gentamicin is toxic to the macula,[35] and there is little if any justification for its use now as an intravitreal drug except where no other alternative is available or positive intraocular cultures mandate its use. If gentamicin administration proves necessary, then it is essential to obtain written, fully informed consent from the patient beforehand explaining

the risks of this agent. Amikacin is also associated with a risk of macular toxicity, but this is much less than with gentamicin.[36] Alternative treatment with intravitreal ceftazidime provides a similar range of antibacterial cover without this additional risk, but without the synergistic activity of vancomycin and amikacin against Staphylococcus, Streptococcus, and Enterococcus spp.[37,38]

If fungal infection is considered a possibility, then amphotericin B 5 µg in 100 µl should be administered in addition to antibacterial therapy.

Systemic antibiotics The Endophthalmitis Vitrectomy Study did not show any additional benefit from intravenous administration of amikacin or ceftazidime. Ceftazidime has been shown to achieve therapeutic levels within the vitreous, particularly in aphakic, vitrectomised, or inflamed eyes, but not in normal eyes.[33] Ciprofloxacin has been shown to cross the blood–retina barrier in normal eyes, but the levels achieved may be insufficient to treat the common spectrum of infecting organisms.[39–41]

Topical and subconjunctival antibiotics It is unlikely that these routes of administration confer any additional clinical benefits when intravitreal antibiotic injections have been performed. Neither route provides good ocular penetration even in an inflamed eye, and intensive topical therapy or uncomfortable subconjunctival injections may only increase the distress and discomfort for the patient. If used, the choice of topical antibiotics, should be the same as the intravitreal and systemic antibiotics which usually requires antibiotic eye drops to be specially prepared by the hospital pharmacy.

Steroid therapy

Endophthalmitis is usually associated with severe intraocular inflammation that may persist even when the infecting organism is successfully eradicated by antibiotic therapy. It is uncertain how much ocular damage may result from the inflammatory process as distinct from infection mediated ocular injury, but systemic steroids have been used empirically in combination with antibiotic therapy in endophthalmitis. For example, a course of oral prednisolone commencing 24 hours after intravitreal antibiotic injection starting with a dose of 60 mg/day (and rapidly tapered). Unfortunately, the perceived benefits from the use of systemic steroids in endophthalmitis have not been reliably confirmed by randomised clinical trials.

The Endophthalmitis Vitrectomy Study did not investigate the value of systemic steroids or intravitreal steroid injection in endophthalmitis. Shah et al.[42] showed that the use of intravitreal steroids was associated with a poorer visual outcome than when steroids were not used, whereas Das et al.[43] showed that intravitreal dexamethasone administration resulted in less intraocular inflammation but without any beneficial effect on visual outcome. Animal studies of intravitreal steroids in experimental endophthalmitis have shown a reduction in intraocular inflammation and a reduction in retinal injury.

Topical steroids may be administered after antibiotic therapy has been commenced. Although intensive (hourly or more frequent) administration is often advocated, there is little published evidence of significant clinical benefit, and it is suggested that the steroid dose be managed according to clinical progress. It is likely that steroid drop frequency of more than every two hours by day has little clinical value, particularly when fibrinolytic therapy is utilised to treat intraocular fibrin (see below).

Mydriatic treatment

Miosis is a major management problem in eyes with endophthalmitis, and the use of subconjunctivally administered mydriatics such as Mydricaine® (Moorfields Eye Hospital) or equivalent may be helpful, especially when combined with fibrinolytic therapy (see below). This can then be followed by use of a regular topical mydriatic.

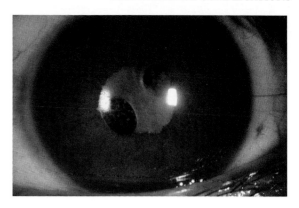

Figure 12.8 Pupillary membrane following endophthalmitis. This can be prevented by recombinant tissue plasminogen activator.

Fibrinolytic therapy

The management of intraocular fibrin deposition (Figure 12.8) has been revolutionised by the availability of recombinant tissue plasminogen activator (TPA).[44] Intracameral administration of 10–25 µg leads to rapid dissolution of fibrin, allowing dilatation of the pupil, lysis of synechiae, and improved visualisation of the posterior segment. Although expensive, recombinant tissue plasminogen activator may be aliquotted into insulin syringes ready for use and stored frozen at −30°C.

Postoperative management

Postoperative management is tailored to the individual and according to clinical progress. In general, once there is evidence of clinical improvement, antibiotic and anti-inflammatory therapy can be tapered down, usually over a period of weeks.

Failure to improve or documented deterioration may necessitate repeat ocular sampling and intravitreal antibiotics. Other factors that might contribute to increasing visual failure such as retinal detachment should be considered, and B-scan ultrasound may be very helpful.

Persistent opacification of ocular media such as pupillary membranes, lens capsule thickening,

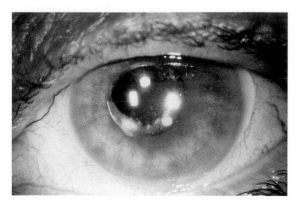

Figure 12.9 *Propionibacterium acnes* endophthalmitis with capsular infiltrates and central capsulotomy.

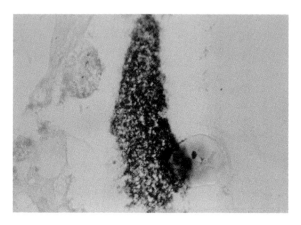

Figure 12.10 Viable *Propionibacterium acnes* organisms in lens capsule after vancomycin treatment.

and vitreous turbidity may require specific surgical intervention when the intraocular infection has been controlled and the eye is quiet. As a general principle, it is best to defer any further surgery until all signs of cellular activity have settled, although this may not always be possible.

Delayed postoperative endophthalmitis

This condition has been increasingly recognised during the past two decades as a significant cause of postoperative inflammation and visual morbidity in eyes with otherwise uncomplicated surgery. It is characterised by low grade inflammation with keratic precipitates, aqueous cells, and white plaques on the posterior lens capsule (Figure 12.9). Hypopyon is uncommon but may occur after yttrium aluminium garnet (Nd:YAG) laser capsulotomy, when the diagnosis is likely to be obvious.

The most common pathogen causing this syndrome is *Propionibacterium acnes*, but the clinical picture may also be caused by coagulase negative *Staphylococcus epidermidis* and, less commonly, by other organisms such as *Bacillus licheniformis*. Fungal endophthalmitis after cataract surgery is typically indolent but without the typical capsular changes seen in *P. acnes* infection, and may be caused by *Candida* spp. or *Peicilomyces* spp. The major difference in

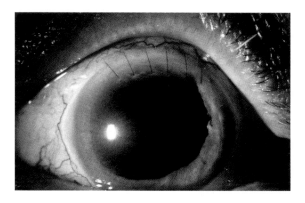

Figure 12.11 Lens removal and capsulectomy from patient in Figure 12.9.

management between acute and delayed endophthalmitis is that vitrectomy with capsular biopsy is often required to confirm the diagnosis in the delayed pattern and to treat the condition effectively.[45] Viable organisms can be sequestered in the lens capsule (Figure 12.10) despite intravitreal vancomycin therapy, to which the responsible organisms are almost invariably susceptible in vitro. For this reason, as much capsule as possible should be removed at the primary vitrectomy to minimise the risk of recurrence. Should recurrence occur, it is advisable to remove the IOL implant and perform a complete capsulectomy (Figure 12.11), following which an IOL can be replaced in the

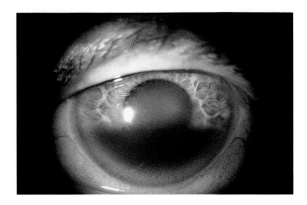

Figure 12.12   Postoperative hyphaema.

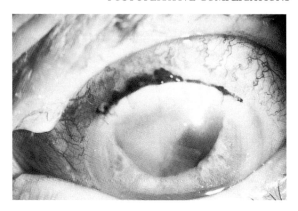

Figure 12.13   Suprachoroidal haemorrhage with iris incarcerated in the wound.

form of an anterior chamber lens or a suture supported lens either as a primary or secondary procedure.

Haemorrhage

Hyphaema and uveitis–glaucoma–hyphaema syndrome (Figure 12.12)

Hyphaema following cataract surgery is commonly a result of iris root bleeding from a deep posterior corneoscleral incision. Patients with Fuchs' heterchromic cyclitis have abnormal angle blood vessels that may cause a hyphaema, either after cataract extraction or following anterior chamber paracentesis.[46] In most cases postoperative hyphaema is mild and resolves spontaneously, but the intraocular pressure (IOP) should be monitored. Failure to respond to medical treatment may require an anterior chamber washout to prevent corneal blood staining. Low dose recombinant tissue plasminogen activator (TPA) can be successful in treating persistent hyphaema with uncontrolled IOP.[47]

Hyphaema that occurs many months after cataract surgery is usually caused by wound vascularisation or erosion of the iris by the IOL. Wound vascularisation may be detected by gonioscopy and is treated with argon laser.[48] Erosion or chaffing of the iris by the IOL is unusual with modern lenses. Hyphaema in these circumstances is often present with uveitis and glaucoma as part of the uveitis–glaucoma–hyphaema (UGH) syndrome.[49] Iris supported lenses and rigid anterior chamber lenses used in the past that were poorly finished and underwent warpage were commonly associated with the UGH syndrome. Contact between the iris and the sharp irregular edges of the IOL causes erosion of the iris, breakdown of the blood–aqueous barrier, and chronic inflammation. Modern lenses have much better surface qualities and UGH syndrome is now rare, although it has been reported as a complication of an unstable sulcus supported IOL.[50] Medical treatment with pressure lowering and topical corticosteroids may succeed in the short term, but ultimately lens removal or exchange is usually required.

Suprachoroidal haemorrhage

Fortunately, sudden bleeding into the space external to the choroid (i.e. suprachoroidal haemorrhage) is an infrequent complication of cataract extraction, occurring in 0·1% of operations in a large UK series.[51] The process may progress very rapidly, causing an expulsive haemorrhage in which much of the ocular contents may be expelled with disastrous results (Figure 12.13). Warning signs of suprachoroidal haemorrhage include loss of the red reflex, shallowing of the anterior chamber, iris prolapse, and vitreous loss. Rapid wound closure with 7/0 or stronger sutures is required, and if this proves impossible then relieving sclerostomies may be required. These are made over the site of the haemorrhage or 5–7 mm posterior to the ora serrata.

Suprachoroidal haemorrhage is thought to result from sudden hypotony, which causes bending and then rupture of sclerotic arteries as they cross the suprachoroidal space. During extracapsular and intracapsular surgery, the large incision rapidly decompresses the anterior chamber with loss of IOP. In contrast, the small self-sealing incision used in phacoemulsification permits the maintenance of positive pressure in the anterior chamber during surgery, therefore reducing the risks and effects of suprachoroidal haemorrhage. Other risk factors associated with suprachoroidal haemorrhage include glaucoma, myopia, intraocular inflammation, age, and hypertension.

Delayed suprachoroidal haemorrhage is less common than intraoperative suprachoroidal haemorrhage, and presents with pain, loss of vision, and shallowing of the anterior chamber. Its aetiology is unclear, but it may be the result of a sudden episode of hypotony or choroidal effusion. Choroidal effusion, usually a result of low IOP, is caused by exudation of fluid from vessels of the choroid, which may place tension on suprachoriodal veins or arteries that finally rupture.

The management of suprachoroidal haemorrhage depends on its site, size, and timing. Delayed suprachoroidal haemorrhage is typically smaller and generally has a better visual prognosis.[52] In these circumstances, careful observation, topical steroids, and treatment to control IOP may be all that is required. As mentioned above, scleral incisions may be indicated during an acute haemorrhage. Large collections that cause apposition between the retina ("kissing choroidals") have a poor prognosis and require surgery. This is typically performed seven to ten days after presentation using a three-port pars plana vitrectomy with silicone oil tamponade and scleral incisions to drain the blood.

Raised intraocular pressure and glaucoma

Open angle glaucoma

Rises in IOP are common within 48 hours following cataract surgery, occurring in nearly 8% of patients.[51] Typically, these are transient and related to retained viscoelastic (see Chapter 7). In patients with a compromised trabecular meshwork, such as primary open angle glaucoma, the pressure rise may be accentuated. In such cases, prophylactic treatment with either a topical β-blocker or an oral carbonic anhydrase inhibitor is advisable.

The topical steroids routinely used following cataract surgery can cause an increased IOP in susceptible individuals (typically two to three weeks after commencing treatment). Patients at higher risk include those with primary open angle glaucoma or a family history of it. Because the pressure rise is determined by the frequency and efficacy of the steroid,[53] these cases may benefit from a less potent steroid following surgery. However, in the majority of patients the IOP will return to normal on cessation of treatment.

Retained lens matter may also cause an increase in IOP after surgery. This is usually associated with uveitis and may result from incomplete cortical clean up or, more commonly, posterior capsule rupture and a dropped nucleus or lens fragment. As discussed above, this cause of uveitis should be distinguished from endopthalmitis. In mild cases medical treatment may suffice; however, surgery may be required to remove residual lens matter (see Chapter 11).

A postoperative hyphaema may occasionally cause an increased IOP by red blood cell blockage of the trabecular meshwork. In these circumstances medical treatment is usually all that is required, although occasionally an anterior chamber washout is necessary. Vitreous haemorrhage can cause ghost cell glaucoma, and treatment in these patients may also require a vitrectomy.

An increase in IOP is common following intracapsular cataract extraction in which α-chymotrysin has been used.[54] This is thought to be caused by zonule fragments blocking the trabecular meshwork and may be prevented by irrigation of the anterior chamber before lens cryoextraction. Use of a low volume and concentration of α-chymotrysin also reduces the risk of a postoperative pressure rise.[55]

Narrow angle glaucoma

The majority of closed or narrow angle glaucoma following cataract extraction is the result of pupil block. Nonetheless, it is a rare complication, occurring in only 0·03% of cataract extractions.[51] Aqueous that is unable to pass through the pupil is trapped in the posterior chamber and forces the peripheral iris against the cornea, blocking the angle. On examination, the IOP is typically increased and the anterior chamber shallowed with iris bombe. Pupil block is an unusual complication following posterior chamber IOL implantation but is more common with anterior chamber lens implants or aphakia (in which the hyaloid face or posterior capsule blocks the pupil).[56] It may also occur if a substantial volume of air is left in the anterior chamber at the end of surgery. A prophylactic periperal iridectomy should always be performed as part of an intracapsular cataract extraction or where an anterior chamber IOL is used (see Chapter 8). Pupil block may still occur, however, if inflammatory exudate, vitreous, or a ciliary body process blocks the iridectomy. Pupil block is treated initially with medical management followed by neodymium Nd:YAG laser peripheral iridotomy or a surgical iridectomy. In long-standing cases of pupil block, permanent peripheral anterior synechiae (PAS) may develop and the IOP may not be controlled, requiring long term topical medication or glaucoma drainage surgery.

Table 12.3   Causes of post-operative anterior chamber shallowing

Cause	Typical IOP	Diagnostic features
Wound leak	Low	Seidel positive
Pupil block	Raised	Iris bombe
Suprachoroidal haemorrhage	Raised	Altered red reflex
Malignant glaucoma (aqueous misdirection)	Raised	Lack of iris bombe Luscent zone in anterior vitreous

IOP, intraocular pressure.

Alternative causes of raised IOP and a shallow anterior chamber should be considered in the differential diagnosis of pupil block glaucoma (Table 12.3). Malignant glaucoma is a rare complication of cataract surgery and is more often associated with trabeculectomy or combined cataract and glaucoma surgery. Also known as aqueous misdirection syndrome, malignant glaucoma is typically a result of anterior chamber shallowing caused by a wound leak in the early postoperative period. The normal aqueous drainage pathway is disrupted and aqueous is diverted into the vitreous, forcing the lens iris diaphagrm anteriorly. This further shallows the anterior chamber, closing the angle and perpetuating the aqueous misdirection. Like pupil block glaucoma, the anterior chamber is shallow but there is a lack of iris bombe and there may be a luscent zone of sequestered aqueous visible behind the capsule or hyaloid face. Treatment of malignant glaucoma is initially with mydriasis and medical treatment to reduce the IOP. Breaking the capsule and anterior hyaloid with a Nd:YAG laser is then usually effective,[57] but a vitrectomy may be necessary.[58]

Narrow angle glaucoma following cataract surgery may also follow the formation of PAS, which can occur in chronic uveitis, rubeosis, or epithelial down-growth. As discussed in Chapter 10, rubeosis or iris new vessels can affect diabetics following cataract surgery. PAS have also been associated with anterior vaulted posterior chamber lens implants placed in the

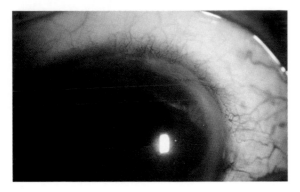

Figure 12.14 Epithelial down-growth following phacoemulsification complicated by a wound leak.

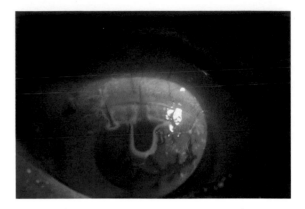

Figure 12.15 A Seidel positive wound leak.

ciliary sulcus.[59] Epithelial down-growth is a rare complication of cataract extraction that is usually the result of a postoperative aqueous wound leak. This allows ocular surface epithelial cells to grow into the anterior chamber, which may be seen as a translucent membrane with a slowly advancing edge on the iris surface and endothelium (Figure 12.14). Epithelial down-growth is usually associated with a chronic uveitis and, although the angle is open at first, PAS rapidly form causing a rise in IOP. The down-growth may be difficult to see, but unlike normal iris tissue a blanching response occurs when argon laser is applied to it.[60] An anterior chamber paracentesis[61] and specular microscopy may also be helpful in establishing the diagnosis.[62] Management is difficult, often requiring a combination of excision of affected tissue[63] and cryotherapy.[64]

Wound related complications

Wound leak/dehiscence

Compared with a well constructed phacoemulsification, which is extremely strong,[65] the large incision used in extracapsular or intracapular surgery is less robust and watertight. If the eye is subjected to significant blunt trauma, or if suturing technique is poor, then a large wound may either dehisce, with prolapse of intraocular contents, or allow aqueous

Table 12.4 Causes of post-operative hypotony

Cause	Diagnostic features
Wound leak	Seidel positive
Filtering bleb	Seidel negative
Ciliary body disdisinsertion	
Cyclodialysis	Gonioscopic cleft
Choroidal effusion	Indirect ophthalmoscopy
(anterior)	or B-scan ultrasound appearance
Retinal detachment	Indirect ophthalmoscopy or B-scan ultrasound appearance

leak.[66] This increases the risk of endophthalmitis and, in the long term, intractable glaucoma due to epithelial down-growth. In a large UK study,[51] wound leak or dehiscence was noted in 1·2% of cases during the first two days after cataract extraction.

All patients who have undergone large incision cataract surgery should be examined using 2% fluorescein and a cobalt blue light in the early postoperative period (Figure 12.15). Leaking aqueous dilutes the fluorescein, which then fluoresces (a positive Seidel test). A wound leak may be intermittent, and a low IOP after surgery should be distinguished from other conditions associated with hypotony (Table 12.4). If the incision is posterior to the limbus, then examination may reveal a conjunctival filtering bleb. Gonioscopy, indirect ophthalmoscopy, and

B-scan ultrasound are useful in detecting ciliary body disinsertion or retinal detachment. The latter is particularly important because it may be confused with a choroidal detachment caused by a low IOP after cataract surgery.

The treatment of a wound leak depends on its severity, the anterior chamber depth, and the time elapsed after surgery. If the anterior chamber is formed, then padding the eye or inserting a large diameter bandage contact lens may resolve a slow or moderate aqueous leak. Reducing aqueous production using a carbonic anhydrase inhibitor or topical β-blocker can reduce leakage, and minimising steroid use may also promote healing. A persistent or severe leak should be treated with early wound resuturing, whereas anterior chamber loss with lens–corneal touch or iris tissue prolapsed into the wound requires immediate intervention. In the absence of hypotony, infection, or a shallow anterior chamber, a filtering bleb can usually be observed. If this is not the case, then wound revision or manoeuvres to promote scarring can be attempted, such as those used to reduce over-drainage from a trabeculectomy bleb. Following traumatic wound dehiscence, early wound repair is ideal. Prolapsed iris tissue should be reposited or excised, and vitrectomy may be required.

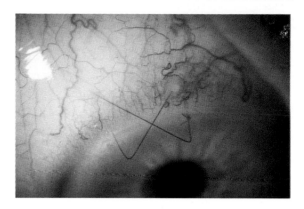

Figure 12.16   Suture inflammation.

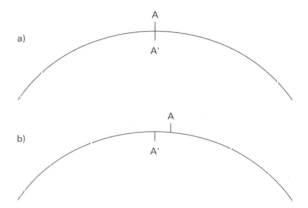

Figure 12.17   Translational malposition. (a) Correct. (b) Incorrect.

Suture complications and surgically induced astigmatism

Following large incision cataract surgery, non-absorbable corneal sutures, particularly those made of nylon, are best removed once the wound is stable (typically ten weeks after surgery).[67] This is performed with a needle and forceps under topical anaesthesia at the slit lamp, and followed by a one week course of topical antibiotics.[68] Broken sutures give rise to a foreign body sensation, and if suture track inflammation develops then pain may occur in association with localised infiltration and hyperaemia (Figure 12.16). If sutures are left in situ long term, presentation to eye casualty many months or years after surgery is common. If neglected, this may cause bacterial keratitis or endopthalmitis.

Incision type, site, and size are the key determinants of surgically induced astigmatism (SIA) following phacoemulsification, which is discussed in detail in Chapter 2. Suture placement and suture tension are additional factors that account for the relatively high incidence of astigmatism after large incision cataract surgery.[69] Inaccurate suture placement may permit translational malposition of the wound (Figure 12.17); however, this can be reduced by using preplaced sutures. Loose or tight sutures may give rise to areas of wound gape (Figure 12.18) or bunching with corneal

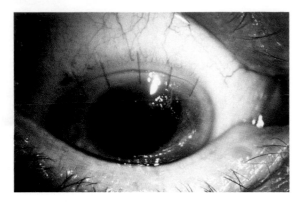

Figure 12.18 Loose sutures in a gaping wound (as seen in Figure 12.15).

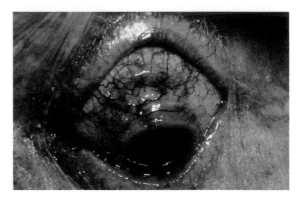

Figure 12.19 Surgically induced necrotising sclerokeratitis (SINS).

striae, respectively. Both alter the normal corneal shape and may predispose to wound leakage. A tight suture causes steepening of the cornea with increased corneal power in the same meridian as the suture. A superior incision closed with tight sutures therefore typically causes "with the rule" astigmatism (plus cylinder at 90°). Removal of a tight suture or sutures, approximately ten weeks after surgery, can reduce excessive with the rule SIA. Refraction and the position of corneal tension lines act as guides to the location of tight sutures, although corneal topography may be required in more complex cases. In contrast, loose sutures cause flattening of the cornea, a minus cylinder, and usually "against the rule" astigmatism (plus cylinder at 180°). These sutures may require removal before ten weeks because of the potential for suture track inflammation and intraocular infection. Unfortunately, any against the rule SIA is likely to become worse after suture removal. If this is excessive and cannot easily be corrected with spectacles, then the wound may need to be resutured or a refractive surgical technique may be required, for example astigmatic keratotomy.

Sclerokeratitis/corneal melt

Surgically induced necrotising sclerokeratitis (SINS) is a rare, potentially devastating complication of cataract surgery (Figure 12.19).[70]

It is unusual for it to present in the immediate postoperative period, and it typically occurs many months after surgery. The aetiology of SINS is thought to be an autoimmune hypersensitivity reaction that causes a vasculitis. It is often associated with systemic collagen diseases and is more common in eyes that have undergone more than one surgical procedure. Corneal or scleral necrosis commences in close proximity to the ocular wound, but the inflammatory process may progress to include the entire globe. Although SINS is usually treatable, late diagnosis is associated with poor visual outcome. Occasionally, patients respond to treatment with non-steroidal anti-inflammatory drugs, but more commonly, high dose systemic steroids are required. Typically these are then used as maintainance therapy for months or years, and other cytotoxic immunosuppression may be necessary. In severe cases of SINS, ocular perforation may occur and this requires excision of affected tissue with tectonic repair. Prophylactic steroid treatment should be used when any further ocular surgery is performed.

Corneal complications

Epithelial and stromal oedema

During cataract surgery several mechanisms may lead to endothelial injury, including direct trauma from instruments, ultrasound energy from phacoemulsification, and irrigation fluid

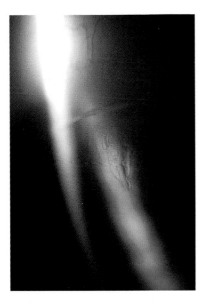

Figure 12.20   Postoperative corneal oedema.

turbulence. Despite the use of viscoelastics, corneal oedema is one of the commonest complications after cataract extraction, affecting approximately 10% of patients.[51] It is particularly common in eyes with endothelial disease, such as Fuchs' endothelial dystrophy, in which oedema may not resolve and may require penetrating keratoplasty. More typically, corneal thickening and oedema is localised to the area of the incision, where most endothelial trauma occurs (Figure 12.20). In the absence of endothelial disease, oedema involving the entire cornea may clear, starting in the periphery, in a matter of weeks.

Chronic trauma to the endothelium from an unstable IOL causes late corneal decompensation and oedema. In these cases IOL explantation or exchange is required. Vitreous contact or "touch" on the endothelium may have a similar effect and require a vitrectomy.

Brown–McLean syndrome is an unusual condition that typically occurs after intracapsular cataract extraction, but may also occur following extracapsular cataract extraction or phacoemulsification.[71] It is characterized by peripheral corneal oedema that commences inferiorly and progresses circumferentially. Corneal guttata are frequently present and punctate orange-brown pigmentation may underlie the oedema. It is more frequent in eyes that have suffered surgical complications or undergone multiple intraocular procedures.

Descemet's membrane detachment

Descemet's membrane detachment typically occurs in the region of the incision, where instruments entering the eye cause localised stripping of the membrane from the underlying stroma. This is usually detected during surgery and is reported to affect 0·1% of eyes.[51] An additional cause of Descemet's membrane detachment occurs when fluid injection takes place without the cannula tip fully inside the eye. This mechanism accounts for the extensive Descemet's membrane detachments that occur with poorly positioned anterior chamber maintainers. After surgery a Descemet's membrane detachment causes stromal oedema, and a large detachment may give a double anterior chamber appearance on slit lamp examination. To prevent Descemet's membrane detachment, instruments should be carefully inserted under direct vision. Similarly, when fluid is injected into the eye, the cannula tip must be fully inside the eye before injection commences.

A small Descemet's membrane detachment noted at the end of surgery will usually resolve spontaneously and requires no treatment. Alternatively, viscoelastic can be used to position the detachment or, if the detachment is superior, a bubble of air can be left in the eye. There is a risk of an IOP rise with both of these approaches and the patient should be carefully monitored. In place of air, sulphur hexafluoride may be used but this long acting gas is usually reserved for larger Descemet's membrane detachments that do not resolve.[72] Full thickness sutures have also been described to reposition the detached Descemet's membrane and tissue fibrinogen glue can be placed into the space between the stroma and Descemet's membrane. If reattachment completely fails, then it may be necessary to resort to a penetrating keratoplasty.[73]

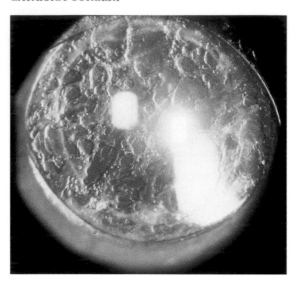

Figure 12.21   Posterior capsule opacification.

Table 12.5   Intraocular lens and surgical factors that reduce the incidence of posterior chamber opacification

Factors	Examples
Intraocular lens	Rectangular optic edge profile
	Posterior haptic angulation
	Optic–capsular adherence
	Biocompatibility (low lens
	epithelial cell growth)
Surgical technique	Rhexis size smaller than optic
	Capsular bag placement
	Hydrodissection and
	complete cortical clean up

Intraocular lens implant related complications

The details of postoperative refractive error are discussed in Chapter 6.

Capsule opacification

Posterior capsule opacification

Central to the pathogenesis of posterior capsule opacification (PCO) is the concept that, following cataract surgery, lens epithelial cells (LECs) migrate from the equator of the capsular bag and undergo fibroblastic-like change behind the optic of the IOL (Figure 12.21). The clinical failure of pharmacological intervention to reduce PCO has directed attention toward other solutions (Table 12.5). The importance of the IOL as a factor affecting the incidence of PCO is well recognised.[74,75] Several aspects of surgical technique have also been highlighted as particularly relevant in reducing PCO.[76] Thorough cortical cleaving hydrodissection in combination with careful cortical clean up decreases the volume of residual LECs and

hence PCO.[77] Also of importance are precise "in the bag" IOL placement and the dimensions of the capsulorhexis. The optic out or partially out of the capsular bag is associated with an increase in PCO.[78] Care should therefore be taken to ensure that the IOL is fully within the capsular bag and that the rhexis overlaps the optic.[79] This allows the anterior and posterior capsule to fuse around the lens edge, reducing the migration of LECs from the anterior capsule onto the posterior capsule, and behind the lens optic.

A central factor in reducing PCO is the geometrical shape of the IOL optic edge. It has been shown that migrating LECs are inhibited at a sharp discontinuous bend.[80] IOLs with sharp rectangular optic edges produce a sharp discontinuous bend in the capsule and hence have low incidence of PCO, irrespective of lens optic material.[81–83] The AcrySof lens (Alcon) has a dramatically low PCO rate and a sharp rectangular edge.[84] Although a rectangular IOL optic edge profile is advantageous in reducing PCO, it may cause glare and halos.[85] This problem is mimimised in lenses with an equi-biconvex optic design constructed from a material with a low refractive index.[86]

Other lens related factors that influence the development of PCO include posterior convexity of the lens optic and the haptic loop angle.[87] These may influence the degree of capsule discontinuity and hence the incidence of

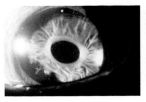
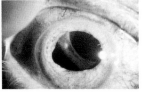

a)   b)

Figure 12.22 Anterior capsule opacity and contraction (capsulophimosis). (a) Encroaching on the visual axis. (b) Associated with intraocular lens subluxation.

PCO. The finding that different lens materials show differing degrees of adhesion to the lens capsule[88] illustrates a further factor that alters the lens–capsule interaction and may affect PCO rate. The role of other aspects of biocompatibility, such as facility to allow LEC growth on the lens optic, remains to be fully explained.[89] However, in conjunction with surgical technique, recent changes in IOL materials and design have the potential to reduce the incidence of PCO to a rare complication of cataract surgery.[76]

Anterior capsule opacification and contraction (capsulophimosis)

Anterior capsular contraction sydrome was first described in 1993 and is characterised by reduction in diameter of the anterior capsular rhexis that may cause opacification over the visual axis (Figure 12.22a) and IOL decentration (Figure 12.22b).[90,91] It is associated with eyes that have weak zonules,[90–92] for example those with pseudoexfoliation, high myopia, myotonic dystrophy, pars planitis, or uveitis. It is likely that the efficiency of hydrodissection and cortical clean up influence the pathogenesis of anterior capsule opacification and phimosis. Polishing and removing LECs from the anterior capsule may be advantageous,[93] particularly when using IOL types that are associated with anterior capsule opacification and capsulophimosis. IOL material, haptic rigidity, and haptic configuration are all

factors affecting their development. Rhexis contraction with silicone lenses has been reported to be more common in those with a plate haptic design as compared with polymethylmethacrylate (PMMA) loop haptics[94] but less common when a plate haptic is compared with polypropylene loop haptics.[95] Postmortem studies suggest that anterior capsule opacification is more prevalent in silicone plate haptic lenses than in silicone loop haptic lenses, and is least common in those with an acrylic optic.[96] Rhexis movement over time is less when an acrylic lens is compared with a silicone lens,[97] and this may reflect the adhesive quality of acrylic material.[88] The high level of biocompatibility and LEC growth with hydrogel lenses has been implicated in the marked capsule contraction observed with these lenses.[93] Implantation of a capsule tension ring[98] or rings[99] may reduce capsule contraction; however, bag shrinkage[100] and complete phimosis may still occur.[101]

If phimosis affects the visual axis, then Nd:YAG anterior capsulotomy may be undertaken. Several radial cuts are made in the rhexis edge using minimum laser energy and no posterior defocus.[91,92,102] Lens decentration associated with capsule fibrosis is a common indication for IOL explantation and insertion of a sulcus positioned lens (see below). An alternative is to reopen the capsular bag with blunt dissection and viscodissection, via two to three paracenteses, and reposition the lens.[103]

Nd:YAG laser capsulotomy

Hydrogel lenses have been reported as Nd:YAG laser resistant.[104] Comparison of the effects of Nd:YAG laser on acrylic, silicone, and PMMA shows that silicone has the lowest threshold for laser induced damage and greater linear extension of damage than PMMA and acrylic lenses.[105] In practice, the minimum possible laser energy and careful focus should

a)

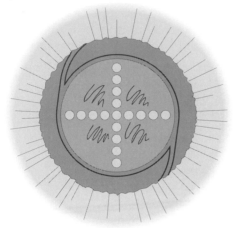

b)

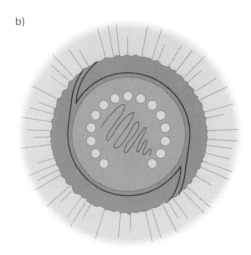

Figure 12.23 Nd:YAG posterior capsulotomy: laser technique. (a) Cruciate pattern. (b) Circular pattern.

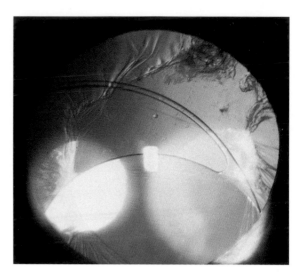

Figure 12.24 Inferior displacement of posterior chamber intraocular lens due to deficiency of capsular support after posterior capsule rupture.

complication.[108] However, it is recommended that Nd:YAG capsulotomy be delayed in this lens type until at least six months after surgery.

Intraocular lens subluxation and dislocation

Lens implant stability is discussed in Chapter 7.

Intraocular lens explantation

The most common indications for postoperative lens explantation are IOL decentration/dislocation (Figures 12.22b and 12.24), incorrect lens power, optic related glare or optical aberrations, and chronic inflammation.[109] This procedure is more technically complex than explanting an IOL intraoperatively but good visual outcomes have been reported.[110] It may be possible to open the original incision with a blunt cannula, although explantation may require construction of a new incision. The anterior chamber is then filled with a viscoelastic and the capsular bag is released from the lens by a combination of viscodissection and blunt dissection. Where anterior phimosis has occurred, it may be necessary to enlarge the anterior capsulorhexis first to facilitate removal

always be used when performing a Nd:YAG posterior capsulotomy. If optic damage is anticipated then a circular capsulotomy, which avoids the optical axis, is preferable over a technique that creates a cruciate pattern (Figure 12.23). Unlike loop haptic lenses, those with plate haptics constructed of silicone or hydrogel[106] may sublux or dislocate posteriorly into the vitreous following Nd:YAG laser capsulotomy. This may be an immediate event or delayed.[107] Large dial holes were introduced in silicone plate haptic lenses (Figure 7.2) to improve capsular fixation and reduce the incidence of this

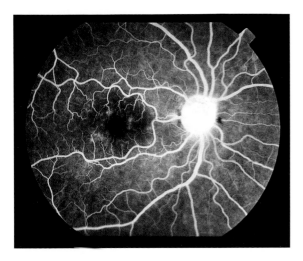

Figure 12.25 Fluorescein angiogram of macular oedema following cataract surgery (Irvine–Gass syndrome). There is hyperfluorescence at the optic disc and around the fovea (perifoveal capillary leakage).

of the lens. If a lens is strongly adherent to the capsule, as may occur with an acrylic lens, then a sharp needle or instrument may be required to first release the capsulorhexis. The IOL can then usually be rotated out the bag, although it may be necessary to cut the haptics from the optic. If the haptic fragments cannot be easily removed, they may be left in situ.[111] If the lens can be "dialled" in the anterior chamber then it can be removed using one of the techniques described in Chapter 7 to explant a foldable lens intraoperatively, or the incision may be enlarged as necessary.

Retinal complications

Cystoid macula oedema

Cystoid macular oedema (CMO) following cataract surgery, also know as Irvine–Gass syndrome, is typically self-limiting and occurs three to twelve weeks after surgery. It is a more frequent complication of intracapsular than of extracapsular cataract surgery.[112] CMO may be asymptomatic or cause profound central visual loss, but in the absence of vitreous complications it rarely causes persistent loss of visual acuity, and usually resolves spontaneously within a

year of surgery. Its exact aetiology is unclear but among its risk factors are vitreous loss (vitreous traction) and uveitis (postoperative inflammation). Extracelluar fluid accumulates in the inner nuclear and outer plexiform layers of the foveal retina, and this may form cystic spaces that coalesce to form a lamellar or full thickness retinal hole. Optic disc swelling and intraretinal haemorrhages can also occur.[113]

The presence of CMO can be difficult to detect by fundoscopy, and a subtle change in the foveal reflex may be more obvious using red free light or a contact lens during slit lamp biomicroscopy. In many cases CMO is only identifiable with fluorescein angiography (Figure 12.25).[114] Fluoroscein angiography also helps to distinguish CMO from other conditions that can become apparent after cataract surgery, such as diabetic maculopathy (see Chapter 10), a stage 1 macular hole, or age related macular degeneration. In psuedophakic eyes prostaglandin based glaucoma medication may also cause macular oedema.[115]

Treatment for postcataract surgery CMO is complicated by its self-limiting nature and the lack of randomised controlled trials. Furthermore, data derived from uveitis related macular oedema is often applied to the treatment of CMO. Corticosteroids administered by topical or systemic routes, or by periocular injection appear to be effective, but these are usually used in combination with topical or oral non-steroidal anti-inflammatory drugs.[116] Combined topical medication is usually considered first line treatment, and the use of systemic treatment or periocular injection is reserved for those who do not respond.[117] The roles of acetazolamide[118] and hyperbaric oxygen,[119] both of which have been explored as alternative treatments, are uncertain. Where vitreous is adherent to the incision (Figure 12.26), chronic CMO may improve by cutting the vitreous by either Nd:YAG laser[120] or three-port pars plana vitrectomy.[121] Prophylaxis for CMO with topical non-steroidal anti-inflammatory drugs and corticosteroids is effective but, given that the

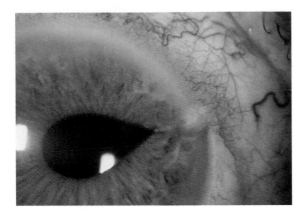

Figure 12.26 Vitreous strand to a paracentesis distorting the pupil.

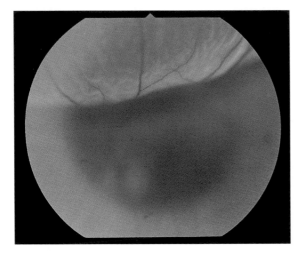

Figure 12.27 Pseudophakic superior retinal detachment.

incidence of symptomatic CMO is relatively low and often resolves spontaneously, it is probably best used in those individuals at high risk.

Retinal detachment

Retinal detachment is rare after cataract surgery, and when it does occur it is usually associated with intraoperative vitreous complications, myopia (axial length of 24 mm or greater[122]), or predisposing retinal lesions (Figure 12.27). It is more common following intracapsular surgery than extracapsular surgery

and is least frequent after phacoemulsification. In one large series, 0·1% of patients developed a retinal detachment or retinal tear within three months of cataract surgery.[51] The increased risk of retinal detachment following cataract extraction means that all patients should, if the lens opacity permits, have a full fundal examination before surgery. A history of previous retinal detachment or a family history of it is also relevant in assessing an individual's risk. Careful fundal examination after surgery is particularly important in those identified as at risk. Prophylactic treatment of retinal holes with argon laser photocoagulation has been recommended for retinal tears recognised either before surgery or after surgery.[123] Following Nd:Yag laser capsulotomy, there is an added significant increase in the risk of retinal detachment, particularly in patients with longer axial lengths, who should be carefully assessed.

Retinal light toxicity

Operating microscope light induced phototoxicity remains a recognised cause of permanent retinal damage after cataract surgery.[124] It is more common when surgical time is prolonged, for example following complicated surgery or when learning. In addition to minimising surgical time, there are several ways in which retinal light exposure can be reduced during cataract surgery (Box 12.1). The microscope light

---

Box 12.1 Methods to reduce the incidence of phototoxicity from operating microscope illumination

- Use minimal illumination
- Turn light off between manoeuvres
- Minimise surgical time
- Tilt the microscope toward the surgeon★
- Use ultraviolet filter in the microscope
- Use oblique or non-coaxial illumination (unless red reflex required)

★Depending on surgical approach: ≥ 10° superior; ≥ 15° temporal.

---

should be turned down as far as possible without reducing the view of the anterior segment (this is also more comfortable for the patient when operating under topical anaesthesia). The light can also be switched off or the eye shielded during pauses between surgical manoeuvres.

Tilting the microscope toward the surgeon moves the area of light exposed retina away from the fovea. It is calculated that to avoid foveal exposure, the angle of tilt when the surgeon is sitting superiorly should be at least 10° and increased to 15° or more when sitting temporally.[125,126] However, the exact angle of tilt also depends on the microscope illumination system, the degree of centration over the pupil, and the axial length of the operated eye (increased axial length requires greater tilt). A further method of reducing phototoxicity is to use an oblique light, in place of coaxial illumination, which is not focused on the retina. Oblique light does not produce a red reflex but can be used when this is not required, for example during suturing. Because short wavelength light is known to cause retinal damage, an ultraviolet light filter within the microscope may also reduce retina light toxicity.

References

1 Christy NE, Lall P. Postoperative endophthalmitis following cataract surgery. *Arch Ophthalmol* 1973;**90**: 361–6.
2 Kattan HM, Flynn HW, Pflugfelder S, *et al.* Nosocomial endophthalmitis survey. *Ophthalmology* 1991;**98**:227–38.
3 Sherwood DR, Rich WJ, Jacob JS, *et al.* Bacterial contamination of intraocular and extraocular fluids during extracapsular cataract extraction. *Eye* 1989;**3**:308–12.
4 Speaker MG, Milch FA, Shah MK, *et al.* Role of external bacterial flora in the pathogenesis of acute postoperative endophthalmitis. *Ophthalmology* 1991;**98**:639–49.
5 Stern WH, Tamura E, Jacobs RA, *et al.* Epidemic postsurgical *Candida parapsilosis* endophthalmitis. *Ophthalmology* 1985;**92**:1701–9.
6 Pettit TH, Olson RJ, Foos RY, *et al.* Fungal endophthalmitis following intraocular lens implantation. *Arch Ophthalmol* 1980;**98**:1025–39.
7 Vafidis G, Marsh RJ, Stacey AR. Bacterial contamination of intraocular lens surgery. *Br J Ophthalmol* 1984;**68**: 520–3.
8 Zaluski S, Clayman HM, Karsent G, *et al.* Pseudomonas aeruginosa endophthalmitis caused by contamination of the internal fluid pathways of a phacoemulsifier. *J Cataract Refract Surg* 1999;**25**:540–5.
9 Norregaard JC, Thoning H, Bernth-Petersen P, Andersen TF, Javitt JC, Anderson GF. Risk of endophthalmitis after cataract extraction: results from the International Cataract Surgery Outcomes study. *Br J Ophthalmol* 1997;**81**:102–6.
10 Burns RP, Oden M. Antibiotic prophylaxis in cataract surgery. *Trans Am Ophthalmol Soc* 1972;**70**:43–57.
11 Allansmith MR, Anderson RP, Butterworth M. The meaning of preoperative cultures in ophthalmology. *Trans Am Acad Ophthalmol Otolaryngol* 1969;**73**: 683–90.
12 Chitkara DK, Manners T, Chapman F, *et al.* Lack of effect of preoperative norfloxacin on bacterial contamination of anterior chamber aspirates after cataract surgery. *Br J Ophthalmol* 1994;**78**:772–4.
13 Apt L, Isenberg SJ, Yoshimori R, *et al.* Chemical preparation of the eye in ophthalmic surgery: III. Effect of povidone-iodine on the conjunctiva. *Arch Ophthalmol* 1984;**102**:728–79.
14 Isenberg SJ, Apt L, Yoshimori R, *et al.* Chemical preparation of the eye in ophthalmic surgery: IV. Comparison of povidone-iodine on the conjunctiva with a prophylactic antibiotic. *Arch Ophthalmol* 1985;**103**: 1340–2.
15 Speaker MG, Menikoff JA. Prophylaxis of endophthalmitis with topical povidone-iodine. *Ophthalmology* 1991;**98**:1769–75.
16 Feys J, Salvanet-Bouccara A, Emond JP, Dublanchet A. Vancomycin prophylaxis and intraocular contamination during cataract surgery. *J Cataract Refract Surg* 1997;**23**:894–7.
17 Beigi B, Westlake W, Chang B, Marsh C, Jacob J, Riordan T. The effect of intracameral, per-operative antibiotics on microbial contamination of anterior chamber aspirates during phacoemulsification. *Eye* 1998;**12**:390–4.
18 Manners TD, Turner DP, Galloway PH, Glenn AM. Heparinised intraocular infusion and bacterial contamination in cataract surgery. *Br J Ophthalmol* 1997;**81**:949–52.
19 Kohnen T, Dick B, Hessemer V, *et al.* Effect of heparin in irrigating solution on inflammation following small incision cataract surgery. *J Cataract Refract Surg* 1998;**24**:237–43.
20 Okhravi N, Towler HMA, Hykin P, *et al.* Assessment of a standard treatment protocol on visual outcome following presumed bacterial endophthalmitis. *Br J Ophthalmol* 1997;**81**:719–25.
21 Montan PG, Koranyi G, Setterquist HE, Stridh A, Philipson BT, Wiklund K. Endophthalmitis after cataract surgery: risk factors relating to technique and events of the operation and patient history: a retrospective case-control study. *Ophthalmology* 1998; **105**:2171–7.
23 Endophthalmitis Vitrectomy Study Group. Results of the Endophthalmitis Vitrectomy Study. A randomized trial of immediate vitrectomy and of intravenous antibiotics for the treatment of postoperative bacterial endophthalmitis. *Arch Ophthalmol* 1995;**113**:1479–96.
23 Wisniewski SR, Capone A, Kelsey SF, *et al.* Characteristics after cataract surgery or secondary lens implantation among patients screened for the Endophthalmitis Vitrectomy Study. *Ophthalmology* 2000;**107**:1274–82.
24 Johnson MW, Doft BH, Kelsey SF, *et al.* The Endophthalmitis Vitrectomy Study. Relationship

between clinical presentation and microbiologic spectrum. *Ophthalmology* 1997;**104**:261–72.

25 Driebe WT, Mandelbaum S, Forster RK, *et al*. Pseudophakic endophthalmitis. *Ophthalmology* 1986;**93**:442–8.

26 Han DP, Wisniewski SR, Kelsey SF, *et al*. Microbiologic yields and complication rates of vitreous needle aspiration versus mechanized vitreous biopsy in the Endophthalmitis Vitrectomy Study. *Retina* 1999;**19**:98–102.

27 Joondeph BC, Flynn HW, Miller D, *et al*. A new culture method for infectious endophthalmitis. *Arch Ophthalmol* 1989;**107**:1334–7.

28 Hykin PG, Tobal K, McIntyre G, Matheson MM, Towler H, Lightman S. The diagnosis of delayed post-operative endophthalmitis by polymerase chain reaction of bacterial DNA in vitreous samples. *J Med Microbiol* 1994;**44**:408–15.

29 Okhravi N, Adamson P, Mant R, *et al*. Polymerase chain reaction and restriction fragment length polymorphism mediated detection and speciation of *Candida* spp causing intraocular infection. *Invest Ophthalmol Vis Sci* 1998;**39**:859–66.

30 Okhravi N, Adamson P, Carroll N, *et al*. PCR-based evidence of bacterial involvement in eyes with suspected intraocular infection. *Invest Ophthalmol Vis Sci* 2000;**41**:3474–9.

31 Jaeger EE, Carroll NM, Choudhury S, *et al*. Rapid detection and isolation of *Candida*, *Aspergillus*, and *Fusarium* species in ocular samples using nested PCR. *J Clin Microbiol* 2000;**38**:2902–8.

32 Okhravi N, Adamson P, Matheson MM, Towler HMA, Lightman S. PCR-RFLP-mediated detection and speciation of bacterial species causing endophthalmitis. *Invest Ophthalmol Vis Sci* 2000;**41**:1438–47.

33 Aguilar HE, Meredith TA, Shaarawy A, *et al*. Vitreous cavity penetration of ceftazidime after intravenous administration. *Retina* 1995;15:154–9.

34 Shaarawy A, Meredith TA, Kincaid M, *et al*. Intraocular injection of ceftazidime. Effects of inflammation and surgery. *Retina* 1995;15:433–8.

35 Conway BP, Campochiaro PA. Macular infarction after endophthalmitis treated with vitrectomy and intravitreal gentamicin. *Arch Ophthalmol* 1986;**104**:367–71.

36 D'Amico DJ, Caspers-Velu L, Libert J, *et al*. Comparative toxicity of intravitreal aminoglycoside antibiotics. *Am J Ophthalmol* 1985;**100**:264–75.

37 Doft BH, Barza M. Ceftazidime or amikacin: choice of intravitreal antimicrobials in the treatment of postoperative endophthalmitis [letter]. *Arch Ophthalmol* 1994;**112**:17–8.

38 Yay WM, Fishman P, Aziz M, Shockley RK. Intravitreal ceftazidime in a rabbit model: dose- and time-dependent toxicity and pharmacokinetic analysis. *J Ocul Pharmacol* 1987;**3**:257–62.

39 el-Baba FZ, Trousdale MD, Gauderman WJ, Wagner DG, Liggett PE. Intravitreal penetration of oral ciprofloxacin in humans. *Ophthalmology* 1992;**99**:483–6.

40 Lesk MR, Ammann H, Marcil G, Vinet B, Lamer L, Sebag M. The penetration of oral ciprofloxacin into the aqueous humor, vitreous, and subretinal fluid of humans. *Am J Ophthalmol* 1993;**115**:623–8.

41 Kowalski RP, Karenchak LM, Eller AW. The role of ciprofloxacin in endophthalmitis therapy. *Am J Ophthalmol* 1993;**116**:695–9.

42 Shah GK, Stein JD, Sharma S, *et al*. Visual outcomes following the use of intravitreal steroids in the treatment of postoperative endophthalmitis. *Ophthalmology* 2000;**107**:486–9.

43 Das T, Jalali S, Gothwal VK, *et al*. Intravitreal dexamethasone in exogenous bacterial endophthalmitis: results of a prospective randomised study. *Br J Ophthalmol* 1999;**83**:1050–5.

44 Heiligenhaus A, Steinmetz B, Lapuente R, *et al*. Recombinant tissue plasminogen activator in cases with fibrin formation after cataract surgery: a prospective randomised multicentre study. *Br J Ophthalmol* 1998;**82**:810–5.

45 Aldave AJ, Stein JD, Deramo VA, Shah GK, Fischer DH, Maguire JI. Treatment strategies for postoperative *Propionibacterium acnes* endophthalmitis. *Ophthalmology* 1999;**106**:2395–401.

46 Jones NP. Fuch's heterochromic uveitis: an update. *Surv Ophthalmol* 1993;**37**:253–72.

47 Kim MH, Koo TH, Sah WJ, Chung SM. Treatment of total hyphema with relatively low-dose tissue plasminogen activator. *Ophthalmic Surg Lasers* 1998;**29**:762–6.

48 Petrelli EA, Wiznia RA. Argon laser photocoagulation of inner wound vascularization after cataract extraction. *Am J Ophthalmol* 1977;**84**:58–61.

49 Ellingson FT. Complications with the Choyce Mark VIII anterior chamber lens implant (uveitis-glaucoma-hyphaema). *Am Intraocular Implant Soc J* 1977;**3**:199–201.

50 Aonuma H, Matsushita H, Nakajima K, *et al*. Uveitis-glaucoma-hyphema syndrome after posterior chamber intraocular lens implantation. *Jap J Ophthalmol* 1997;**41**:98–100.

51 Desai P, Minassian DC, Reidy A. National Cataract Surgery Survey 1997-8: a report of the results of the clinical outcomes. *Br J Ophthalmol* 1999;**83**:1336–40.

52 Scott IU, Flynn HW Jr, Schiffman J, *et al*. Visual acuity outcomes among patients with appositional suprachoroidal haemorrhage. *Ophthalmology* 1997;**104**:2039–46.

53 Podos SM, Krupin T, Asseff C, Becker B. Topically administered corticosteroid preparations. Comparison of intraocular pressure effects. *Arch Ophthalmol* 1971;**86**:251–4.

54 Galin MA, Barasch KR, Harris LS. Enzymatic zonulolysis and intraocular pressure. *Am J Ophthalmol* 1966;**61**:690–6.

55 Kirsch RE. Dose relationship of alpha chymotrypsin in production of glaucoma after cataract extraction. *Arch of Ophthalmol* 1966;**75**:774–5.

56 Sugar HS. Pulpillary block and pupil-block glaucoma following cataract extraction. *Am J Ophthalmol* 1966;**61**:435–43.

57 Little BC, Hitchings RA. Pseudophakic malignant glaucoma: Nd:YAG capsulotomy as a primary treatment. *Eye* 1993;7:102–4.

58 Tsai JC, Barton KA, Miller MH, Khaw PT, Hitchings RA. Surgical results in malignant glaucoma refractory to medical or laser therapy. *Eye* 1997;**11**:677–81.

59 Evans RB. Peripheral anterior synechia overlying the haptics of posterior chamber lenses. Occurrence and natural history. *Ophthalmology* 1990;**97**:415–23.

60 Stark WJ, Michels RG, Maumenee AE. Cupples H. Surgical management of epithelial ingrowth. *Am J Ophthalmol* 1978;**85**:772–80.

61 Calhoun FP. An aid to the clinical diagnosis of epithelial downgrowth into the anterior chamber following cataract extraction. *Am J Ophthalmol* 1966;**61**:1055–9.

62 Smith RE, Parrett C. Specular microscopy of epithelial downgrowth. *Arch Ophthalmology* 1978;**96**:1222–4.

63 Rice TA, Michels RG. Current surgical management of the vitreous wick syndrome. *Am J Ophthalmology* 1978;**85**:656–61.

64 Taylor HR, Michels RG, Stark WJ. Vitrectomy methods in anterior segment surgery. *Ophthalmic Surg* 1979;**10**:25–58.

65 Ernest PH, Lavery KT, Kiessling LA. Relative strength of scleral corneal and clear corneal incisions constructed in cadaver eyes. *J Cataract Refract Surg* 1994;**20**:626–9.

66 Chowers I, Anteby I, Ever-Hadani P, Frucht-Pery J. Traumatic wound dehiscence after cataract extraction. *J Cataract Refract Surg* 2001;**27**:1238–42.

67 Danjoux JP, Reck AC. Corneal sutures: is routine removal really necessary? *Eye* 1994;**8**:339–42.

68 Heaven CJ, Davison CR, Cockcroft PM. Bacterial contamination of nylon corneal sutures. *Eye* 1995;**9**:116–8.

69 Minassian DC, Rosen P, Dart JK, Reidy A, Desai P, Sidhu M. Extracapsular cataract extraction compared with small incision surgery by phacoemulsification: a randomised trial. *Br J Ophthalmol* 2001;**85**:822–9.

70 O'Donoghue, Lightman S, Tuft S, Watson P. Surgically induced necrotising sclerokeratitis (SINS) – precipitating factors and response to treatment. *Br J Ophthalmol* 1992;**76**:17–21.

71 Gothard TW, Hardten DR, Lane SS, *et al.* Clinical findings in Brown-McLean syndrome. *Am J Ophthalmol* 1993;**115**:729–37.

72 Kremer I, Stiebel H, Yassur Y, Weinberger D. Sulfur hexafluoride injection for Descemet's membrane detachment in cataract surgery. *J Cataract Refract Surg* 1997;**23**:1449–53.

73 Macsai MS. Total detachment of Descemet's membrane after small-incision cataract extraction. *Am J Ophthalmol* 1992;**114**:365–7.

74 Nishi O. Incidence of posterior capsule opacification in eyes with and without posterior chamber intraocular lenses. *J Cataract Refract Surg* 1986;**12**:519–22.

75 Born CP, Ryan DK. Effect of intraocular lens optic design on posterior capsular opacification. *J Cataract Refract Surg* 1990;**16**:188–92.

76 Apple DJ, Peng Q, Visessook N, *et al.* Eradication of posterior capsule opacification. *Ophthalmology* 2001;**108**:505–18.

77 Apple D, Peng Q, Visessook N, *et al.* Surgical prevention of posterior capsule opacification. *J Cataract Refract Surg* 2000;**26**:188–97.

78 Hayashi K, Hayashi H, Fuminori N, *et al.* Capsular capture of silicone intraocular lenses. *J Cataract Refract Surg* 1996;**22**(suppl 2):1267–1271.

79 Ravalico G, Tognetto D, Palomba M-A, *et al.* Capsulorhexis size and posterior capsule opacification. *J Cataract Refract Surg* 1996;**22**:98–103.

80 Nishi O. Update/review: posterior capsule opacification. *J Cataract Refract Surg* 1999;**25**:106–117.

81 Nishi O, Nishi K, Akura J, *et al.* Effect of round edged acrylic intraocular lenses on preventing posterior capsule opacification. *J Cataract Refract Surg* 2001;**27**:608–13.

82 Schauersberger J, Abela C, Schild G, Amon M. Two year results: sharp versus rounded optic edges on silicone lenses. *J Cataract Refract Surg* 2000;**26**:566–70.

83 Nagata T, Watanabe I. Optic sharp edge or convexity: comparison of effects on posterior capsule opacification. *Jpn J Ophthalmol* 1996;**40**:397–403.

84 Kohnen T, Magdowski G, Koch DD. Surface analysis of acrylic and hydrogel IOLs. *J Cataract Refract Surg* 1996;**22**(suppl 2):1342–50.

85 Masket S. Truncated edge design, dysphotopsia, and inhibition of posterior capsule opacification. *J Cataract Refract Surg* 2000;**26**:145–7.

86 Erie JC, Bandhauer MH, McLaren JW. Analysis of postoperative glare and intraocular lens design. *J Cataract Refract Surg* 2001;**27**:614–21.

87 Apple DJ, Solomon KD, Tetz MR. Posterior capsule opacification. *Surv Ophthalmol* 1992;**37**:73–116.

88 Oshika T, Nagata T, Ishii Y. Adhesion of lens capsule to intraocular lenses of poly methymethacrylate, silicone, and acrylic foldable materials: an experimental study. *Br J Ophthalmol* 1998;**82**:549–553.

89 Hollick EJ, Spalton DJ, Ursell PG. Surface cytologic features on intraocular lenses: can increased biocompatibility have disadvantages? *Arch Ophthalmol* 1999;**117**:872–8.

90 Hansen SO, Crandall AS, Olson RJ. Progressive constriction of the anterior capsular opening following intact capsulorhexis. *J Cataract Refract Surg* 1993;**19**:77–82.

91 Davison JA. Capsule contraction syndrome. *J Cataract Refract Surg* 1993;**19**:582–9.

92 Young DA, Orlin SE. Capsulorhexis contracture in phacoemulsification surgery. *Ophthalmic Surg* 1994;**25**:477–8.

93 Joo CK, Shin JA, Kim JH. Capsular opening contraction after continuous curvilinear capsulorhexis and intraocular lens implantation. *J Cataract Refract Surg* 1996;**22**:585–90.

94 Gonvers M, Sickenberg M, van Melle G. Change in capsulorhexis size after implantation of 3 types of intraocular lens. *J Cataract Refract Surg* 1997;**23**:231–8.

95 Patel CK, Ormonde S, Rosen P, Bron AJ. Post-operative changes in the capsulorhexis aperture: a prospective, randomised comparison between loop and plate haptic silicone intraocular lenses. *Eye* 2000;**14**:185–9.

96 Werner L, Pandey SK, Escobar-Gomez M, Visessook N, Peng Q, Apple DJ. Anterior capsule opacification: a histopathological study comparing different IOL styles. *Ophthalmology* 2000;**107**:463–71.

97 Ursell PG, Spalton DJ, Pande MV. Anterior capsule stability in eyes with intraocular lenses made of polymethyl methacrylate, silicone, and AcrySof. *J Cataract Refract Surg* 1997;**23**:1532–8.

98 Gimbel HV. Role of capsular tension rings in preventing capsule contraction. *J Cataract Refract Surg* 2000;**26**:791–2.

99 Liu C, Eleftheriadis H. Multiple capsular tension rings for the prevention of capsule contraction syndrome. *J Cataract Refract Surg* 2001;**27**:342–3.

100 Stren K, Menapace R, Vass C. Capsular bag shrinkage after implanation of an open-loop silicone lens and PMMA capsule tension ring. *J Cataract Refract Surg* 1997;**23**:1543–7.

101 Fashinger CW, Eckhardt M. Complete capsulorhexis opening occlusion despite capsular tension ring implantation. *J Cataract Refract Surg* 1999;**25**:1013–5.

102 Martinez Toldos JJ, Artola Roig A, Chipont Benabent E. Total anterior capsule closure after silicone intraocular lens implantation. *J Cataract Refract Surg* 1996;**22**:269–71.

103 Fine IH, Hoffman RS. Late reopening of fibrosed capsular bags to reposition decentered intraocular lenses. *J Cataract Refract Surg* 1997;**23**:990–4.

104 Skelnik DL, Lindstrom RL, Allarakhia L, *et al.* Neodymium: YAG laser interaction with Alcon IOGEL intraocular lenses: an in vitro toxicity assay. *J Cataract Refract Surg* 1987;**13**:662–8.

105 Newland TJ, McDermott ML, Eliott D, *et al.* Experimental neodymium:YAG laser damage to acrylic, poly(methyl methacrylate), and silicone intraocular lens materials. *J Cataract Refract Surg* 1991;**25**:72–6.

106 Levy JH, Pisacano AM, Anello RD. Displacement of bag-placed hydrogel lenses into the vitreous following neodymium: YAG laser capsulotomy. *J Cataract Refract Surg* 1990;**16**:563–6.

107 Tuft SJ, Talks SJ. Delayed dislocation of foldable plate-haptic silicone lenses after Nd:YAG laser anterior capsulotomy. *Am J Ophthalmol* 1998;**126**:586–8.

108 Whiteside SB, Apple DJ, Peng Q, Isaacs RT, Guindi A, Draughn RA. Fixation elements on plate intraocular lens: large positioning holes to improve security of capsular fixation. *Ophthalmology* 1998;**105**:837–42.

109 Price FW Jr, Whitson WE, Collins K, Johns S. Explantation of posterior chamber lenses. *J Cataract Refract Surg* 1992;**18**:475–9.

110 Mamalis N. Complications of foldable intraocular lenses requiring explanation or secondary intervention: 1998 survey. *J Cataract Refract Surg* 2000;**26**:766–72.

111 Rao SK, Sharma T, Parikh S, *et al.* Explantation of silicone plate haptic intraocular lenses. Ophthalmic Surg Lasers 1999;**30**:575–8.

112 Stark WJ, Maumenee AE, Fagadau W, *et al.* Cystoid macular edema in pseudophakia. *Surv Ophthalmology* 1984;**28**(suppl):442–51.

113 Bovino JA. Kelly TJ. Marcus DF. Intraretinal hemorrhages in cystoid macular edema. *Arch Ophthalmol* 1984;**102**:1151–2.

114 Jaffe NS, Luscombe SM, Clayman HM, Gass JD. A fluorescein angiographic study of cystoid macular edema. *Am J Ophthalmol* 1981;**92**:775–7.

115 Callanan D, Fellman RL, Savage JA. Latanoprost-associated cystoid macular edema. *Am J Ophthalmol* 1998;**126**:134–5.

116 Mackool RJ. Anti-inflammatory regimen for cystoid macular edema after cataract surgery. *J Cataract Refract Surg* 2000;**26**:474.

117 Abe T, Hayasaka S, Nagaki Y, Kadoi C, Matsumoto M, Hayasaka Y. Pseudophakic cystoid macular edema treated with high-dose intravenous methylprednisolone. *J Cataract Refract Surg* 1999;**25**:1286–8.

118 Wolfensberger TJ. The role of carbonic anhydrase inhibitors in the management of macular edema. *Doc Ophthalmol* 1999;**97**:387–97.

119 Pfoff DS, Thom SR. Preliminary report on the effect of hyperbaric oxygen on cystoid macular edema. *J Cataract Refract Surg* 1987;**13**:136–40.

120 Katzen LE, Fleischman HA, Trokel S. YAG laser treatment of cystoid macular edema. *Am J Ophthalmol* 1983;**95**:589–92.

121 Fung WE. Vitrectomy for chronic aphakic cystoid macular edema. Results of a national, collaborative, prospective, randomized investigation. *Ophthalmology* 1985;**92**:1102–11.

122 Olsen G, Olson RJ. Update on a long-term, prospective study of capsulotomy and retinal detachment rates after cataract surgery. *J Cataract Refractive Surg* 2000;**26**:1017–21.

123 Fan DS, Lam DS, Li KK. Retinal complications after cataract extraction in patients with high myopia. *Ophthalmology* 1999;**106**:688–91.

124 Postel EA, Pulido JS, Brynes GA, *et al.* Long-term follow-up of iatrogenic phototoxicity. *Arch Ophthalmol* 1998;**116**:753–7.

125 Brod RD, Olsen JR, Ball SF, Packer AJ. The site of operating microscope light-induced injury on the human retina. *Am J Ophthalmol* 1989;**107**:390–7.

126 Pavilack MA, Brod RD. Site of potential operating microscope light-induced phototoxicity on the human retina during temporal approach eye surgery. *Ophthalmology* 2001;**108**:381–5.

13 Cataract surgery in the Third World

The World Health Organisation (WHO) estimates that there are 20 million people blinded by cataract, which is approximately 45% of all blindness (Figure 13.1). At present this number is growing by about one million per year as the world's population increases and ages. Around 80% of these people live in the poor countries of the developing world.[1] If present trends continue, it is estimated that by 2020 there will be 75 million blind people in the world, of whom 50 million will be blind from cataract.[2] Currently, there are approximately ten million cataract operations per year, of which about four million are carried out in Third World countries.[3] To avoid a massive increase in cataract blindness, the number of operations must grow to 32 million per year.[2] This requires an increase in the number of cataract operations of about 7% per year. Virtually all of this increase must take place in Third World countries.

As well as extracting a terrible cost in terms of human suffering, cataract has major economic implications. It has been estimated that the cost of blindness in India is more than four billion dollars every year. Approximately half of this cost is due to cataract.[4]

The cataract surgical rate (CSR; namely the number of operations per million people per year) is a simple measure of the delivery of cataract surgery to a population. Currently the CSR varies from over 5000 in parts of North America to less than 100 in some African

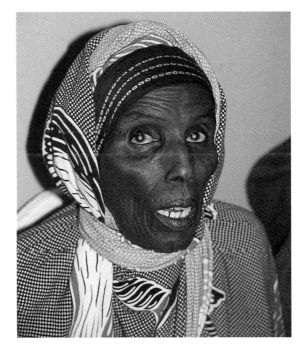

Figure 13.1   This woman had been blind for at least two years when she came to an eye clinic in Beletwein, Somalia. She had travelled for more 200 km in order to have cataract surgery. Her situation is typical of the millions who are blind from cataract today.

countries. The CSR needed to eliminate cataract blindness will vary according to the number of elderly people in a population and the perceived visual requirements of that population, but it is thought that the minimum required is about 2000 operations per million people per year.

Global situation

Africa

Africa has the highest prevalence of blindness in the world, estimated by WHO to be approximately 1%. Half of this is due to cataract. Africa also has the fewest resources with which to combat blindness. There is, on average, only one ophthalmologist for one million people. Although simple cataract surgery may cost only $30 per procedure, this is more than ten times the annual per capita health budget of many African countries. The CSR is 100–500 in most African countries.

Asia

The prevalence of blindness in Asia is 0·75%, of which about two thirds is due to cataract. Most Asian countries are better equipped to deal with the problems of cataract blindness, having approximately one ophthalmologist per 100 000 people. However, these resources are at risk of being overwhelmed by the sheer scale of the problem. There are now about 3 500 000 cataract operations performed annually in India alone, representing a CSR of about 3 500. Unfortunately, this has not yet eliminated the backlog of cataract blind patients. In China it is difficult to obtain accurate figures, but it appears that no more than 250 000 operations are carried out each year for a population of more than one billion, yielding a CSR of less than 300.

Latin America

Latin America has a relatively smaller population, with a prevalence of blindness of around 0·5%, of which about half is due to cataract. There is no shortage of ophthalmologists, but cataract blindness remains a serious problem. Many ophthalmologists practise in large towns and cities, where services are of a high standard. However, these services are inaccessible to rural people and urban slum dwellers.

Barriers to cataract surgery

Modern cataract surgery is one of the most successful medical interventions of all time. Why is cataract still the world's leading cause of blindness? The explanation lies in the barriers that prevent blind people from coming for surgery. These can be divided into patient related (i.e. motivation, mobility, and money) and provider related factors (i.e. manpower, materials, management, and marketing).

- Motivation. Patients who have a different understanding of health and disease may be reluctant to come for surgery because they do not believe that cataract is a curable disease. Cataract blindness may be regarded as a normal part of ageing. Alternatively, they may not believe the surgeon's claims that surgery will cure their disability.

- Mobility. Travel is difficult in developing countries. For a blind person it is almost impossible. In Africa many blind people live over 100 km from the nearest eye surgeon. Because cataract blind patients are relatively immobile, they cannot reach eye clinics.

- Money. Many Third World countries now require patients to pay for their treatment. This constitutes a significant barrier for blind patients, who are already impoverished because of their disability.

- Manpower. A lack of trained personnel means that many cataract patients never meet an eye surgeon. Their condition may not be recognised by a rural health worker who has little ophthalmic expertise.

- Materials. Shortages of essential materials are a recurrent problem for all types of health care in the Third World. This has been addressed by encouraging the local manufacture of essential supplies such as sutures, eye drops, glasses, and even intraocular lenses (IOLs).

- Management. Mismanagement and poor marketing of scarce health care resources are further problems. Resources are concentrated in the capital cities of most Third World countries, although most blind people are found elsewhere.

With the knowledge and techniques available to us today, it should be possible to eliminate cataract blindness. The failure to achieve this suggests that the problem is not technical but managerial. It has been suggested that ophthalmologists might learn from the MacDonald's fast food outlets. If cataract surgery was as universally available, as effectively marketed, and as efficiently delivered as a "Big Mac", then the cataract backlog would rapidly disappear.[5]

Essential resources for cataract surgery

Human resources

Innovative strategies have been devised to overcome the lack of trained ophthalmic personnel in most of the Third World, particularly in Africa, where the deficit is most severe.

In many African countries, non-physician health workers have been trained to deliver basic eye care, including the diagnosis and referral of cataract patients. In east and southern Africa, selected ophthalmic assistants have been trained to perform cataract surgery. Prospective studies have shown that, with uncomplicated senile cataracts, non-physician cataract surgeons can obtain excellent results.[6]

Although training programmes are effective at providing basic instruction for ophthalmologists and cataract surgeons, human resources development is ineffective unless it also includes mechanisms for providing supervision, continuing education, and adequate material resources. If these are not incorporated, then the value of the training is severely compromised.

At the village level, ordinary members of the community, and traditional healers, have been trained to identify blindness. These community based field workers visit blind people and their families, and encourage them to come for surgery. Because those individuals are already known to the patients, they are more effective at communicating the benefits of cataract surgery than are eye care professionals, who may have no link to the patients' own communities.[7] However, because the community perceives blindness as a chronic disability associated with ageing, rather than as an eye disease that can be cured, patients may not come to an eye clinic, which is perceived as treating eye diseases. Most Third World eye surgeons have had the experience of finding a patient, blind from cataract for many years, living within a few hundred metres of their clinic.

Material resources

Great efforts have been made during the past two decades to develop simple and appropriate solutions to overcome the lack of locally manufactured ophthalmic surgical resources. In Africa, for example, many centres now make their own eye drops. It is possible for a small pharmacy to produce 60 000 bottles of eye drops per year, at an average cost of about $0·30 per bottle. This not only saves money but also ensures a reliable supply of effective topical medications.[8]

High quality, single piece polymethylmethacrylate lenses are currently made in Eritrea, Nepal, and India. They are sold for $7–10 each, and have been found to be of a standard equivalent to that of similar designs of lens manufactured in industrialised countries. The availability of well manufactured, inexpensive lens implants has had an enormous impact on Third World cataract surgery.

A lack of inpatient accommodation has been addressed by "eye camps", in which cataract operations are performed outside the usual eye hospital setting. Although conditions for surgery are not ideal, eye camps provide cataract surgery for patients who cannot get to a hospital (Figure 13.2).

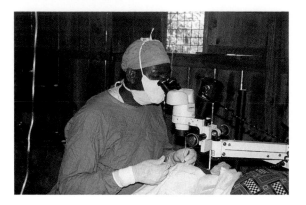

Figure 13.2 A non-physician cataract surgeon operating in a refugee camp in Kenya. The operating theatre is a wooden hut, with a corrugated iron roof. More than 600 successful cataract operations have been performed here since 1992. The operating microscope weighs less than 20 kg and can be carried in a suitcase.

Intraocular lenses

The use of IOLs in the Third World has been controversial.[9-11] However, there is now widespread agreement that IOLs represent the best solution to cataract blindness in developing countries.[12] Aphakic spectacles are safe and inexpensive. Unfortunately, they are frequently lost or broken. The distortion and magnification associated with aphakic glasses also militate against their use.[13] Cataract surgery with aphakic glasses reduces the number of cataract blind but increases the number blind from uncorrected aphakia, leading to little change in the overall prevalence of blindness.[14]

When the other eye sees well, spectacle correction of unilateral aphakia leads to intolerable anisometropia, and aniseikonia, and so surgery must be deferred until the patient has bilateral visual impairment. With bilateral loss of vision, travel becomes even harder. The patient's remaining savings will have been spent on food and other essentials, so that there is nothing left for luxuries such as medical care. The use of an IOL makes it possible to intervene much earlier, before the patient is blind in both eyes; this in effect prevents cataract blindness, with all of its associated human, social, and economic costs.

Surgical techniques

Intracapsular cataract extraction and anterior chamber intraocular lenses

Intracapsular cataract extraction (ICCE) remains popular in parts of the Third World. The surgery does not require complex equipment or expensive irrigating fluids. The use of loupes with four- to fivefold magnification gives results that are comparable to those obtained with an operating microscope.

However, ICCE is associated with serious posterior segment complications, such as retinal detachment. The larger incision required leads to greater astigmatism and prolongs recovery. In poor countries there are relatively few centres that can manage aphakic detachments, and astigmatic spectacle lenses are too expensive for many people.

Early designs of anterior chamber lens implants, particularly those with closed loop haptics, were associated with unacceptably high complication rates. This has given anterior chamber IOLs a poor reputation in the developed world. Recently, it has been shown that open loop designs, with three or four point fixation, have fewer complications.[15] The lack of posterior capsule opacification following ICCE and anterior chamber IOL implantation is a distinct advantage in a Third World setting, where follow up is limited and there are few neodymivm : yttrium aluminium garnet (Nd: YAG) lasers. A prospective study conducted in Nepal has demonstrated the safety and efficacy of this operation.[16]

However, although modern designs of open loop anterior chamber lenses are safer than their predecessors, many surgeons are reluctant to use them in young people for fear of long term damage to the endothelium and trabecular meshwork. Moreover, so long as anterior chamber IOLs are not regarded as the optimum treatment for aphakia in developed nations, they will not be received enthusiastically in the Third World.

Extracapsular cataract extraction and posterior chamber intraocular lenses

Uncomplicated extracapsular cataract extraction (ECCE) carries a much lower risk of posterior segment complications. However, there is a significant risk of posterior capsule opacification. This can easily be treated with a Nd:YAG laser, but these lasers are expensive and are not available in most Third World eye clinics. This is important in developing countries. It can be difficult for a blind person to travel once to an eye clinic for surgery. To make the journey twice may be impossible.

The risk of posterior capsule opacification can be minimised by good surgical technique, and by the IOL material and design.[17] Most patients presenting for surgery in the Third World have mature cataracts, and the risk of capsule opacity may be lower in these eyes.[18] Furthermore, although capsule opacification may occur, it rarely reduces vision to below 6/60, following uncomplicated extraction of a senile cataract. If the capsule does become opaque, then in the absence of a Nd:YAG laser a surgical capsulotomy can be performed through the pars plana.

To obtain good results with extracapsular surgery, an operating microscope is essential. Until recently these have been prohibitively expensive for most eye clinics in poor countries. It is now possible to obtain a good quality coaxial microscope, which can be packed in a suitcase and taken to outlying clinics, for around $3000.

Despite the risk of posterior capsule opacity, the use of ECCE, with a posterior chamber IOL, is increasing in Third World countries. The advent of low cost coaxial microscopes, inexpensive IOLs, and a desire to achieve the same standard of care as in developed countries have all played a role in this trend.

Phacoemulsification and small incision surgery

Phacoemulsification equipment is costly, complex, and difficult to maintain. Because many patients do not present until they are completely blind, a high proportion of Third World cataracts are mature or hypermature and are less amenable to phacoemulsification.

However, small incision surgery offers real advantages for developing countries. The small incision causes less inflammation and leaves a strong eye. Visual rehabilitation is faster, and there is minimal induced astigmatism. This means that follow up beyond the immediate postoperative period is not essential, which is even more desirable in the Third World than in an industrialised country.

Unfortunately, foldable IOLs remain too expensive for most patients in the Third World. This will change, and there will be intense efforts to develop safe and reliable methods of removing the nucleus through a small incision without the cost or complexity of phacoemulsification.

Cataract surgical outcomes

Although hospital based studies have shown excellent results from both ICCE and anterior chamber IOL,[16] and ECCE and posterior chamber IOL,[19,20] studies in the community suggest that too many patients have a poor outcome,[21,22] with as many as 40% of operated eyes having an acuity of less than 6/60.[21] The main reasons for the poor outcome are preexisting eye disease, complications of surgery, and uncorrected refractive error. Although the use of IOLs will reduce the latter, it will not affect the other causes.

The same studies have shown that quality of life and visual function measurements are closely correlated with postoperative visual acuity.[21] If patients have a poor outcome, it will have an adverse effect on their quality of life. This will in turn affect the community's perception of the effectiveness of cataract surgery, reducing demand and raising the barriers to surgery.

The WHO has recently suggested that at least 90% of operated cataract eyes should have a best corrected acuity of 6/18 or better, and that fewer than 5% should be worse than 6/60.[23] These targets are low compared with expected outcomes in wealthy countries, but are ambitious for most Third World eye clinics. Whether or not the WHO targets are achieved, it is essential for cataract surgeons to monitor their outcomes as well as their output, and to set goals for regular quality control and continuous improvement.

The aim of outcome monitoring is not primarily to compare one clinic or surgeon with another, but to assist all surgeons to identify why they have poor outcomes and to take the necessary corrective measures. This will lead to improved outcomes for all patients.

Cost of surgery

Cataract extraction is thought to be one of the most cost effective interventions in modern medicine.[24] However, the communities in greatest need of surgery are also the least able to pay for it.

The cost of cataract surgery can be divided into the cost of consumables (such as the IOL, drugs, and sutures) and fixed costs (salaries, depreciation, etc.). The cost of consumables can be minimised by bulk purchase from suppliers in Third World countries. However, it is unlikely to be less than $20–$25 per operation. Fixed costs remain the same whether the clinic does 10 operations or 100. The best way of minimising the fixed cost per operation is to increase the number of operations. If a clinic does 500 operations per year, then the cost per operation is $20 + (total fixed costs/500). If the clinic works more efficiently, and doubles its output, then the cost per operation will be $20 + (total fixed costs/1000).

Ideally, a clinic should aim to achieve self-sufficiency, from generating sufficient income from patient fees and sale of glasses, among other sources, to cover all their costs. The only way this can be accomplished in a Third World situation is to have tiered pricing. Poor patients, who may have been blind for years, must be treated for free. Other patients can only pay a small proportion of the total cost of surgery. Others can pay the full cost. A minority will be willing to pay more than the true cost of surgery if they receive preferential treatment, for example a private or air conditioned room. This approach has been very successful in some hospitals in Nepal and India.

The future

The problem of cataract blindness in the Third World is so large that there is no single simple answer. Different circumstances will require different solutions. In all situations the quality of the surgery and of the overall patient care will influence outcome more than variations in the type of operation.

In training surgeons for developing countries, the ideal is probably "complete eye surgeons", who are equally at home performing high volume surgery in an eye camp and small incision surgery at the base hospital. However, in addition to having technical proficiency, Third World eye surgeons must be aware that the patients on whom they operate represent only a fraction of those in need. The surgeon's objective should be to increase the numbers of sight restoring operations by minimising the barriers that prevent people from obtaining surgery. This can be accomplished by actively involving local communities in the elimination of cataract and by providing high quality surgery with a good visual outcome at an affordable price.

References

1 World Health Organisation. *The World Health Report. Life in the 21st century: a vision for all.* Geneva: World Health Organisation, 1998.
2 World Health Organisation. *Vision 2020, the global initiative for the elimination of avoidable blindness.* Geneva: World Health Organisation, 1999.
3 Foster A. Cataract: a global perspective: output, outcome and outlay. *Eye* 1999;**13**:449–53.
4 Shamanna BR, Dandona L, Rao GN. Economic burden of blindness in India. *Indian J Ophthalmol* 1998;**46**: 169–72.
5 Venkataswamy G. Can cataract surgery be marketed like hamburgers in developing countries? *Arch Ophthalmol* 1993;**111**:580.

6 Foster A. Who will operate on Africa's 3 million curably blind people? *Lancet* 1991;**337**:1267–9.

7 Yorston D. *Accessible eye care: primary health care and community-based rehabilitation*. In: Proceedings of the Fifth General Assembly. International Agency for Prevention of Blindness, 1994.

8 Taylor J. Appropriate methods and resources for third world ophthalmology. In: Tasman W, Jaeger EA, eds. *Duane's clinical ophthalmology*, vol 5. Hagerstown: Lippincott, 1984.

9 Taylor HR, Sommer A. Cataract surgery. A global perspective [editorial] *Arch Ophthalmol* 1990;**108**:797–8.

10 World Health Organisation. Use of intraocular lenses in cataract surgery in developing countries: memorandum from a WHO meeting. *Bull World Health Organ* 1991;**69**:657–66.

11 Young PW, Schwab L. Intraocular lens implantation in developing countries: an ophthalmic surgical dilemma. *Ophthalmic Surg* 1989;**20**:241–4.

12 Yorston D. Are intraocular lenses the solution to cataract blindness in Africa? *Br J Ophthalmol* 1998;**82**:469–71.

13 Hogeweg M, Sapkota YD, Foster A. Acceptability of aphakic correction. Results from Karnali eye camps in Nepal. *Acta Ophthalmol* 1992;**70**:407–12.

14 Cook CD, Stulting AA. Impact of a sight-saver clinic on the prevalence of blindness in northern KwaZulu. *S Afr Med J* 1995,**85**.28–9.

15 Auffarth GU, Wesendahl TA, Brown SJ, Apple DJ. Are there acceptable anterior chamber intraocular lenses for clinical use in the 1990's? *Ophthalmology* 1994;**101**:1913–22.

16 Hennig A, Evans JR, Pradhan D, *et al*. Randomised controlled trial of anterior chamber intra-ocular lenses. *Lancet* 1997;**349**:1129–33.

17 Spalton DJ. Posterior capsular opacification after cataract surgery. *Eye* 1999;**13**:489–92.

18 Argento C, Nunez E, Wainsztein R. Incidence of post-operative posterior capsular opacification with types of senile cataracts. *J Cataract Refract Surg* 1992;**18**:586–8.

19 Yorston D, Foster A. Outcome of ECCE & PC-IOL in adults in E. Africa. *Br J Ophthalmol* 1999;**83**:897–901.

20 Prajna NV, Chandrakanth KS, Kim R, *et al*. The Madurai Intraocular Lens Study II: clinical outcomes. *Am J Ophthalmol* 1998;**125**:14–25.

21 Zhao J, Sui R, Jia L, Fletcher AE, Ellwein LB. Visual acuity and quality of life outcomes in patients with cataract in Shunyi county, China. *Am J Ophthalmol* 1998;**126**:582–5.

22 Limburg H, Foster A, Vaidyanathan K, Murthy GVS. Monitoring visual outcome of cataract surgery: results from India. *Bull World Health Organ* (in press).

23 World Health Organisation. *Informal consultation on analysis of blindness prevention outcomes*. Geneva: World Health Organisation WHO/PBL/98·68, 1998.

24 Marseille E. Cost-effectiveness of cataract surgery in a public health eye care programme in Nepal. *Bull World Health Organ* 1996,**74**.319–24.

14 Cataract surgery: the next frontier

When Kelman[1] introduced phacoemulsification over 30 years ago, he revolutionised cataract surgery not only by introducing small incision surgery but also by spurring the development of new lens technology, namely the foldable intraocular lens (IOL). The results of these new developments have greatly improved patient outcomes by decreasing induced astigmatism and decreasing wound complications, and thus enabling quicker rehabilitation.[2] However, this technique is not without its problems. Issues of safety related to the release of excess energy at the probe tip, and the consequent effects on non-target tissues such as the iris, cornea, and posterior capsule remain a concern. The excessive heat generated around the phaco tip mandate that a sleeve be present to provide a water bath to prevent subsequent corneal burns and wound distortion. Until recently this has limited the incision size to between 2·2 and 3·2 mm (see chapter 4). Thus, there is a drive to study and develop newer and better technologies to circumvent these problems. Other techniques that are currently under investigation include the use of lasers, warm water jet technology (to melt the lens), and mechanical instruments such as Catarex and phacotmesis. The Catarex machine uses a small impellar to break up the lens, whereas phacotmesis involves a spinning needle. Smaller incisions require new solutions to lens implantation. Development has been directed toward capsular filling techniques, which may also provide the answer to restoring accommodation following surgery.

Lasers for cataract removal

Evolution

In 1975 Kasnov[3] reported the technique of laser phacopuncture, the first laser procedure for cataract removal. With a Q switched ruby laser, microperforations were made in the anterior capsule, thus enabling gradual reabsorption of the lens material over time. This technique had very limited applications because it was only effective for very soft cataracts. There was also the problem of induced uveitis. In the ensuing years, focus was shifted toward four ultraviolet wavelengths: 193 nm (argon fluoride), 248 nm (krypton fluoride), 308 nm (xenon chloride), and 351 nm (xenon fluoride).[4–6] Of these, the 308 nm excimer laser appeared most promising because of both efficacy of ablation and transmissibility through fibreoptics.[4–6] However, the cataractogenic effects of the 308 nm laser posed a threat to the eyes of the surgeon,[7–9] and questions of possible retinal toxicity and carcinogenic effects arose.[7,8,10] Attention was then redirected toward the infrared wavelengths, namely the erbium : yttrium aluminium garnet (Er:YAG)[11–14] and the neodymium : yttrium aluminium garnet (Nd:YAG)[15–17] lasers.

In 1980, Aron-Rosa and others reported the use of the Nd:YAG (pulsed 1064 nm) laser for performing posterior capsulotomy,[18–20] peripheral iridotomy,[20–22] and cutting of pupillary membranes.[20,21,23] This then evolved into the next stage in the use of lasers for cataract removal, namely laser anterior capsulotomy

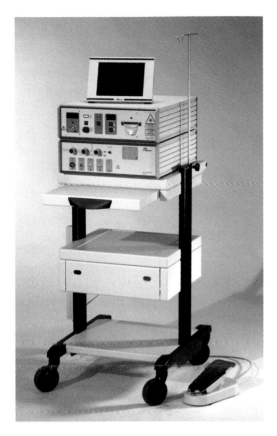

Figure 14.1   Dodick laser photolysis unit.

before cataract extraction.[24] This technique never gained widespread acceptance because of problems of intraocular pressure rise, inflammation, and poor mydriasis at the time of surgery, and the need to perform surgery promptly after the laser treatment.[25,26]

The next procedure to come along in this evolution was laser photofragmentation,[27–31] which involved the use of the Nd:YAG laser to photodisrupt the lens nucleus before phacoemulsification. By firing the laser into the substance of the lens nucleus while leaving the anterior and posterior capsules intact, the nucleus is softened, thus making subsequent phacoemulsification easier. Although several studies did demonstrate less phaco time and power needed in those cases pretreated with laser, this procedure does carry the risk of inadvertent perforations of the anterior/posterior

capsules and potential increase in intraoperative complications. This also had the inconvenience of a two staged procedure.

Nd:YAG laser systems

Dodick photolysis (ARC Lasers; Figure 14.1)

Since the early 1990s, Dodick has been studying the use of the Q switched, pulsed 1064 nm Nd:YAG laser for one stage, direct photolysis of cataractous lenses.[15] The probe, similar to a standard irrigation and aspiration hand piece, consists of an irrigation and aspiration port chamber, which contains a 300 µm quartz clad fibre. The proximal portion of the 300 µm fibre is attached via a standard laser connector to the laser source. The fibre enters the probe through the infusion cannula and terminates approximately 2 mm in front of a titanium target inside the probe tip. The pulsed laser energy is transmitted via the quartz fibre and is focused on the titanium target, thus enabling optical breakdown and plasma formation to occur at very low energy levels. This in turn causes the emanation of shock waves, which propagate within the aspiration chamber toward the mouth of the probe, where the nuclear material is held in place by the suction created by the aspiration port. The shock waves disrupt the nuclear material and the fragments are aspirated.[15,32]

The titanium target is the key element of this device because the metal target, with its low ionization potentials, acts as a transducer in converting light energy to shock waves at low laser energy levels. Because there is no direct contact between the laser energy and the target tissues, the shock waves generated here are more controlled, so that only the area in contact with the tip of the device is disrupted. In effect, the titanium target shields the non-target tissues such as the endothelium and the retina, as well as the surgeon's eyes, from direct laser light.[33,34] The quartz clad fibre and the titanium targets are relatively inexpensive, making disposable hand pieces a possibility. The same tip may be used for irrigation and aspiration.

Photon (Paradigm Medical Industries)

This is a Nd:YAG system that is partnered with the manufacturer's conventional ultrasonic phaco system. The probe consists of a titanium tip with a fused silica fibre. It currently has a repetition rate of 10–50 Hz, which will eventually be increased to above 50 Hz to increase its ability to fragment tissue. Its fluidics system also allows for surge control at all vacuum levels up to 500 mmHg. It is a uni-manual unit in which the irrigation and aspiration system is incorporated into the laser probe. The probe has a tip diameter ranging from 1·2 to 1·7 mm, and passes through a 3·0–3·5 mm incision. The unit uses a peristaltic system with up to 500 mmHg vacuum. The company has completed phase I US Food and Drug Administration trials and is currently in phase II trials, which are being conducted at seven clinical sites across the USA. To date, over 100 procedures have been performed using this system, and the results demonstrate quieter eyes on postoperative day one compared with ultrasound phaco cases. The reported endothelial cell loss is 7·6% at 3 months of follow up for all sites.

Er:YAG laser systems

Another laser currently being developed for cataract removal is the Er:YAG system.[11–14] Er:YAG emits energy in the mid-infrared region (2940 nm), and may be transmitted through a 150 μm fibreoptic probe.[13] One advantage of the erbium system is that the 2940 nm wavelength corresponds to the maximum peak of water absorption. This translates into low penetration (~1 mm), with excess energy absorbed by water without dispersion to surrounding non-target tissues. The laser is focused directly into the lens nucleus to create an optical breakdown in the

nucleus, leading to microfractures of the lens without heat generation. Fragmentation rate per pulse is related not only to pulse energy but also to the repetition frequency. With high pulse frequency, longitudinal chains of cavitation bubbles form at the probe tip. Depending on the pulse energy, these bubbles may extend up to 3 mm or more in water and up to 1 mm in nuclear material. Because the bubbles allow the laser energy to travel further than the penetration depth of the laser radiation (energy travelling through bubbles rather than absorbed by water), they facilitate the fragmentation of denser nuclei. However, this also increases the risk to damage of adjacent structures (i.e. the posterior capsule).

There are three companies currently developing the Er:YAG laser for cataract removal. All systems presently available use a conventional irrigation and aspiration system to remove tissue and debris from the capsular bag. In addition, because the laser is focused directly into the lens and not onto a metal target, there is some exposure of the patient's and surgeon's eyes to direct laser light.

A number of systems are under trial, including the following:

- Phacolase (Aesculap-Meditec)
- Centauri (EyeSys-Premier)
- Adagio (WaveLight).

Advantages of laser cataract removal

Currently, several laser systems are available in Europe, while clinical trials continue in the USA. Although laser is unlikely to replace ultrasound phaco systems in the near future, laser phaco systems do have several advantages over ultrasound systems. Because the laser probes produce no clinically significant heat, there is no risk of corneal and scleral burns. Studies have demonstrated that after 30 seconds of continual use in standard conditions, a

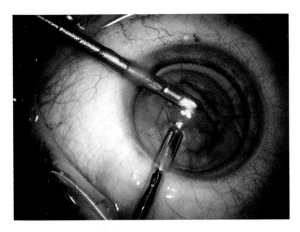

Figure 14.2 Bimanual laser photolysis procedure. Probe on right delivers infusion. Probe on left delivers laser and aspiration.

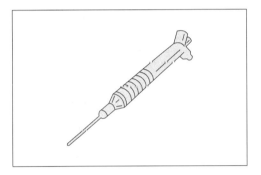

Figure 14.3 Laser photolysis probe: a lightweight disposable probe made of injection molded plastic.

temperature increase of 2·6°C was noted with a laser probe, as compared with an increase of 30°C with an ultrasound probe. Furthermore, the water temperature in a 2·5 cc closed chamber increased by 1°C with a laser probe versus 9·5°C with an ultrasound probe. The minimal heat generated by the laser probes eliminates the need for a water bath around the probe, thus enabling the separation of irrigation from laser/aspiration, thereby reducing probe and incision size (Figure 14.2).

Unlike ultrasound phaco hand pieces, the laser probes do not house motors and do not require electrical voltage to drive vibrating needles, both of which are subject to wear and tear. In addition to being lighter and easier to handle, the components of the laser probes are relatively cheap, thus making disposable hand pieces a possibility (Figure 14.3).

A notable problem with the current laser systems is that dense nuclei still present a challenge. One can expect that with further refinements in fluidics and laser parameters, this problem will be overcome in the near future.

New lens technology

Just as the introduction of ultrasound phacoemulsification spurred the development of foldable IOLs, laser phaco systems have already brought about revolutions in lens technology. In July 1999, the first case of IOL insertion through a 1·8 mm incision was reported by Kanellopoulos in Greece.[35] The new lens was developed by Dr Christine Kreiner, of Acritec (Berlin, Germany). The acrylic IOL has a 6 mm optic, is 12·5 mm in total length, and was prefolded by 27% dehydration. The folded lens has a width of 1·2–1·3 mm and can be implanted through an incision of less than 2 mm. Once in the capsular bag, the lens slowly unfolds over 25–30 minutes. In the future, we can look forward to the next generation of IOLs to be made of injectable substances such as silicone, hydrogel, or collagen that could be used to refill the capsular bag through the same small opening that is used to evacuate the cataract. This would facilitate true endocapsular surgery and enable us to preserve accommodation.

Accommodative lens technology

In addition to the restoration of accommodation, the goals of this lens technology comprise the following:

- A small incision/capsulorhexis

- Injection of a biocompatible material with appropriate refractive indices/transparency/elasticity

- Control of posterior capsule opacification.

In the 1960s, Kessler[36] and Agarwal et al.[37] were among the first to report lens refilling with silicone oil in rabbits. However, silicone oil leakage from the capsular bag was noted to be a major problem in these cases.

Use of polymeric gels

In the 1980s, in order to overcome the problem of leakage, several investigators attempted to refill lens capsules using precured silicone polymeric gels, commonly known as silicone elastomers or silicone rubbers.[38–40] Haefliger et al.[40] found evidence to suggest that the injected silicone gel undergoes accommodative change when the ciliary body is stimulated by pilocarpine. Although the actual amplitude of accommodation could not be directly measured because of posterior capsule opacification, observations such as the forward movement and increase in curvature of the anterior lens capsule, and the decrease in anterior chamber depth by an amount comparable to that of the natural lens suggested preservation of accommodation in these eyes. While the use of a precured silicone gel simplifies the surgical procedure, it is difficult to prepare a gel with viscosity that is high enough to prevent leakage and low enough to enable injection through a small needle. An alternative method would be to inject liquid silicone that polymerises in situ. This approach would, in turn, require some means of sealing the capsular opening.

The endocapsular balloon

In the late 1980s, Nishi and coworkers[41,42] developed an inflatable endocapsular balloon for the purpose of lens refilling. In this technique, lens extraction is performed via a 1·2–1·5 mm minicapsulorhexis. The capsular bag is then treated with ethylenediaminetetraacetic acid (EDTA) to remove any lens epithelial cells (LECs). The deflated balloon is inserted into the empty capsular bag, and a mixture of two liquid silicone polymers is injected into the balloon. The liquid silicone polymerises in situ in 2 hours, and the resultant inflated balloon fills the capsular bag. Problems encountered with this technique included fibrin deposition and capsular fibrosis. It was also observed that the postoperative amplitude of accommodation was a small fraction of that present preoperatively, and that the amplitude subsequently decreased over time. A possible explanation for this finding was that the capsular tension was not effectively transmitted to the balloon because of discrepancies in size, shape, and other physical properties. Progressive capsular fibrosis, which decreases capsular pliability, may in turn account for the gradual decrease in postoperative accommodative amplitude. These studies also demonstrated that the final shape and the degree of filling of these endocapsular balloons are important factors in determining not only the transmission of capsular tension but also the amplitude of accommodation. In studies on young monkey eyes, Nishi et al. reported a mean accommodation amplitude of $4·6 \pm 0·5$ diopters (D). Using the same technique several years later, Sakka et al.[43] reported an average accommodative change of 6·74 D after instillation of 4% pilocarpine.

Endocapsular polymerisation

An alternative approach to injecting liquid polymers into an endocapsular balloon is to inject the materials directly into the capsular bag and allow endocapsular polymerisation. This eliminates the need for a containment device such as a balloon. However, such a process may be associated with endogenous heat production, which may secondarily affect the lens capsule and zonules. Hettlich et al.[44] examined this issue with studies on an acrylate copolymer, and found that the maximal temperature recorded was at the posterior capsule (45·1°C) for several seconds. This temperature rise was not believed to be significant in causing damage to the capsular collagen. This study also confirmed an earlier observation reported by Haefliger et al.[40] that the degree of capsular refilling is inversely related to the degree of posterior capsule opacification.

Direct capsular filling: capsular plug

Of the materials studied to date, silicone compounds appear to the best currently available substances for lens refilling because of their transparency, biocompatibility, refractive index, and elasticity. After studies on the endocapsular balloon, Nishi and coworkers[45–51] went on to develop a direct lens refilling technique, in which a silicone plug is used to seal the minicapsulorhexis of 1·2–1·5 mm. The plug consists of a silicone double plate through which a thin delivery tube provides access to the capsular bag. Two liquid silicone polymers are injected via the delivery tube, which is then cut at its root. A soft silicone gel is then used to fill the remaining tube stump, thus preventing reflux. The injected mixture then polymerises in the capsular bag within 2 hours. Problems encountered with this technique include capsular tears during plug insertion into the capsular bag. In some cases, mild leakage occurred at the capsular opening during silicone injection because of difficulty in maintaining the stability of the plug–syringe connection. In instances of leakage, it was noted that the liquid silicone remained cohesive in aqueous because of its hydrophobic nature, and that no adhesions to adjacent tissues occurred. Silicone leakage occurring at the time of injection was washed out of the anterior chamber with ease, and that which had polymerised (detected after surgery) was removed surgically without difficulty on postoperative day one. In a series conducted by Nishi and Nishi,[47] postoperative accommodative amplitude ranged from 1 to 4·5 D with mean of 2·3 ± 1·3 D (while preoperative accommodative amplitude ranged from 5·75 to 11·25 D with mean of 8·0 ± 2·0 D). This demonstrated that refilling the lens capsule was feasible, although the postoperative amplitude of accommodation was only a fraction of that present before surgery.

Determining lens power

Postoperative refraction using the lens refilling technique is determined by two main factors: the refractive index of the injected material and the anterior capsular curvature, which is determined by the degree of capsular filling. The greater the degree of capsular filling, the steeper the anterior capsular curvature and the greater the power of the implant. However, the degree of capsular filling also determines the amplitude of accommodation. At low volumes, the accommodation amplitude increases as the degree of capsular refilling increases. The accommodative amplitude then reaches a maximum value, after which any further increase in volume results in a decrease in accommodative amplitude. Nishi and coworkers[45–47] observed that the optimal accommodation amplitude with silicone polymers is achieved by filling the capsular bag to 60–70% capacity. However, postoperative emmetropia is not achieved when the capsule is under-filled to this extent, and optimal accommodation amplitude is attained at the expense of refractive outcome. In Nishi's series, with capsule filling of 60–70%, an average accommodation amplitude of 2·3 ± 1·3 D was achieved, but with a mean hyperopic shift of +6·4 D in postoperative refraction. This hyperopic shift is probably due to the relatively low refractive index (1·405) of injected silicone, as well as a flatter anterior capsule curvature secondary to the under-filling. Methods of correcting the residual refractive error may include corneal refractive surgery or IOL implantation. The ideal solution would, of course, be the development of new injectable materials with different refractive indices that would enable the achievement of emmetropia along with optimal accommodation amplitude.

Posterior capsule opacification

A common finding among all studies, regardless of the technique of lens refilling, is posterior capsule opacification in the early postoperative period. Haefliger et al.[40] noted proliferation of LECs on the posterior capsule as early as two weeks postoperatively, with the equatorial region being the most prominent. In several other series,[40,47] posterior capsule opacification precluded refraction at three months. Histopathological studies demonstrated a thick layer of LECs that had migrated posteriorly between the lens capsule and the injected silicone. In Nishi's series,[46] YAG laser capsulotomy was performed. Although no silicone leakage or herniation was noted with the procedure, it may negate the accommodation attained previously. To date, various methods of removing LECs have been reported. Nishi and coworkers studied the use of ultrasound aspiration,[48] as well as the use of a high concentration of a proteolytic enzyme,[49,50] to loosen LECs at their junction complexes. Humphrey et al.[51] had described the use of EDTA and trypsin for the removal of LECs. Thus far, no method has proven ideal. The problem of posterior capsule opacification must be solved before any lens refilling technology may be introduced clinically. Nevertheless, with further advances in research and development of new products, the 21st century promises to be a very exciting era for cataract surgery.

References

1 Kelman CD. Phaco-emulsification and aspiration: a new technique of cataract removal, a preliminary report. *Am J Ophthalmol* 1967;**64**:23–35.

2 Leaming DV. Practice styles and preferences of ASCRS members: 1987 survey. *J Cataract Refract Surg* 1988;**14**:552–9.

3 Krasnov MM. Laser phakopuncture in the treatment of soft cataracts. *Br J Ophthalmol* 1975;**56**:96–8.

4 Maguen E, Martinez M, Grundfest W, et al. Excimer laser ablation of the human lens at 308 nm with a fiber delivery system. *J Cataract Refract Surg* 1989;**15**:409–14.

5 Nanevicz T, Prince MR, Gawande AA, et al. Excimer laser ablation of the lens. *Arch Ophthalmol* 1986;**104**:1825–9.

6 Puliafito CA, Steinert RF, Deutsch TF, et al. Excimer laser ablation of the cornea and lens: experimental studies. *Ophthalmology* 1985;**92**:741–8.

7 Marshall J, Sliney DH. Endoexcimer laser intraocular ablative photodecomposition [letter]. *Am J Ophthalmol* 1986;**101**:130–1.

8 Zuclich JA. Ultraviolet-induced photochemical damage in ocular tissues. *Health Phys* 1989;**56**:671–82.

9 Borkman RF. Cataracts and photochemical damage in the lens. *Ciba Found Symp* 1984;**106**:88–109.

10 Kochevar IE. Cytotoxicity and mutagenicity of excimer laser radiation. *Lasers Surg Med* 1989;**9**:440–5.

11 Colvard DM. *Erbium:YAG laser removal of cataracts.* Presented at the American Society of Cataract and Refractive Surgery Annual Meeting, Seattle, May 1993.

12 Margolis TI, Farnath DA, Destro M, Puliafito CA. Erbium-YAG laser surgery on experimental vitreous membranes. *Arch Ophthalmol* 1989;**107**:424–8.

13 Peyman GA, Katoh N. Effects of an erbium:YAG laser in ocular ablation. *Int Ophthalmol* 1987;**10**:245–53.

14 Tsubota K. Application of erbium:YAG laser in ocular ablation. *Ophthalmologica* 1990;**200**:117–22.

15 Dodick JM. Laser phacolysis of the human cataractous lens. *Dev Ophthalmol* 1991;**22**:58–64.

16 Dodick JM, Sperber LTD, Lally JM, Kazlas M. Neodymium-YAG laser phacolysis of the human cataractous lens. *Arch Ophthalmol* 1993;**111**:903–4.

17 Dodick JM, Christiansen J. Experimental studies on the development and propagation of shock waves created by the interaction of short Nd:YAG laser pulses with a titanium target: possible implication for Nd:YAG laser phacolysis of the cataractous human lens. *J Cataract Refract Surg* 1991;**17**:794–7.

18 Aron-Rosa D, Aron J, Griesemann M, et al. Use of the neodymium:YAG laser to open the posterior capsule after lens implant surgery: a preliminary report. *Am Intraocul Implant Soc J* 1980;**6**:352–4.

19 Dodick JM. Nd:YAG laser treatment of the posterior capsule. *Trans New Orleans Acad Ophthalmol* 1988;169–78.

20 Fankhauser F, Roussel P, Steffen J, et al. Clinical studies on the efficiency of high power laser radiation upon some structures of the anterior segment of the eye: first experiences of the treatment of some pathological conditions of the anterior segment of the human eye by means of a Q-switched laser system. *Int Ophthalmol Clin* 1981;**3**:129–39.

21 Fankhauser F. The Q-switched laser: principles and clinical results. In: Trokel SL, ed. *YAG laser ophthalmic microsurgery.* Norwalk, CT: Appleton-Century-Crofts, 1983.

22 Klapper RM. Q-switched neodymium:YAG laser iridotomy. *Ophthalmology* 1984;**91**:1017–21.

23 Fankhauser F, Rol P. Microsurgery with the Nd:YAG laser: an overview. *Int Ophthalmol Clin* 1985;**25**:55–8.

24 Aron-Rosa D. Use of a pulsed neodymium-YAG laser for anterior capsulotomy before extracapsular cataract extraction. *J Am Intraocul Implant Soc* 1981;**7**:332–3.

25 Aron-Rosa DS, Aron JJ, Cohn HC. Use of a pulsed picosecond Nd:YAG laser in 6,654 cases. *Am Intra-Ocular Implant Soc J* 1984;**10**:35–9.

26 Chambless WS. Neodymium:YAG laser anterior capsulotomy and a possible new application. *J Am Intraocul Implant Soc* 1985;**11**:33–4.

27 Chambless WS. Neodymium:YAG laser phacofracture: an aid to phacoemulsification. *J Cataract Refract Surg* 1988;**14**:180–1.

28 L'Esperance FA Jr. *Ophthalmic lasers,* vol. 2, ed 3. St. Louis: CV Mosby, 1989.

29 Levin ML, Wyatt KD. Prospective analysis of laser photophacofragmentation. *J Cataract Refract Surg* 1990;**16**:96–8.

30 Ryan EH Jr, Logani S. Nd:YAG laser photodisruption of the lens nucleus before phacoemulsification. *Am J Ophthalmol* 1987;**104**:382–6.

31 Zelman J. Photophaco fragmentation. *J Cataract Refract Surg* 1987;**13**:287–9.

32 Dodick JM. Can cataracts be removed using laser technology? *Ophthalmol Clin N Am* 1991;**4**:355–64.

33 Dodick JM, Lally JM, Sperber LTD. Lasers in cataract surgery. *Curr Opin Ophthalmol* 1993;**4**:107–9.

34 Dodick JM, Sperber LTD. The future of cataract surgery. *Int Ophthalmol Clin* 1994;**34**:201–10.

35 Charters L. Two-mm incision barrier is broken in Greece. *Ophthalmology Times* July 1, 1999;**1**:24.

36 Kessler J. Experiments in refilling the lens. *Arch Ophthalmol* 1964;**71**:412–7.

37 Agarwal LP, Narsimhan EC, Mohan M. Experimental lens refilling. *Orient Arch Ophthalmol* 1967;**5**:205–12.

38 Gindi JJ, Wan WL, Schanzlin DJ. Endocapsular cataract surgery, I. *Cataract* 1985;**2**:6–10.

39 Parel J-M, Gelender H, Trefers WF, Norton EW. Phaco-ersatz: cataract surgery designed to preserve accommodation. *Graefes Arch Clin Exp Ophthalmol* 1986;**224**:165–73.

40 Haefliger E, Parel J, Fantes F, *et al.* Accommodation of an endocapsular silicone lens (Phaco-Ersatz in the non-human primate. *Ophthalmology* 1987;**94**:471–7.

41 Nishi O, Hara T, Hara T, *et al.* Refilling the lens with an inflatable endocapsular balloon: surgical procedure in animal eyes. *Graefes Arch Clin Exp Ophthalmol* 1992;**230**:47–55.

42 Nishi O, Nakai Y, Yamada Y, Mizumoto Y. Amplitudes of accommodation of primate lenses filled with two types of inflatable endocapsular balloons. *Arch Ophthalmol* 1993;**111**:1677–84.

43 Sakka Y, Hara T, Yamada Y, Hara T, Hayashi F. Accommodation in primate eyes after implantation of refilled endocapsular balloon. *Am J Ophthalmol* 1996:**121**:210–2.

44 Hettlich H, Lucke K, Asiyo-Vogel MN, Schulte M, Vogel A. Lens refilling and endocapsular polymerization of an injectable intraocular lens: in vitro and in vivo study of potential risks and benefits. *J Cataract Refract Surg* 1994;**20**:115–23.

45 Nishi O, Nishi K, Mano C, Ichihara M, Honda T. Controlling the capsular shape in lens refilling. *Arch Ophthalmol* 1997;**115**:507–10.

46 Nishi O, Nishi K, Mano C, Ichihara M, Honda T. Lens refilling with injectable silicone in rabbit eyes. *J Cataract Refract Surg* 1998;**24**:975–82.

47 Nishi O, Nishi K. Accommodation amplitude after lens refilling with injectable silicone by sealing the capsule with a plug in primates. *Arch Ophthalmol* 1998;**116**:1358–61.

48 Nishi O. Removal of lens epithelial cells by ultrasound in endocapsular cataract surgery. *Ophthalmic Surg* 1987;**18**:577–580.

49 Nishi O, Nishi K. A new approach to remove lens epithelial cells: dispersion aspiration. *Journal of the Eye* 1990;7:605–610.

50 Nishi O, Nishi K, Hikida M. Removal of lens epithelial cells by dispersion with enzymatic treatment followed by aspiration. *Ophthalmic Surgery* 1991;**22**:444–450.

51 Humphry RC, Davies EG, Jacob TJ, Thompson GM. The human anterior capsule: an attempted chemical debridement of epithelial cells by ethylenediaminetetraacetic acid (EDTA) and trypsin. *Br J Ophthalmol* 1988;**72**:406–8.

Index

Page numbers in **bold** refer to figures and those in *italic* type refer to tables or boxed material. Abbreviations used in sub entries include; IOL, intraocular lens; PCR, polymerase chain reaction.

INDEX